Pediatric Oncology 1

Cancer Treatment and Research

WILLIAM L. McGUIRE, *series editor*

Volume 2

1. R.B. Livingston, ed., Lung Cancer 1. 1980. ISBN 90-247-2394-9.
3. J.J. De Cosse and P. Sherlock, eds., Gastrointestinal Cancer 1. 1981. ISBN 90-247-2461-9.

series ISBN 90-247-2426-0.

Pediatric Oncology 1

with a special section on

Rare Primitive Neuroectodermal Tumors

edited by

G. BENNETT HUMPHREY
Oklahoma Children's Memorial Hospital and University of Oklahoma Health Sciences Center

LOUIS P. DEHNER
University of Minnesota Medical School

GERALD B. GRINDEY
New York State University at Buffalo

and

RONALD T. ACTON
University of Alabama in Birmingham

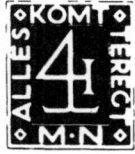

1981

MARTINUS NIJHOFF PUBLISHERS
THE HAGUE / BOSTON / LONDON

Distributors:

for the United States and Canada

Kluwer Boston, Inc.
190 Old Derby Street
Hingham, MA 02043
USA

for all other countries

Kluwer Academic Publishers Group
Distribution Center
P.O. Box 322
3300 AH Dordrecht
The Netherlands

Library of Congress Cataloging in Publication Data   ⊏⊐

Main entry under title:

Pediatric oncology.

  (Cancer treatment and research; v. 2)
  Includes index.
  1. Tumors in children. I. Humphrey, George Bennett, 1934- II. Series.
[DNLM: 1. Neoplasms—In infancy and childhood—Period. W1 CA693 v. 2 etc.]
RC281.C4P43   618.92'994   80-23151

ISBN-13: 978-94-009-8221-5   e-ISBN-13: 978-94-009-8219-2
DOI: 10.1007/978-94-009-8219-2

Contents

I. Selected Topics

II. Rare Tumors of the Central Nervous System

Cancer Treatment and Research

Foreword

Where do you begin to look for a recent, authoritative article on the diagnosis or management of a particular malignancy? The few general oncology textbooks are generally out of date. Single papers in specialized journals are informative but seldom comprehensive; these are more often preliminary reports on a very limited number of patients. Certain general journals frequently publish good indepth reviews of cancer topics, and published symposium lectures are often the best overviews available. Unfortunately, these reviews and supplements appear sporadically, and the reader can never be sure when a topic of special interest will be covered.

Cancer Treatment and Research is a series of authoritative volumes which aim to meet this need. It is an attempt to establish a critical mass of oncology literature covering virtually all oncology topics, revised frequently to keep the coverage up to date, easily available on a single library shelf or by a single personal subscription.

We have approached the problem in the following fashion. First, by dividing the oncology literature into specific subdivisions such as lung cancer, genitourinary cancer, pediatric oncology, etc. Second, by asking eminent authorities in each of these areas to edit a volume on the specific topic on an annual or biannual basis. Each topic and tumor type is covered in a volume appearing frequently and predictably, discussing current diagnosis, staging, markers, all forms of treatment modalities, basic biology, and more.

In Cancer Treatment and Research, we have an outstanding group of editors, each having made a major commitment to bring to this new series the very best literature in his or her field. Martinus Nijhoff Publishers has made an equally major commitment to the rapid publication of high quality books, and world-wide distribution.

Where can you go to find quickly a recent authoritative article on any major oncology problem? We hope that Cancer Treatment and Research provides an answer.

WILLIAM L. McGUIRE
Series Editor

Preface

This book is addressed to those who are involved in the care of children with cancer. The editors hope that physicians with training in surgery, radiation therapy, chemotherapy and pathology will find all or some of these articles of interest and pertinence.

The intent of this volume and those to follow is to focus on aspects of pediatric oncology and related fields not consistently and comprehensively covered in other books or journals. Each volume will have two sections. The first section will pursue concepts in research from the basic sciences that the editors feel are applicable to human malignancies. Unique approaches in the clinical management of cancer are also described, as are controversial treatments for specific tumors. We would like to stress that this section will not only report on progress in the treatment of cancer, but will also include topics such as tumor biology, genetics, diagnosis, detection, prevention, psychosocial rehabilitation, etc. All four editors have participated in the planning of this section and all are responsible for its content.

The editors feel that much needs to be learned about specific rare tumors, so it is their intention that the second part of each volume in this series serves as an informal tumor registry with specific malignancies chosen each year. Neoplasms will be selected that occur at a rate such that major centers may encounter only a few examples each year which means that the smaller institution may see one or two cases in a decade. Such low rates of occurrence make treatment difficult since the number of cases does not justify time and effort involved in creating a treatment protocol for each rare tumor; nor do the numbers generate results that will have statistical significance. To compound the problem further, most journals are reluctant to give space to articles reporting fewer than ten patients or in which statistical analysis cannot be undertaken. This inaugural section has taken on the enigmatic problem of the small cell neoplasms in the central nervous system designated by some as the 'primitive neuroectodermal tumor of the CNS.'

In the belief that children and their physicians are bound to benefit from shared knowledge, we have invited some of the major institutions in Japan, Australia, Europe, and the Americas to report their recent experience with specific rare tumors. So that there will be some consistency to the data, we have asked them to limit their reviews to cases treated within the last 10 to 15 years under the assumption that management was probably multimodal and that some of the current antitumor chemotherapeutic agents would have been used. After all the case material was received by the editors, the entire collection was sent back to all participating investigators for their comments. Finally, these have been incorporated by the editors into an overview on the management of that particular tumor group. The editors realize that there are many pitfalls to this approach, primarily caused by inconsistencies in diagnosis and treatment. In spite of these inconsistencies, the editors hope some insight will be gained into the clinical characteristics, overall prognosis, period of greatest risks of relapse for patients who respond to initial therapy, and perhaps also into therapeutic approaches.

In future volumes, a multi-institutional pathological review may be initiated. Two of the editors (GBH, LPD) assume responsibility for this section.

We would like to express our thanks to Dr. William L. McGuire, the series editor for advice and consultation throughout the preparation of this volume. We would also like to thank Dr. M.L.N. Willoughby, Dr. P.A. Voute, and Dr. Donald Metcalf for serving as consultants to the editors. We would also like to express our thanks to Jeffrey K. Smith, Publisher in the Medical Division of Martinus Nijhoff Publishers B.V. for his advice and guidance, and finally to Ms. Lucia Lane and Ms. Leslie Alexander for editorial assistance, and Ms. Terry Kazimir and Ms. Peggy Devinish for secretarial and administrative assistance in preparation of this volume.

We anticipate that *Pediatric Oncology* will be an annual publication. We would like to encourage additional institutions to participate in the recording of rare tumors in the future. Interested parties are encouraged to contact either Dr. Humphrey or Dr. Dehner. All of the editors would also welcome any suggestions for topics that should be reviewed in the future.

List of Contributors

ACTON, Ronald T., Diabetes Research & Training Center, University of Alabama in Birmingham, 1808 Seventh Avenue South, University Station, Birmingham, AL 35291, U.S.A.

BANKS, W.L., Jr., Department of Biochemistry, Medical College of Virginia (VCU), Richmond, VA 23298, U.S.A.

BARGER, Bruce O., Tissue Typing Laboratory, Diabetes Research and Training Center, University of Alabama in Birmingham, 1808 Seventh Avenue South, University Station, Birmingham, AL 35294, U.S.A.

BARNES, Patrick D., University of Oklahoma Health Sciences Center, Oklahoma Children's Memorial Hospital, P.O. Box 26901, Oklahoma City, OK 73190, U.S.A.

BARON, S., Department of Microbiology, The University of Texas Medical Branch, Galveston, TX 77550, U.S.A.

BAUM, Edward S., The Children's Memorial Hospital, The McGaw Medical Center of Northwestern University, 2300 Children's Plaza, Chicago, IL 60614, U.S.A.

BRODER, Samuel, Metabolism Branch, National Cancer Institute, National Institutes of Health, Bethesda, MD 20205, U.S.A.

BRUNO, Leonard A., Division of Neurosurgery, Children's Hospital of Philadelphia, 34th and Spruce Streets, Philadelphia, PA 19104, U.S.A.

CAMPBELL, P.E., Royal Children's Hospital, Flemington Road, Parkville, Victoria 3052, Australia.

CANGIR, Ayten, The University of Texas System Cancer Center, M.D. Anderson Hospital and Tumor Institute, Department of Pediatrics, 6723 Bertner Drive, Houston, TX 77025, U.S.A.

CHOW, C.W., Royal Childen's Hospital, Flemington Road, Parkville, Victoria 3052, Australia.

DAL CANTO, Mauro C., The Children's Memorial Hospital, The McGaw Medical Center of Northwestern University, 2300 Children's Plaza, Chicago, IL 60614, U.S.A.

DEHNER, Louis P., University of Minnesota Medical School, Department of Laboratory Medicine and Pathology, Division of Surgical Pathology, Box 609, Mayo Memorial Building, 420 Delaware Street, S.E., Minneapolis, MN 55455, U.S.A.

EDWARDS, Michael S., Departments of Radiation Oncology and Neurological Surgery, University of California, San Francisco, CA 94143, U.S.A.

FLEISCHMANN, W. Robert, Jr., Department of Microbiology, The University of Texas Medical Branch, Galveston, TX 77550, U.S.A.

HEPPNER, Gloria H., Michigan Cancer Foundation, Wayne State University, Detroit, MI 48201, U.S.A.

HUMPHREY, G. Bennett, University of Oklahoma Health Sciences Center, Oklahoma Children's Memorial Hospital, P.O. Box 26901, Oklahoma City, OK 73190, U.S.A.

ISAACS, Hart, Jr., University of Southern California School of Medicine, Children's Hospital of Los Angeles, P.O. Box 60850, Terminal Annex, Los Angeles, CA 90060, U.S.A.

JENKIN, Derek, Ontario Cancer Institute, Department of Radiation Oncology, 500 Sherbourne Street, Toronto, Canada M4X 1K9.

JENKIN, R.D.T., University of Oklahoma Health Sciences Center, Oklahoma Children's Memorial Hospital, P.O. Box 26901, Oklahoma City, OK 73190, U.S.A.

JENNINGS, S.S., Medical College of Virginia (VCU), Richmond, VA 23298, U.S.A.

KAPLAN, A.M., Medical College of Virginia (VCU), Richmond, VA 23298, U.S.A.

KAPLAN, Ralph J., University of Oklahoma Health Sciences Center, Oklahoma Children's Memorial Hospital, P.O. Box 26901, Oklahoma City, OK 73190, U.S.A.

KROUS, Henry F., University of Oklahoma Health Sciences Center, Oklahoma Children's Memorial Hospital, P.O. Box 26901, Oklahoma City, OK 73190, U.S.A.

LEVIN, Victor A., Department of Radiation Oncology and Neurological Surgery, University of California, San Francisco, CA 94143, U.S.A.

MARTON, Laurence J., Department of Laboratory Medicine, School of Medicine, University of California, San Francisco, CA 94143, U.S.A.

MORGAN, Elaine R., The Children's Memorial Hospital, The McGaw Medical Center of Northwestern University, 2300 Children's Plaza, Chicago, IL 60614, U.S.A.

NESBIT, Mark E., University of Minnesota Medical School, Department of Pediatrics, Division of Oncology, Box 609, Mayo Memorial Building, 420 Delaware Street, S.E., Minneapolis, MN 55455, U.S.A.

NORRIS, Donald G., University of Pennsylvania School of Medicine, Department of Neurosurgery, 34th and Spruce Streets, Philadelphia, PA 19104, U.S.A.

KNAPP, John, The University of Texas System Cancer Center, M.D. Anderson Hospital and Tumor Institute, Department of Pediatrics, 6723 Bertner Drive, Houston, TX 77025, U.S.A.

PRIEST, John, University of Minnesota Medical School, Department of Pediatrics, Division of Oncology, Box 609, Mayo Memorial Building, 420 Delaware Street, S.E., Minneapolis, MN 55455, U.S.A.

RANKIN, Joan K., Michigan Cancer Foundation, Wayne State University, Detroit, MI 48201, U.S.A.

RORKE, Lucy B., Children's Hospital of Philadelphia, University of Pennsylvania School of Medicine, 34th and Spruce Streets, Philadelphia, PA 19104, U.S.A.

SEIDENFELD, Jerome, Brain Tumor Research Center, School of Medicine, University of California, San Francisco, CA 94143, U.S.A.

SEXAUER, Charles L., University of Oklahoma Health Sciences Center, Oklahoma Children's Memorial Hospital, P.O. Box 26901, Oklahoma City, OK 73190, U.S.A.

SHAPIRO, William R., Michigan Cancer Foundation, Wayne State University, Detroit, MI 48201, U.S.A.

SHELINE, Glenn E., Departments of Radiation Oncology and Neurological Surgery, University of California, San Francisco, CA 94143, U.S.A.

SIEGEL, Stuart E., University of Southern California School of Medicine, Children's Hospital of Los Angeles, P.O. Box 60850, Terminal Annex, Los Angeles, CA 90060, U.S.A.

STANLEY, Philip, University of Southern California School of Medicine, Children's Hospital of Los Angeles, P.O. Box 60850, Terminal Annex, Los Angeles, CA 90060, U.S.A.

SUNG, Joo-Ho, University of Minnesota Medical School, Department of Pediatrics, Division of Oncology, Box 609, Mayo Memorial Building, 420 Delaware Street, S.E., Minneapolis, MN 55455, U.S.A.

SURTI, Nergesh R., Departments of Radiation Oncology and Neurological Surgery, University of California, San Francisco, CA 94143, U.S.A.

VAN EYS, Jan, The University of Texas System Cancer Center, M.D. Anderson Hospital and Tumor Institute, Department of Pediatrics, 6723 Bertner Drive, Houston, TX 77025, U.S.A.

WALD, Barton, University of Southern California School of Medicine, Children's Hospital of Los Angeles, P.O. Box 60850, Terminal Annex, Los Angeles, CA 90060, U.S.A.

WARA, William M., Department of Radiation Oncology, University of California, San Francisco, CA 94143, U.S.A.

WATERS, K.D., Royal Children's Hospital, Flemington Road, Parkville, Victoria 3052, Australia.

WEST, Patrice M., The Children's Memorial Hospital, The McGaw Medical Center of Northwestern University, 2300 Children's Plaza, Chicago, IL 60614, U.S.A.

WILSON, Charles B., Departments of Radiation Oncology and Neurological Surgery, University of California, San Francisco, CA 94143, U.S.A.

YOUNG, H.F., Medical College of Virginia (VCU) and The MCV/VCU Cancer Center, Richmond, VA 23298, U.S.A.

I. Selected Topics

1. Abnormal Immunoregulation in Pediatric Cancer and Immunodeficiency

SAMUEL BRODER

1. NORMAL DIFFERENTIATION AND THE CELLULAR CONTROL OF IMMUNITY

Immune responses require an intricate interplay of negative as well as positive regulatory influences [1–3]. It is thought that early bone marrow lymphocyte precursors may develop according to two pathways of maturation: one involving B cells, which ultimately become plasma cells via a process of mitosis and clonal expansion and mediate humoral immune reactions, and another involving T cells, which mediate cellular immune reactions. The first precursor cell that can be identified as having a unequivocal commitment to the B-cell/plasma cell series contains *trace* amounts of cytoplasmic IgM without easily detectable surface membrane immunoglobulin. These special precursor cells, which have been referred to as pre-B cells, make an early appearance in fetal liver liver and later tend to reside predominantly in bone marrow [4, 5]. The pre-B cells develop in a clonal fashion into immature B cells, which have a single immunoglobulin isotype (IgM) on their cell surface, and then into mature B cells. Mature B cells exhibit a profile of surface membrane receptors including binding sites for antigen–antibody complexes, complement components, and certain plant lectins (such as pokeweed mitogen). Characteristically, mature B cells express membrane-bound immunoglobulin molecules (often IgM and IgD) which have the same antigen-binding portions (variable regions) as the immunoglobulin molecules ultimately synthesized and secreted by their plasma-cell, clonal progeny.

The cells of the immune system involved in cellular immune responses undergo differentiation in the microenvironment of the thymus and are referred to as T cells. In certain animal models, thymic epithelial cells play a direct role in selecting the ulimate recognition capacity of maturing T cells [6]. T cells mediate the classical reactions of cellular immunity, including delayed cutaneous hypersensitivity, allograft rejection, graft-versus-host reactions, and direct tumor-cell-killing.

G.B. Humphrey et al. (eds.), Pediatric oncology 1, 3–45. All rights reserved.
Copyright © 1981 Martinus Nijhoff Publishers bv, The Hague/Boston/London.

In man, mature T cells form spontaneous rosettes with sheep red cells and may be killed by heterologous antisera raised against thymic lymphocyte antigens. Although some T-cell subsets may express antigen-binding receptors which have the same (or very similar) variable regions as the variable regions which may be associated with immunoglobulin heavy chains [7–9], T cells do not produce conventional immunoglobulin molecules. However, T cells, either directly or through soluble factors, do play a crucial role in the regulation of humoral immune responses by acting to augment or impair the B-cell transition into immunoglobulin-secreting plasma cells. Those cells which augment this B-cell transition are referred to as helper cells, and those that inhibit it are referred to as suppressor T cells. Help and suppression appear to be mediated by distinct cellular subsets, genetically committed to mediate only one of these two functions [10–12]. Both antigen-specific and nonspecific (polyclonal) regulatory cells exist.

Regulatory cells that are not of T-cell origin may also exert positive and negative influences on immune responses. One of the most important cells in immune functions is the macrophage [13–15]. Cells which belong to the monocyte–macrophage series may be exceedingly important as phagocytic effector cells in the defense against microbial pathogens and neoplastic cells. Furthermore, macrophages play an indispensable role in antigen-processing as well as antigen-presentation to both T cells and B cells. Macrophages may enhance immune responses both *in vivo* and *in vitro*. Moreover, there is evidence that macrophages (or at least certain macrophage subclasses) can suppress *in vitro* and *in vivo* immune reactions. In certain instances, the apparent regulatory effect of suppressor T cells is in reality mediated by macrophages as the final modulator of immunity [14–16]. There are data to suggest that T cells may produce soluble 'suppressor-arming' factors which bind to the surface of macrophages. 'Armed' macrophages may have an important intermediary role in the transfer of suppressor signals between T-cell subsets [17].

Many lymphoproliferative diseases can be classified as malignancies of either B-cell or T-cell origin [18]; moreover, neoplastic cells from some children and adults with leukemia or lymphoma may behave as though they are trapped (in an operational sense) at defined points in the schema for normal lymphocyte differentiation and regulation.

Although a complete classification of childhood lymphoproliferative diseases on the basis of immunologic and biochemical markers is beyond the scope of this chapter, it might be worthwhile to briefly discuss one special area in pediatric oncology—acute lymphoblastic leukemia (ALL)—where an immunologic classification of membrane markers has proven to be of both clinical and theoretical revelance. ALL may be divided into at least four subcategories on the basis of immunologic membrane markers. Most pediatric oncologists recognize a so-called 'common' type, a T-cell type, a B-cell type, and a null or unclassified type. The 'null' category is an entirely unsatisfactory designation, which is constantly influenced by the immunologic, and biochemical, reagents available. Leukemic cells from patients with the common type of ALL (roughly 80% of the cases studied) do not form spontaneous rosettes with sheep erythrocytes or express easily detectable surface membrane immunoglobulin determinants. It is possible to raise heterologous antibodies that can identify antigen(s) present on common type leukemic cells, but are absent on normal circulating lymphocytes [19, 20]. Common type ALL cells express what are termed Ia-like antigens. (These antigens are taken up in a more basic science context later in this chapter.) The common type of ALL occurs most frequently in young children, with no apparent predilection for either sex. The common type of ALL is generally not associated with a mediastinal mass or leukemic count greater than 10^5 cells/mm^3. A majority of these patients can achieve a long remission with modern therapy, available at many medical centers. The total leukemic count at initial presentation appears to be a significant prognostic factor [19].

Certain cases of 'common'-type ALL probably represent leukemias of pre-B cell origin [21]. As mentioned earlier, the pre-B cell appears to be an early stage in the maturation of normal B cells in which small quantities of *cytoplasmic* IgM are detectable, but surface immunoglobulins are not identifiable. There are strong data to suggest that neoplastic cells from some patients with what otherwise would be classified as common type ALL have the properties of pre-B cells. (B-cell ALL is discussed below.) Although the data are still preliminary, it appears the patients with pre-B-cell ALL respond favorably to combination chemotherapy.

In roughly 20% of ALL cases, the leukemic cells form spontaneous sheep erythrocyte rosettes or react with antisera raised against human T-cell associated antigens [22–24]. Patients whose leukemic cells exhibit these properties fall into the category of T-cell ALL, and such patients may have clinical courses which are dramatically different from those with common-type ALL. T-cell ALL should probably be viewed as a clinical spectrum which overlaps with what has been termed childhood lymphoblastic lymphoma associated with mediastinal mass (a T-lymphoma). Both clinical entities occur in patients who are somewhat older than patients with common ALL, and appear to occur more frequently in males [25, 26]. Patients with T-cell ALL commonly have very high leukemic counts at presentation, and such patients very often have anterior mediastinal masses. Both T-cell ALL and lymphoblastic lymphoma patients have a high risk of developing meningeal involvement, and the overall prognosis tends to be quite poor.

T-cell neoplasms in adults may take the form of cutaneous lymphomas (e.g. mycosis fungoides or the Sezary syndrome), which represent totally different clinopathologic entities.

In a small fraction of children with ALL (less than 5%), the leukemic cells express monoclonal surface membrane immunoglobulin determinants [19, 27]. These comprise the B-cell category of ALL. The leukemic cells in the category have cytologic features which resemble Burkitt's lymphoma. These patients do not have mediastinal involvement; their prognosis is poor. It is likely that some cases which are classified as B-cell ALL represent forms of Burkitt's lymphoma.

The last category of patients with ALL represents a small subset referred to as null-cell or unclassified ALL because the leukemic cells lack B-cell or T-cell surface membrane markers and, by contrast to the common form of ALL, fail to react with the anti-ALL antisera described above. In many ways, the term 'unclassified' ALL would be preferable to the term 'null-cell' ALL. The term 'null-cell' has had different meanings to different pediatric oncologic researchers. Some authors have used the term 'null-cell' leukemia in referring to the so-called *common* form of ALL, which is somewhat misleading because *common-type* ALL cells do have a characteristic profile of cell-surface markers (and in some cases can be definitively characterized as neoplastic pre-B cells.) Patients with unclassified-type ALL represent a heterogeneous clinical population in terms of presentation and response to chemotherapy. Those who present with mediastinal masses probably have a poorer prognosis than those who do not. In principle, as the science of characterizing human neoplasms according to their immunologic marker status progresses, the number of patients who fit into the unclassified-type of ALL should markedly decline. It is now possible to produce monoclonal (hybridoma) antibodies with unprecedented specificity against human lymphocyte membrane antigens [28]. Clinical oncologists should expect an application of this technology in the classification of human neoplasms soon.

In the future, attempts to understand the maturational status of neoplastic lymphocytes may lend themselves to totally new therapeutic approaches based on a manipulation of the physiological forces that govern lymphocyte differentiation. Certain lessons learned from the study of multiple myeloma might provide a useful reference frame for pediatric oncologists in approaching a variety of lymphoproliferative disorders. Multiple myeloma is an adult-disease which represents the monoclonal proliferation of malignant plasma cells. Most patients with multiple myeloma have so-called paraproteins in their serum and/or urine. In general, myeloma paraproteins may be viewed as homogeneous immunoglobulin end-products or immunoglobulin subunits, such as light chains. The immunoglobulins evoked in a conventional immune response are a heterogeneous mixture of antibody molecules that originate from multiple clones, and are therefore termed *polyclonal*. In many cases, the myeloma paraproteins are essentially indistinguishable from conventional antibodies except for their extreme homogeneity due to a monoclonal origin [29]. Indeed, a number of myeloma proteins from patients and mice have antigen-binding activity, sometimes with extremely high affinity. Furthermore, even though the monoclonal plasma cells found in multiple myeloma are the products of a neoplastic process, they may still arise as part of a linear maturation from primitive lymphocytoid precursors (including pre-B cells) which at some point have the same cytoplasmic and cell surface-membrane immunoglobulin receptors as those ultimately secreted by the malignant plasma cells [30, 31]. In certain animal models, there may be T-cell and macrophage-mediated helper and suppressor influences which regulate neoplastic plasma cell proliferation and immunoglobulin secretion in a manner which greatly resembles the T-cell and macrophage control of antigen-driven normal B-cell differentiation [32]. In an analogous fashion, it has been shown that neoplastic B cells obtained from certain patients with chronic lymphocytic leukemia may undergo terminal differentiation to immunoglobulin-secreting plasma cells if provided with the appropriate helper T-cell influence [33]. The concept that the functional status of neoplastic cells may still be, at least partially, influenced by physiologic interaction with normal cells will be taken up again later in this chapter.

2. INTRODUCTION TO GENETIC REGULATION OF IMMUNITY AND SUPPRESSOR T-CELL FUNCTION

The major histocompatibility complex is a chromosomal region found in mammalian species countaining genes that control the strongest allo-transplantation antigens [34]. Genes located within this region (so-called immune-response genes) also profoundly affect several functions of the immune system, including the capacity to generate immune responses to certain well-defined antigens [35–37]. In humans, this gene complex is found on the sixth chromosome and carries information for the synthesis of human leukocyte antigens (*HLA*) clinically useful in transplantation typing. These include the serologically defined *HLA-A, HLA-B,* and *HLA-C;* as well as the *HLA-D*-related antigens, which were initially detected by their capacity to elicit mixed lymphocyte reactions and more recently by serologic techniques. *HLA-D* antigens are detected primarily on B cells and macrophages, whereas *HLA-A, HLA-B* and *HLA-C* can be detected on both B cells and T cells. However, there is recent proof that *HLA-D*-related markers are expressed on T cells under certain conditions of activation [38].

Much of what is known about the cellular control of immune function, and especially the genetics of immunoregulation, is derived from the study of certain carefully defined genetic strains of mice. Since many of the concepts relating to immunoregulation and cancer are based on work done in these murine systems, it is worth reviewing some of the observations in mice which are shaping thinking regarding human systems.

The major histocompatibility complex in mice is called *H-2*. A variety of immune response genes are clustered within this region. It is known that several T-cell helper and suppressor regulatory activities are associated with the so-called *I* region of the *H-2* complex. By using murine strains with recombinant events within this region, it has been possible to define five *I* subregions. These are now designated *I-A*, *I-B*, *I-J*, *I-E*, and *I-C*. The genetic information for a number of distinct immune functions can be assigned to one (or more) specific subregions of the *I* complex. Cell surface antigens encoded by genes which map within this major histocompatibility region involved in the control of immune reactions are called *Ia*-(immune response associated) antigens. *Ia* antigens are readily detected on B cells and macrophages. There is evidence that at least some of the structural information for soluble helper T-cell factors may be encoded in the *I-A* subregion [39–41]. Other *I* subregions participate in suppressor cell function. For example, Rich and Rich have found that suppressor T cells capable of inhibiting mixed-lymphocyte reactions release a factor that depresses the reactivity of responding cells sharing the same *I-C* subregion genotype [42]. Furthermore, the *I-J* subregion contains the genetic information for surface-membrane markers found on suppressor T cells (and on a special subclass of helper T cells) [37, 43–46]. The *I-J* subregion encodes information for determinants found on soluble inhibitory factors derived from certain types of suppressor T cells. Under certain conditions, it is possible to establish continuous culture lines of cells which synthesize and secrete large quantities of these *I-J* related suppressor factors [47, 48]. *I-J* related suppressor T-cell factors may profoundly depress both humoral and cellular immune reactions. Under some conditions, such suppressor factors work only in *I-J* compatible systems [43], and in other circumstances, these factors may work across such histocompatibility barriers [49].

I-J associated suppressor factors are antigen-specific and lack immunoglobulin constant regions. Their molecular weight is approximately 50,000 daltons. It appears that the capacity to generate such suppressor factors is encoded by a gene (or set of genes) different from the gene(s) that determine whether an appropriate target cell will actually be able to accept the suppressor signal conveyed by these factors [50].

It has been shown that the intravenous injection of alloantisera directed against *I-J* determinants can augment certain immune responses by diminishing suppressor-cell function [51]. Indeed, the administration of alloantisera raised against appropriate *I-J*-related antigens can actually reverse a form of genetic nonresponsiveness to certain synthetic antigens, which is mediated by suppresssor cells. Thus, genetically nonresponder mice can be made to acquire immune reactivity to the relevant antigen, presumably as a direct consequence of the serologic disruption of their suppressor T-cell system. Later in this chapter we shall return to the *I-J* subregion and the implications of studies showing the antisera to *I-J* encoded products can actually potentiate certain immune responses.

An understanding of immune response genes, *Ia* antigens, and the genetic regulation of suppressor T-cell function in humans is still in an early stage. It is thought that the *HLA-D* region in man corresponds to the *I* region of mice. There is recent evidence that *HLA-D* associated products may serve as structures permitting certain types of suppressor T cells to recognize appropriate target cells for exertion of inhibitory activity [52]. A glycoprotein antigen complex of 23,000 and 30,000 dalton subunits (referred to as p23,30) is probably one human counterpart to murine *Ia* antigens. This *Ia*-like antigen is present on normal human B cells, macrophages, and activated T cells [38, 53]. As already discussed, in part, it is possible to classify a variety of human leukemias based on their expression of *Ia*-like molecules [53]. Thus, most chronic lymphocytic leukemia cells are *Ia*-like antigen positive. In roughly 80% of the cases studied, acute lymphoblastic leukemia cells are *Ia*-like antigen-positive. Essentially all cases of acute myeloblastic leukemia, but not typical cases of chronic myelogenous leukemia, are *Ia*-like antigen-positive.*

We have data that antibodies to human *Ia* can activate suppressor cells [54]. During the next few years the genetics of human immunoregulation and the relationship between the surface antigenic products of immune response genes and the clinical outcome of certain neoplasms will undoubtedly prove to be one of the most exciting areas of oncologic research.

3. THE CONCEPT OF ABNORMAL REGULATORY CELLS AS CONTRIBUTORS TO TUMOR GROWTH

Oncogenesis is accompanied by the appearance of tumor-associated neoantigens in a number of systems. Whether these tumor-associated antigens may be characterized as truly 'tumor-specific' is controversial. However, it appears that the immunocompetent cells of the host can often recognize these antigens as 'non-self' and, under certain conditions, can actually inhibit neoplastic growth. Nevertheless, in a number of instances, the tumor grows in

---

* There are recent data indicating that cells from solid (non-lymphoid) tumors may also express *Ia*-like antigens, and there may be subtle differences between the *Ia*-determinants on such tumor cells and those expressed on autologous B cells or monocytes due to glycosylation.

spite of the 'non-self' antigens it expresses. There have been many explana-
tions for the ineffectual immune response of tumor bearing hosts. For a
number of years, circulating-blocking factors were thought to impede the
elimination of tumor cells by the immune system [55, 56]. In the beginning,
workers categorized such blocking factors as serum antibodies. However,
antibody fragments [57, 58], soluble antigens shed by tumor cells, or antig-
en–antibody complexes [59, 60] might all have a role in the enhancement of
tumor growth.

More recently, it has been proposed that host suppressor cells and their
factors may undermine effective antitumor immune responses and enhance
tumor growth. This concept is worth exploring in detail. Recent studies have
demonstrated that interventions which at first glance look like active immunization may paradoxically reduce the host's resistance to neoplastic cell
growth. One very carefully studied system illustrating this point involves the
use of 3-methylcholanthrene-induced sarcomas transplanted in A/J-strain
mice [61]. A critical parameter favoring tumor growth in this syngeneic system is the development of suppressor T cells [61–65]. Tumor cells inoculated
into normal mice caused death with 40 days, whereas tumor cells inoculated
into mice previously rendered immune to this tumor were rejected in about
two weeks. Mice were made immune to the tumor by implanting small
numbers of tumor cells subcutaneously and then completely excising the
tumor mass seven days after initial implantation followed by several
additional cycles of immunizations with such cells. When thymocytes or
splenic cells from animals bearing progressive tumors were injected intravenously into *immune* mice at the same time that they received live tumor
cells, tumor growth was enhanced. Therefore, the thymus glands and spleens
of hosts with growing tumors contained suppressor cells. Moreover, such
suppressor cells could actually counteract host immune defenses when
injected into immune mice during a time of ongoing tumor rejection. These
suppressor cells were detectable and remained fully effective for as long as
active tumor growth occurred. However, suppressor-cell activity disappeared
rapidly after surgical extirpation of the tumor.

The suppressor activity of these tumor-bearing hosts was neutralized *in vitro*
by treatment with antisera against T cells. These studies were extended by
testing the effect of *in vivo* antithymocyte serum on the growth of primary
transplantable syngeneic tumors. Repeated injections of antithymocyte serum
at various times after tumor-cell challenge markedly reduced primary-tumor
growth. This reduction of tumor growth probably occurred because suppressor
T cells had been interfering with the capacity of host effector cells to halt
tumor growth. Therefore, the elimination of such suppressor cells could
promote tumor regression. It should be noted that the suppressor T cells
involved in the enhancement of tumor growth in this system were specific. In

other words, these suppressor cells did not affect the growth of unrelated tumors. However, it is worth emphasizing that both specific and nonspecific suppressor cells are known to exist in a variety of other experimental systems.

In further studies, a soluble factor with essentially the identical tumor growth promoting effect as the intact suppressor T cells was extracted from the lymphoid cells of tumor-bearing mice [61, 64]. This soluble suppressor T cell factor bore strikingly similar immunochemical and biologic features to the *I-J* encoded suppressor factors, which were discussed earlier in this chapter as potent inhibitors of humoral and cellular immunity in other systems.

Recent studies involving the use of antisera directed against *I-J* subregion gene products to inhibit tumor growth deserve special emphasis since they provide an important rationale for certain approaches in the future experimental treatment of human neoplasms. We have already discussed studies proving that the *in vivo* administration of antisera directed against antigenic products of the *I-J* subregion can increase immune responses by impairing suppressor-cell function [51]. Greene and his co-workers [66] took this concept one step further and tested the hypothesis that *in vivo* administration of antisera directed against *I-J*-encoded determinants would reduce the function of suppressor T cells in tumor-bearing animals. The net expected effect of such a maneuver would be to inhibit tumor growth. These workers, in fact, found a major retardation of tumor growth in mice treated daily with *anti-I-J* antisera in microliter quantities. Spleens from tumor-bearing mice given *anti-I-J* antisera no longer contained specific suppressor cells. These experiments provide an important model for the serologic inactivation of suppressor T cells in neoplastic states. They provide an important precedent for inducing the host to mount a more effective immune response against lethal tumors by a process of selective T-cell depletion.

It is important to re-emphasize the indispensable role of the T-cell system as a whole in host defenses against microorganisms and tumor cells in a number of situations. Maneuvers that nonselectively impair overall T-cell function will not necessarily contribute to the survival of tumor-bearing hosts. However, the data discussed above demonstrate that a subset of host T cells may contribute to neoplastic growth and, for this reason, such regulatory cells might be profitable targets for certain therapeutic maneuvers. This is an exceedingly important area for clinical investigation.

4. ADDITIONAL SYSTEMS IN WHICH SUPPRESSOR CELLS MAY PLAY A ROLE IN CERTAIN NEOPLASMS

Suppressor cells may act to interfere with immune cytotoxic effector cells with antitumor activity in some cases. In mice, the generation of cell-mediated toxicity against tumor cels *in vitro* can be inhibited by a subpopulation of cells which adhere to nylon [67]. The overall concept that nylon-adherent T cell may suppress tumor-specific cytotoxic responses *in vitro* has been extended to humans. The peripheral blood of certain patients with osteogenic sarcoma appears to contain both tumor-specific cytotoxic effector cells and suppressor cells [68]. Unfractionated circulating lymphocytes from 12 of 28 patients with osteogenic sarcoma were cytotoxic to cultured osteogenic-sarcoma cells. When lymphocytes from the patients whose unseparated cells were not cytotoxic underwent fractionation on bovine serum albumin gradients, a tumor-specific cytotoxic subset of cells was unmasked in 11 or 13 patients. Lymphocytes capable of suppressing the tumoricidal activity of autologous effector lymphocytes were found in 4 of 10 patients tested. The cells responsible for this suppressor activity formed spontaneous sheep red cell rosettes (indicating a T-cell origin) and adhered to nylon. The suppressor cell activity observed in patients with osteogenic sarcoma was generally not found in the normal population or in parents of the patients. Of the four patients with detectable suppressor cells, three were noted to develop pulmonary tumor metastasis. The fourth patient proved to have pulmonary metastasis shortly after the detection of the suppressor cells under discussion. Only one of the six patients without suppressor T cells was reported to have metastatic disease. These observations provide clues that suppressor cells can affect the clinical presentation of patients with cancer and the final outcome of their malignant disease.

Recent reports have described the presence of non-T suppressor cells in tumor-bearing hosts. Furthermore, there is evidence that certain patients (with malignant melanoma, for example) may have immunosuppressive serum factors that interact with B cells and then secondarily cause such target B cells to activate suppressor cells [69]. In other systems, suppressor cells of non-T cell origin appear to inhibit a series of immune responses [70–79].

Such non-T cell suppressors have been described in human beings and may have a role in the progressive growth of some tumors, or in the overall immunodeficiency state associated with certain cancers. This will be discussed in more detail below.

5. POSSIBLE ROLE OF SUPPRESSOR CELLS IN THE IMMUNODEFICIENCY ASSOCIATED WITH NEOPLASTIC STATES

It is known that certain human tumors, for example, Hodgkin's lymphoma, are associated with significant abnormalities of cellular immunity [80]. Moreover, some neoplastic states, such as the syndrome of thymoma combined with hypogammaglobulinemia and also multiple myeloma [81, 82] are especially associated with abnormalities of humoral immunity that may predispose patients to infection with highly pathogenic organisms even before the underlying tumor is diagnosed.

Suppressor cells probably play a role in the cause or perpetuation of impaired immune function in a subset of patients with congenital or acquired hypogammaglobulinemia [83–85]. Even when suppressor cells cannot readily be linked to the pathogenesis of the hypogammaglobulinemia, excess suppressor activity may conceivably affect certain clinical sequelae, such as persistent echovirus meningoencephalitis [86]. Suppressor cells have also been implicated in the anergy associated with widespread fungal infections [87]. While it is important to recall that the immunodeficiency states associated with certain forms of cancer can be related to a number of factors (including nutritional alterations, nonspecific immunoinhibitory serum factors, hormonal imbalances, etc.), this demonstration of suppressor cells in non-neoplastic diseases has induced a re-evaluation of the factors which are responsible for the immunodeficiency found in patients with cancer.

A number of patients with thymomas (in particular, the spindle-cell subset) have a syndrome characterized by severe B-cell depletion, depressed immunoglobulin levels, eosinopenia, and recurrent infections. There are occasions when this syndrome is further associated with selective red cell aplasia or overt aplastic anemia. A majority of patients with this syndrome of thymoma and hypogammaglobulinemia have circulating suppressor T cells that can block the maturation of lymphocytes which make up the B-cell/plasma cell series [88]. However, it is not known whether such suppressor cells are a primary cause of the hypogammaglobulinemia by acting to inhibit early B-cell development or, perhaps more likely, represent the secondary accumulation of inhibitory T cells in patients with a fundamental B-stem-cell defect.

We have discussed multiple myeloma in our earlier discussion of the concept that neoplastic cells may retain an inherent maturational capacity in spite of their neoplastic status. However, multiple myeloma also provides a very clear example of a neoplasm with clinically significant immune impairments as a consequence of abnormal host regulatory cell activation. Patients with multiple myeloma generally have reduced *in vivo* polyclonal immunoglobulin synthetic rates [82], and, consequently, they may have low titers of antibodies in their serum [89, 90]. They may also have reduced percentages of circulating lymphocytes that bear normal surface-membrane immunoglobulin determinants [91–94].

A number of theories have been devised to explain the impaired B-cell function observed inpatients with multiple myeloma. According to one theory, myeloma tumor cells secrete infective molecules of informational RNA that alter the expression of normal immunoglobulin receptors on the surfaces of host B cells, thereby inhibiting the recognition of foreign antigenic substances and the appropriate humoral immune responses [95–99]. According to another theory, myeloma cells release so-called chalones, which may be thought of as specific mitotic inhibitors that block the critical expansion of normal B-cell clones in response to antigenic confrontation [100].

In the past, most investigators focused on myeloma cells or their direct products as the cause of immune impairment in myeloma. It is now clear that the immunoregulatory cell system of the host must be taken into account because certain patients who have multiple myeloma develop very potent circulating suppressor cells. In patients with multiple myeloma [91], and in mice bearing malignant plasma cell tumors [101], host macrophage-like cells appear to play a role in the immunodeficiency observed. In mice, such cells are especially evident in the spleen and peritoneal cavity [102]. Other investigators have confirmed that suppressor cells of non-T-cell origin (including cells other than macrophages) may play a part in the immunodeficiency state associated with multiple myeloma [103]. Malignant plasma cells do not appear to be directly responsible for the suppressor effect observed, but they very likely initiate a chain of events that leads to immunosuppression via macrophages. These concepts should help frame future clinical investigations into the status of immune function in children with cancer.

Patients with a variety of solid tumors may have impaired delayed hypersensitivity skin reactions to such agents as streptokinase-streptodornase and *Candida* extract. They may also show impaired contact sensitivity to 2,4-dinitro-1-chlorobenzene (DNCB). These depressed cellar immune reactions are, in general, related to large total-body tumor burdens. *In vitro* lymphocyte blastic transformation induced by nonspecific mitogens or specific antigens is also depressed in many such patients. Again, the etiology for this nonspecific immunodepression is multifactorial; however, there is evidence that at least one mechanism relates to a subset of circulating macrophage-like cells [104]. In certain patients, suppressor T cells may be responsible.

Hodgkin's disease is a very interesting lymphoma associated with an acquired *in vivo* and *in vitro* deficiency of cell-mediated immunity. Patients with Hodgkin's disease are often cutaneously anergic and the likelihood of anergy increases with progressive disease [105]. This defect of cellular immune function cannot be corrected by giving leukocytes from normal donors [106]. By contrast, patients with Hodgkin's disease tend to have normal (or even increased) humoral immune function, except in very advanced forms of the lymphoma. Of course, radiotherapy and/or chemotherapy may alter the immune status of patients. Some patients with Hodgkin's disease have a depression of cellular immune function that appears far out of proportion to the apparent total-body tumor burden. Studies from several laboratories indicate that excessive suppressor-cell activity may be one of the factors responsible for the immunodeficiency state associated with this lymphoma. Twomey and his co-workers[107] found that 16 of 30 patients with Hodgkin's disease had circulating suppressor cells (with adherent properties) that inhibited mixed lymphocyte reactions. In a recent study by Engleman and his co-workers, circulating cells which had the capacity to inhibit mixed lymphocyte reactions were detected in 41 of 70 patients with Hodgkin's disease[108]. These authors provided preliminary data showing that this kind of suppressor-cell activity was restricted by gene products associated with the *HLA-D* subregion. Moreover, Hillinger and Herzig found evidence that patients with Hodgkin's disease had increased activity of suppressor T cells and suppressor macrophage-like cells capable of inhibiting mixed lymphocyte reactions, and they reported data favoring a major histocompatibility complex restriction of suppressor activity in some cases[109]. Further work may eventually provide formal proof for the genetic control of suppressor-cell activity in human neoplastic disease.

It has recently been suggested that the *in vitro* hyporesponsiveness found in certain patients with Hodgkin's disease may be due to excessive synthesis of prostaglandin E_2 by glass-adherent mononuclear suppressor cells[110]. Moreover, indomethacin (a prostaglandin synthetase inhibitor), effected a restoration of *in vitro* blastogenic responses by the lymphocytes of certain patients with Hodgkin's disease. These observations may have an important clinical relevance by defining a relatively safe pharmacologic basis for removing undesirable suppressor cell function in selected diseases. In any case, it appears clear that some of the concepts relating to the genetic regulation of immunity and suppressor cell function, which were discussed earlier in this chapter, will eventually be indispensable in understanding the clinical status of certain patients with cancer.

6. RETENTION OF IMMUNOREGULATORY FUNCTION BY CERTAIN NEOPLASMS

A small subset of patients with acute lymphoblastic leukemia have very severe depressions of their serum immunoglobulin levels before therapy[111]. There are now data indicating that some patients, in whom leukemia or lymphoma of T-cell origin develops, may show immunosuppression because their tumors originate from a subclass of T cells committed to mediate suppressor function. We have recently analyzed the suppressor-cell activity of neoplastic T cells from an unusual child with acute lymphoblastic leukemia and hypogammaglobulinemia[112]. We observed that after systematic chemotherapy, this patient's immunoglobulin levels returned to normal during remission of the leukemia and dropped once again during terminal leukemic relapse. The leukemic T cells from this child acted as potent pro-suppressor cells in an *in vitro* system involving polyclonal activation induced by pokeweed mitogen [113]. In addition, Uchiyama *et al.* have reported that three of six Japanese patients with adult T-cell leukemia had neoplastic cells with suppressor-like properties [114]. One feature of the leukemic cells that we studied was their requirement of a radiosensitive *cooperating* subset of normal T cells before a full suppressor effect could be expressed. This observation may indicate that a T–T interaction is necessary in the generation of human suppressor effector cells, perhaps in a fashion similar to what has been proposed for murine suppressor-cell systems [41, 115, 116].

The recognition of suppressor-cell leukemias underscores the principle that neoplasms of T-cell origin may in some cases retain immunoregulatory properties. It is already known that leukemic T-cells from some, but not all, patients with the Sezary syndrome appear to retain helper-like function [117]. Such a helper-like activity may even be retained when the tumor appears to have undergone a morphologically assessed transformation into a more 'undifferentiated' state [118]. Of note, neoplastic cells with helper-like activity have been reported in mice [119], and murine models may prove quite useful in this area of research.

It is perhaps too early to make broad generalizations about the classes of tumors which may retain immunoregulatory properties. There are data to suggest that neoplastic transformation can occur in an early T lymphocyte capable of further maturation along the distinct pathways for both help and suppression. This possibility is supported by observations in a patient with ataxia telengiectasia who developed a chronic T-cell leukemia bearing a characteristic $14 q^+$ chromosomal translocation [120]. The patient's neoplastic T cells appeared to mediate *both* helper and suppressor activity *in vitro* equivalent to that of normal T cells.

Neoplastic T cells with immunoregulatory properties could be used as a crucial resource for the serologic or biochemical characterization of human helper and suppressor cells. In addition, an understanding of the immunoregulatory properties of neoplastic T cells could have implications for the immediate care of selected patients. Patients with functioning neoplasms of suppressor-cell origin will probably fall into a poor prognostic category because the malignant cells can, in principle, subvert host-immune responses against both the neoplasm itself and pathogenic microorganisms.

7. IMMUNODEFICIENCY STATES WHICH RESULT IN A PREDISPOSITION TO CANCER

Every pediatric and medical oncologist should be aware of the strong relationship between certain immunodeficiency states and neoplastic disease. It is clear that immunodeficiency produced in experimental animals often brings about an increased risk of cancer[121, 122]. In humans, a variety of conditions characterized by an impairment of immune function are associated with a higher frequency of certain cancers than age-matched controls[123, 124]. This higher frequency of cancer is also commonly associated with a shorter latency period. In the following portion of this chapter, we will review certain significant immunodeficiency states and discuss their relationship to cancer. The clinical features of the major immunodeficiency diseases are important because of their practical importance to the pediatric oncologist and because of the research opportunities they provide. It will not be possible to cover all immunodeficiency diseases in the chapter.

8. CANCER IN ORGAN ALLOTRANSPLANT RECIPIENTS

There is roughly a 6% incidence of *de novo* cancer in organ allotransplant recipients who receive immunosuppressant therapy. This frequency of cancer represents at least a 100-fold (and possibly much higher) increase in risk compared to an age-corrected general population[125, 126]. A majority of these cancers occur in young adults, and the average time of tumor appearance is 28 months after transplantation. The increased incidence does *not* represent a generalized risk for all histologic forms of cancer. A high percentage of these malignancies are lymphoreticular in origin, and there is a truly striking predisposition of *de novo* lymphomatous brain involvement[127]. There is also a clear increase in epithelial cancers involving skin.

9. GENERALIZATION ABOUT CANCER IN PATIENTS WITH INHERENT ABNORMALITIES OF THE IMMUNE SYSTEM

Before turning to specific immunodeficiency diseases, a few general comments are in order. Although clinical investigation in this field has been underway for many years, much remains to be done. However, certain trends are striking. For example, in some immunodeficiency diseases there may be a 100-fold increase in the risk of developing a lymphoma (reminiscent of the risk in organ transplantation cited above). Spector, Perry, and Kersey have recently compiled data from the Immunodeficiency-Cancer Registry (ICR) which was established to monitor the cancer incidence in patients with genetically determined immunodeficiency diseases both within the United States and abroad[128]. Attempts to analyze the true incidence of cancer in patients with inherent abnormalities of immunity are complicated by at least three potential sources of error: certain kinds of immunodeficiency diseases may be under-reported, certain histologic forms of cancer may be over-reported, and the histopathologic classification of neoplasms (especially non-Hodgkin's lymphoma) has changed in the years that the Registry patients were diagnosed. Nonetheless, much useful information is available, and Spector *et al.* have used the data from the Registry to formulate several generalizations:

(i) Children with inherent immunodeficiency diseases who develop cancer tend to have a non-Hodgkin's lymphoma. Adults with immunodeficiency diseases tend to develop non-Hodgkin's lymphoma and carcinomas in roughly equal proportion. The most common single histologic type of non-Hodgkin's lymphoma is 'histiocytic' lymphoma. (However, it is very important to emphasize that this pathologic designation per se cannot be taken to mean that the tumor has a macrophage origin.)

(ii) Certain immunodeficiency states have an association with a particular type of pattern of neoplastic disease. For example, there appears to be a disproportionate association between the Wiskott-Aldrich syndrome and myelogenous leukemia. This syndrome has other noteworthy associations, which will be taken up later.

(iii) The stomach is a target organ for carcinomas in both adolescent and adult patients with several kinds of genetically determined immunodeficiency diseases.

In addition to these major generalizations, there are preliminary indications that the neoplastic cells in immunodeficient patients with lymphoproliferative malignancies frequently have a B-cell origin, and to a lesser extent, a T-cell or null-cell origin. However, much more research is necessary to resolve this issue.

10. SPECIFIC IMMUNODEFICIENCY DISEASES

Just as the earlier discussion of the pathways of cellular differentiation provides a reference frame for characterizing potential points of neoplastic cell development of expression in certain lymphoproliferative disorders, the earlier discussion in this chapter provides a means for categorizing certain immunodeficiency states as either blocks at specified points in lymphocyte maturation or abnormalities in the cellular regulation of this process.

11. SEVERE COMBINED IMMUNODEFICIENCY (SCID)

Severe combined immunodeficiency represents a fundamental defect of both B-cell and T-cell development. A defect at the stem-cell level or a profound defect of T cells (including a severe deficit of helper cells necessary for adequate B-cell function) could account for the clinical syndrome observed. There are three different modes of inheritance for this entity that give rise to the same ultimate catastrophe of immune system malfunction: sporadic, autosomal-recessive, and sex-linked. There is also an association with deficiency of adenosine deaminase in a subset of patients who have severe combined immunodeficiency, and there is a variant of the syndrome that is associated with dysostosis.

Patients with severe combined immunodeficiency lack both humoral and cellular immune responses. Profound lymphocytopenia is common. Clinically, severe combined immunodeficiency becomes evident soon after birth and is marked by a steady assault of infections with bacteria, fungi (*Candida* infection of the skin and mucous membranes is almost always present), viruses, and protozoa (*Pneumocystis*). Nearly all of these patients have significant diarrhea, and even though *Salmonella* and pathogenic strains of *E. coli* are identified in certain patients, it is common for the cause of the diarrhea to remain undiagnosed. Such patients are at high risk of graft-versus-host reactions if they receive transfusions of unirradiated blood components containing immunocompetent cells. Patients with severe combined immunodeficiency disease can, in principle, be immunologically reconstituted with *HLA*-matched stem cells given in the form of bone marrow transplantation. However, as a practical matter, the prognosis for these patients is quite poor.

The percentage of cancer observed in patients with this disease is about 1.5% with 0.9 years as the median age at diagnosis of the malignancy [128]. The incidence of lymphoreticular cancer (including leukemia, Hodgkin's disease, and non-Hodgkin's lymphoma) is especially noteworthy. Solid lymphoid malignancies are rare in infants, and it must be assumed that the lymphomas did not occur by chance alone in this patient population.

12. DIGEORGE SYNDROME

Pediatric oncologists may be frequently asked to assist in the diagnosis and care of complex patients who appear to have an immune impairment. For this reason, it is useful to discuss the DiGeorge syndrome even though this syndrome does not have an association with cancer that has been recognized to date. Patients with the DiGeorge syndrome have a developmental failure of structures derived from the third and fourth pharyngeal pouches during embryonic life leading to abnormalities of the ear and facial structures, congenital heart disease, abnormalities of the parathyroid glands with hypocalcemic tetany, and hypoplasia of the thymus with an associated cellular immune deficiency state [129–131]. If the patient survives the neonatal period, increased susceptibility to recurrent pneumonias (including *Pneumocystis carinii* pneumonias) is noted.

During the first six to eight weeks of intrauterine life the thymus and parathyroid glands develop from elements of the third and fourth pharyngeal pouches. The thymus begins to migrate caudally during the twelfth week of gestation. During this period the philtrum of lip and ear tubule become differentiated along with the aortic arch structures. Since, with the exception of one family with two affected members [132], the DiGeorge syndrome has been sporadic, it seems likely that some intrauterine insult occurring early in gestation leads to the abnormalities of the parathyroid, thymus, aortic arch, ears, and facial structures that develop during this period. The nonimmunologic features of this syndrome include hypoparathyroidism and hypocalcemic-related tetany (and seizures) during the first week of life. Cardiovascular defects including a right-sided aortic arch, a double arch or tetralogy of Fallot may be present. The patients have a series of facial abnormalities including micrognathia, hypertelorism, low-set ears with notched ear pinnae, shortened philtrum of the lip and antimongoloid-slant eyes. Patients with this syndrome often die very early in life from either hypoparathyroidism or from overwhelming infection with viral, fungal, or protozoan (*Pneumocystis*) pathogens.

DiGeorge syndrome is considered to be the classic example of an isolated T-cell immunological deficiency associated with thymic hypoplasia. The proper thymic microenvironment for the maturation of T lymphocytes is not available in these patients. However, it should be stressed that the thymic abnormalities and the defects of cell-mediated immunity observed are quite variable. While most patients do not have a thymus demonstrable on lateral X-ray examination of the mediastinum, a substantial number of patients have one or more unusually small thymus glands in an ectopic location. These small glands tend to be histologically normal with normal corticomedullary differentiation and Hassall's corpuscles. There is a subset of patients with this syndrome in whom no thymus is identifiable at autopsy.

The absolute lymphocyte count is usually normal, or at times moderately depressed. However, the percentage of B cells (identified by the expression of easily detectable cell-surface immunoglobulin molecules) is markedly increased and the percentage of T cells (identified either by the capacity to form spontaneous sheep red cell rosettes or reactivity with heterologous anti-T-cell antisera) is markedly reduced [133]. There is also a diminution in the thymic dependent regions of lymph nodes, with a reduction in the size and degree of lymphocytoid cellularity of the deep cortical regions. Patients with DiGeorge syndrome may also have profound defects in a range of T-cell functions. These defects include poor *in vitro* blastogenesis of lymphocytes in response to polyclonal lectins and specific antigens, absent delayed cutaneous hypersensitivity reactions to common antigens, failure of effective sensitization to dinitrochlorobenzene, and prolonged skin allograft survival. Gross abnormalities in *humoral* immune function do not generally occur in patients with DiGeorge-like syndromes, although patients with markedly reduced immunoglobulin levels have been reported [134, 135].

It should be reemphasized the patients with the DiGeorge syndrome generally have increased percentages of circulating B cells and normal thymus independent zones in lymph nodes and spleen. The observation that many patients with this syndrome have relatively normal immunoglobulin levels and antibody responsiveness is somewhat difficult to reconcile with the known requirement for T-cell help in a variety of humoral immune responses (discussed at the beginning of this chapter). Perhaps one explanation for the relatively normal humoral immunity observed in these patients is that the majority have small but histologically normal thymus remnants, permitting a sufficient number of helper T cells to develop without permitting subsets of T cells that mediate other critical cellular immune functions to develop.

Incubation of bone marrow cells from patients with the DiGeorge syndrome with thymosin leads to a marked increase in the number of cells that bear surface antigens recognized by heterologous antithymocyte antibodies [136]. Similarly, following incubation with thymosin, there was an increase in the number of peripheral blood lymphocytes that spontaneously form rosettes with sheep red cells [137]. These observations support the view that the immunological defect in patients with the DiGeorge syndrome is not at the level of precursor T-stem cell but is rather in the development of thymus required for the differentiation of stem cells into functioning T cells.

13. ATAXIA TELANGIECTASIA

Ataxia telangiectasia is an autosomal recessive multisystem disorder characterized by degenerative changes in the central nervous system (especially within the cerebellum), oculocutaneous telangiectasis, recurrent sinopulmonary infections, a high incidence of cancer and a complex immunodeficiency state [138–140]. Progressive neurological abnormalities dominated by cerebellar ataxia are usually recognized very early in childhood. However, the characteristic telangiectasis consisting of dilated venules usually appear between the ages of 2 and 8 years (most often appearing on the conjunctivae and exposed areas of skin). This may make the correct diagnosis extremely difficult on clinical grounds alone before two years of age. Other integumental abnormalities include vitiligo, café au lait spots, sclerodermoid changes and gray hair. The patients frequently have significant retardation of growth. Abnormalities of endocrine function have been described, including abnormalities of ovarian histology in some patients or absence of ovaries in others. Over half of the patients have an abnormality of carbohydrate metabolism consisting of glucose intolerance, increased plasma insulin levels and failure of insulin to reduce blood sugar levels. Anti-insulin receptor antibodies have been demonstrated in certain patients with ataxia telangiectasia and insulin resistance [141]. There appears to be a decreased frequency of *HLA*-B8. However, more *HLA* typing studies are necessary.

Using a sensitive double-antibody radioimmunoassay capable of detecting nanogram per millimeter concentrations, Waldmann and McIntire have demonstrated that essentially all patients with ataxia telangiectasia have elevated serum levels of alpha-fetoprotein [142]. This observation has provided an invaluable tool in the diagnosis of this disorder, especially in atypical cases. Normally, only fetal liver cells or regenerating liver cells secrete significant amounts of alpha-fetoprotein. Certain neoplasms, which have a hepatic or germ-cell origin, also secrete substantial amounts of this protein. Elevated levels of alpha-fetoprotein appear to be a special feature of ataxia telangiectasia which is characteristically not found in other immunodeficiency states. The reasons for the fascinating association between ataxia telangiectasia and elevated levels of this oncofetal marker are still not clear, but this disease may conceivably be the result of a generalized defect in mesenchymal–entodermal interactions, leading to thymic and hepatic derangement. This remains speculative.

Recurrent infections, particularly involving the sinopulmonary tree, occur frequently in this patient population. In a large percentage of patients, chronic infections lead to structural lung damage and respiratory insufficiency.

Patients with ataxia telangiectasia exhibit a complex series of immunological impairments which involve both cellular and humoral immune responses. The full extent of these impairments varies from patient to patient, and even varies at different times in any given patient's clinical course. With respect to humoral immune function, approximately 75% of the patients have depressed levels of serum IgA, often with no IgA detectable by conventional quantitative immunodiffusion techniques. This deficiency of IgA is seen in the respiratory and intestinal secretions as well. IgE is also undetectable or reduced in a large percentage of the patients studied [143, 144]. Serum IgG levels are usually normal, while serum IgM levels are often estimated to be high. However, these high estimates for serum IgM often reflect the unusual presence of a low-molecular (monomeric) form of IgM in a large number of patients with ataxia telangiectasia. Such low-molecular weight IgM molecules diffuse more rapidly in immunodiffusion plates than the standard (pentameric) IgM, giving falsely high values.

Most of the patients tested can make antibody responses to blood group substance, the *Vi* antigen of *E. coli* and the Forget tularemia antigen, although the antibody titers achieved are significantly less than normal. The serum antibody responses in the IgA class appear deficient even in those patients whose serum contains circulating IgA immunoglobulins. Moreover, patients with ataxia telangiectasia make relatively poor antibody responses to viral agents, such as polio and influenza virus. Local secretory antibody responses are usually poor.

Patients with ataxia telangiectasia have a variable impairment of cellular immunity [140, 145]. A large number of patients with this disorder are cutaneously anergic to a battery of common skin test antigens, and in some cases, they cannot be sensitized to dinitrochlorobenzene. In an era in which skin transplantation across histocompatibility barriers was employed as a standard test of clinical immune function, it was learned that a number of patients exhibited delayed rejection of skin allografts. It appears that the critical combination of severe cellular and humoral immune defects is a key factor in the predisposition to infection seen in this disease.

The clinical deficiency of cellular and humoral immunity discussed above is reflected in the microscopic architecture of lymphoid tissues. It is common to observe very small lymph nodes with severe lymphocyte depletion. Perhaps one of the most striking histopathologic features is the significant abnormality of thymic structure seen in many patients with this disease. The thymus gland may be absent or very small. It often has an embryonic appearance. The number of thymic lymphocytes is decreased, and the predominant cell-type has a reticuloendothelial-stromal origin. Typically, no differentiation between thymic cortex and medulla is observed. Moreover, in general, Hassall's corpuscles are not seen. It is probably not accurate to characterize the thymus of patients with this disease as truly atrophic; rather, the thymus glands in this disease can perhaps be characterized as being immature or undeveloped. It is plausible that the abnormalities seen are an extension of the defect in proper mesenchymal–entodermal interaction which was discussed as an hypothesis above.

There are extensive data to suggest that patients with ataxia telangiectasia have a defect of DNA repair mechanisms. Patients with this disorder tend to be extremely sensitive to X-ray photons [146, 147]. Fibroblasts from these patients exhibit defective DNA repair following exposure to X-irradiation. (However, unlike patients with xeroderma pigmentosum, patients with ataxia telangiectasia do not appear to have an unusual sensitivity to ultra-violet photons.) A number of patients who have required ionizing radio therapy for an underlying malignancy have developed severe or even fatal reactions. This point will be taken up further below. The lymphocytes of some, but not all, patients have a very high frequency of spontaneous breaks in their chromosomes [148]. These tend to be translocations or deletions among the group D chromosomes, particularly chromosome 14 [149].

Patients with ataxia telangiectasia have a high cancer incidence. The percentage of malignancies observed is approximately 12%, with 9 years as the median age at the time of diagnosis [128]. A large number of the malignancies observed are leukemias or lymphomas. However, these patients appear to have an increased risk of other malignancies as well. Cases of gastric, central nervous system, ovarian, and cutaneous cancer have all been reported. There are examples of malignancies with different histologic patterns in the same individuals occurring sequentially. Many of the malignancies that occur in this disease may well provide special resources for clinical investigaion. As already discussed, it has been shown that a T-cell form of lymphocytic leukemia in a patient with ataxia telangiectasia appeared to retain the capacity to mediate polyclonal helper and suppressor activity [120].

There are instances in which neoplasms have occurred in siblings with ataxia telangiectasia, but not in other siblings without the phenotypic expression of this disease. This could be viewed as yet another indication that the occurrence of these neoplasms is not a mere random phenomenon.

As implied above, patients with ataxia telangiectasia and cancer pose special problems related to their abnormality of DNA repair and unusual reactivity to ionizing irradiation. Whenever radiotherapy is employed in these patients, the physician should be alert to the possibility of excessive radiosensitivity (especially toxic cutaneous reactions).

14. INFANTILE SEX-LINKED HYPOGAMMAGLOBULINEMIA (BRUTON-TYPE)

Bruton-type hypogammaglobulinemia may be thought of as an opposite counterpart to DiGeorge syndrome, in that the B-cell limb of immune cell development is broken. This X-linked immunological deficiency disease is characterized by defective B-cell function and intact T-cell function [150]. It had been thought that this disease resulted from a defect in the bursalequivalent microenvironment necessary for B-cell maturation. Surgical or pharmacologic bursectomy in chickens produces a comparable immune deficit. Recently, it has been suggested that some patients with this disorder actually have the immediate precursors of B cells, but suppressor T cells block the normal maturational process [85]. Further research is necessary to clarify this issue.

Patients with this form of immunodeficiency lack tonsils and generally lack plasma cells in germinal centers, whereas thymic histology is normal. They are generally not lymphocytopenic; however, they do lack mature B cells in their circulation. These patients have very low concentrations of serum immunoglobulins, and they make little or no specific antibodies in response to antigenic challenge. Clinically, patients with infantile sex-linked hypogammaglobulinemia are subject to recurrent infections with high grade pathogens, such as *Hemophilus influenzae* or *Strep-tococcus pneumoniae*. The sinopulmonary tree is a key target for these infections, and crippling lung damage may occur. Parenteral gammaglobulin replacement therapy can improve the clinical course of these patients to a significant degree.

Several cases of malignancy have been described in patients with infantile sex-linked hypogammaglobulinemia. In what might have been the earliest description, Page *et al.* [151] reported a child with agammaglobulinemia and dermatomyositis who was found to have a lymphoma involving lymph nodes, liver, and kidneys at autopsy. The same report described a child with agammaglobulinemia who was noted to have acute lymphoblastic leukemia at approximately 4 years of age. Several other cases of leukemia (one in association with a thymoma) have been described [123].

At one time, the risk of malignancy in patients with infantile sex-linked hypogammaglobulinemia was estimated to be approximately 6%. However, in the recent report from the Immunodeficiency-Cancer Registry (covering a period from the Fall of 1975 to the Spring of 1977) the percentage of patients with cancer was only 0.7% [128]. The true risk of cancer in this disease must, therefore, be considered an issue which requires further research.

15. COMMON VARIABLE IMMUNODEFICIENCY

This is the most common kind of immunodeficiency disease and represents a heterogeneous group of disorders in which the immunodeficiency state may arise after a period of apparently normal immunologic function. Certain cases of what once was termed acquired hypogammaglobulinemia would now be classified as having common variable immunodeficiency. As with Bruton-type immunodeficiency, these patients have depressed serum immunoglobulin levels. They generally make little or no antibodies in response to antigenic challenge, and replacement gammaglobulin therapy is necessary. Near relatives of patients with common variable immunodeficiency have a high incidence of dysgammaglobulinemia and autoimmune phenomena. A large percentage of patients with common variable immunodeficiency also have significant abnormalities of *in vivo* or *in vitro* assays of cellular immune function. Thus, this disease is often associated with significant T-cell dysfunction. In a large subset of patients, circulating B cells can be detected. As already mentioned, there are data to indicate that perhaps one factor in the cause or perpetuation of this disease is the presence of abnormal suppressor T cell which can act to inhibit the terminal maturation of B cells into immunoglobulin synthesizing and secreting plasma cells [2].

Patients with common variable immunodeficiency referred to the Metabolism Branch of the National Cancer Institute have presented with a constellation of symptoms. Perhaps the most common presenting symptoms are related to sinopulmonary infections reminiscent of Bruton-type immunodeficiency. Patients often have recurrent sinusitis, mastoiditis, and otitis media. Even while receiving replacement gammaglobulin therapy, a number of patients develop recurrent pulmonary infections in the form of severe bronchitis and pneumonia, which may lead to bronchiectasis. One problem is that many patients already have significant pulmonary damage by the time their immunodeficiency is diagnosed, and the structurally damaged lung per se is a risk factor for recurrent infections. The pathogens for these infections (at least early in the patient's course) tend to be encapsulated bacteria such as *Streptococcus pneumoniae* and *Hemophilus influenzae*.

A large number of patients with common variable immunodeficiency may also have serious gastrointestinal problems, especially diarrhea and malabsorption. In a small number of patients, gastrointestinal symptoms represent the major manifestations of this disease complex. Some patients with common variable immunodeficiency have giardiasis, frequently in association with nodular lymphoid hyperplasia of the gastrointestinal tract. There is also a subset of patients who develop gastrointestinal bacterial overgrowth, which may be accompanied by partial villous atrophy of the small intestine.

For reasons which are not clear, perhaps 10 to 15% of patients with common variable immunodeficiency have atrophic gastritis in association with pernicious anemia. These patients may have positive Schilling's tests and may show both hematologic and neurologic sequelae of vitamin B_{12} deficiency. Other unexplained features of this syndrome are splenomegaly and idiopathic noncaseating granulomas of visceral organs, including the liver. Some patients with common variable immunodeficiency suffer the paradoxical development of autoimmune hemolysis and may have Coomb's positive hemolytic anemias. Thus, simply because a patient has a humoral immune impairment, it is not justifiable to dismiss the possibility of autoimmune disease. To emphasize this further, a number of patients have arthralgias and arthritis, primarily of smaller joints. Some patients have a syndrome which resembles overt rheumatoid arthritis. Also, serious dermatomyositis and vasculitis-type syndromes can complicate the course of patients with common variable immunodeficiency.

The incidence of malignancy among patients with common variable immunodeficiency seems clearly higher than found in the general population [128]. In those patients in whom the onset of the immunodeficiency appears before 16 years of age, the percentage of cancer observed is approximately 2.5%. In those patients in whom the onset of immunodeficiency occurs at age 16 or older, the percentage of cancer observed is approximately 8.5%. It is worth adding that patients with selective absence of certain immunoglobulin classes (especially IgM), who do not readily fit the diagnosis of common variable immunodeficiency, may also be at increased risk of neoplasia.

Lymphoreticular tumors (especially histocytic and lymphocytic lymphomas) predominate in this patient group. However, approximately 40% of the neoplasms seen are (non-cutaneous) epithelial tumors [128]. Gastric carcinomas comprise a substantial proportion of the neoplasms seen in this patient population, and perhaps the known tendency for certain patients to develop atrophic gastritis is one factor in the association between gastric cancer and common variable immunodeficiency.

As discussed elsewhere, certain patients with immunodeficiency diseases have inherent biologic abnormalities which may impede standard therapeutic approaches. For example, patients with ataxia telangiectasia have DNA repair defects which may severely complicate attempts to provide radiotherapy. As will be discussed further below, patients with the Wiskott-Aldrich syndrome generally have low platelet counts as an inherent feature of their disease. They often have severe chronic herpetic infections or bacterial superinfection of eczematous sites. These may affect the selection of cytotoxic agents, as will as their dosages and timing of administration. However, patients with common variable immunodeficiency who develop cancer (especially lymphomas) may well be candidates for vigorous diagnostic and therapeutic intervention. While there is certainly an added risk owing to the underlying predisposition to infection, the oncologist who manages such patients should ensure that proper staging and histopathologic classification are carried out. In a number of cases, the clinical oncologist can begin intensive combination chemotherapy (and radiotherapy) tailored to fit the histopathologic classification and stage of the patient's tumor. It is clear that certain advanced non-Hodgkin's lymphomas occurring in the general population can be cured in a significant subset of patients by using aggressive combination chemotherapy [152]. When such lymphomas occur in patients with common variable immunodeficiency, simple palliative therapy is not justified unless there are specific contraindications to combination chemotherapy.

16. THE WISKOTT-ALDRICH SYNDROME (IMMUNODEFICIENCY WITH
    THROMBOCYTOPENIA AND ECZEMA)

The Wiskott-Aldrich syndrome encompasses a fascinating sex-linked disorder which is characterized clinically by the triad of thrombocytopenia, eczema, and recurrent infections with all classes of microorganisms. In certain respects, it is one of the most devastating immunodeficiency diseases. This disease was described in the German literature over 40 years ago, but it was not widely recognized until Aldrich et al. described affected males in a large family pedigree [153, 154].

Infection, bleeding requiring platelet support, and—as will be developed in more detail below—malignancies are significant problems in this syndrome. Previously, few patients survived into the second decade, but one should expect longer survivals in the era of modern antibiotics and platelet support. Patients with this syndrome have profound abnormalities of both the humoral and cellular immune systems [124, 155]. In addition, they have functional defects of cells belonging to the monocyte/macrophage series [156]. The constellation of abnormalities seen in this disorder is strikingly different from all other recognized immunodeficiency diseases.

Marked abnormalities in immunoglobulin production occur. These patients may have extremely elevated IgA and IgE serum levels. Using data collected from metabolic turnover studies, it is known that the *in vivo* synthetic rate for IgG is high; however, for reasons that are not fully understood, these patients have an excessive fractional catabolic rate which masks the elevated synthetic rate and leads to an apparently normal serum IgG concentration [124]. Considering the rarity with which monoclonal gammopathies are observed in general pediatric populations, patients with the Wiskott-Aldrich syndrome have an impressive predilection for the development of monoclonal immunoglobulin spikes [157]. These patients generally have very low IgM levels in their serum. Even when these boys synthesize normal or elevated levels or total immunoglobulin, they have decreased titers of a variety of natural antibodies. Patients with this disease characteristically make poor antibody responses following immunization, and antibody responses to polysaccharide antigens are especially poor. This may be one factor for the known risk of patients with this disease to develop recurrent episodes of pneumoccocal sepsis.

Marked abnormalities of delayed cutaneous hypersensitivity (one measure of cellular immunity) are associated with this syndrome. Typically, patients with the Wiskott-Aldrich syndrome have poor or absent delayed reactions in recall skin testing to such agents as *Candida,* purified protein derivative (PPD), *Trichophyton,* mumps, diphtheria, and tetanus toxoid. Patients with this syndrome also have defective delayed hypersensitivity reactions upon primary exposure to new antigens, such as dinitrochlorobenzene and keyhole limpet hemocyanin. Moreover, in the era in which skin allografting was used clinically in the immune evaluation of patients, it was learned that these patients had defective allograft rejection.

Patients with the Wiskott-Aldrich syndrome have a somewhat unusual profile of *in vitro* functions of cellular immunity. Typically, patients with the Wiskott-Aldrich syndrome have adequate numbers of peripheral T cells. Lymphocytes from these patients have a normal (or supra-normal) proliferative response when exposed to nonspecific mitogens, such as phytohemagglutinin [124]. However, when exposed to specific antigenic stimuli, defective proliferation is observed. The patient's lymphocytes respond very poorly to such specific recall antigens as diphtheria or tetanus toxoid, and they generally serve as poor responder cells in one-way mixed-leukocyte-reaction cultures.

Although there is no question about the severity or clinical significance of the immune abnormalities seen in the Wiskott-Aldrich syndrome, it is difficult to provide a simple classification for the immunodeficiency. There are no good animal models for this disease (although sex-linked, B-cell dysfunction exists in mice). It is worth re-emphasizing that the Wiskott-Aldrich syndrome represents a multisystem abnormality of immunity (involving T-cell, B-cell, and monocyte function). It has been suggested that this syndrome represents a disorder of antigen-processing or recognition, with a preservation of immune effector function at a polyclonal level [155]. A resolution of the basic defect(s) in this disease will have far-reaching clinical and theoretical implications.

One of the most impressive features of the Wiskott-Aldrich syndrome is its high association with malignant disease. Patients with this disorder probably have the highest incidence of cancer among the various immunodeficiency diseases. The percentage of patients with neoplastic disease exceeds 15%, with 6 years as the median age at the time of cancer diagnosis [128]. In series of 41 patients seen at the National Cancer Institute, National Institutes of Health, nearly 30% developed cancer (R.M. Blaese, personal communication). The vast majority of these malignancies are poorly differentiated lymphoproliferative or reticuloendothelial tumors. Infiltration of visceral organs is very common. Moreover, patients with the Wiskott-Aldrich syndrome have a marked tendency to develop lymphomatous infiltration of the brain, sometimes as the primary (or only) site of their neoplasm. This is reminiscent of the cancer pattern seen in organ allo-transplant patients. As already mentioned, there also appears to be a predisposition for the development of myelogenous leukemias in these boys.

The clinical course of neoplasms in patients with this disorder is capricious and frustrating. Patients may develop variably aggressive lymphomas at unusual sites and without warning. (Any patient with this syndrome who develops unexplained headaches, nausea, or vomiting should be considered at risk for a neoplasm of the central nervous system). One Metabolism Branch patient underwent laparotomy and resection of a stage I_E malignant lymphoma of the jejunum, without additional chemotherapy or radiotherapy [158]. The patient died nearly five months following the surgical resection from an intracerebral bleed, and postmortem examination did not reveal residual lymphoma. There has also been a report of a patient with primary reticulum cell sarcoma of the brain treated with cobalt radio-therapy and intravenous vinblastine. Approximately four months after diagnosis the patient died of bronchopneumonia, and had no evidence of viable reticulum cell sarcoma at autopsy [159]. However, it is common for the tumors that occur in these patients to be lethally resistant to therapy. Moreover, as already stressed, patients with the Wiskott-Aldrich syndrome who develop neoplasms may present Herculean extra tasks for the pediatric oncologist. Essentially all patients have inherent thrombocytopenia. A large number of patients have virtually continous bacterial or viral infections. Chronic *Herpes* infections are a serious problem. These conditions significantly magnify the risk of therapy-related complications, and make it difficult (or impossible) to deliver full doses of cytotoxic chemotherapy.

For physicians who see these patients, the problem of neoplasia is likely to become even greater. As already implied vigorous platelet-replacement therapy and antibiotic intervention appear to be making an impact aganst the early deaths due to bleeding or sepsis formerly seen in this disorder. It is conceivable that neoplasms will become the major cause of death in patients with this disorder.

17. HYPOTHESES TO ACCOUNT FOR THE RELATIONSHIP BETWEEN IMMUNODEFICIENCY AND MALIGNANCY

While it is clear that patients with certain immunodeficiency states have an increased risk of cancer, especially lymphoproliferative malignancies, the reasons for the association between immunodepressed states and neoplasia have not been established and are matters for further research. It is important to recognize that in some immunodeficient patients—for example, those with ataxia telangiectasia—chromosomal instability as well as other nonimmunological factors may play a role in the development of neoplasms. Several immunological theories have been proposed to explain the relationship between immunodeficiency states and cancer:

17.1 Abnormal Immunological Surveillance

Perhaps one of the most traditional theories to account for the increased incidence of cancer in patients with immunodeficiency diseases is based on the postulate that in mammals, clones of neoplastic cells arise spontaneously and with high frequency. We have already explored the concept that neoplastic cells may express tumor-associated neoantigens which are recognized as 'non-self.' An intact immune system would be expected to play a role in the early detection and elimination (surveillance) of cells which have undergone a malignant transformation [160, 161]. It is entirely possible that those immunodeficiency patients who develop cancer have faulty immune detection or elimination mechanisms for neoplastic clones. The concept of immunological surveillance is interesting and important, but standing alone it unlikely to provide the complete explanation for the association between immunodeficiency states and neoplasia. There is an undeniable predominance for lympho-proliferative types of cancer in children with immunodeficiency disease. If abnormal immune surveillance *per se* was the only factor, one would expect to see a nonselective increase of cancer that encompassed all histopahtologic types.

17.2 Abnormal Susceptibility of Activation of Oncogenic Viruses

There are a variety of animal models in which viruses are thought to play a direct role in oncogenesis. It is conceivable that oncogenic viruses play a significant role in the pathogenesis of certain human tumors, and that patients with immunodeficiency diseases are unable to mount an effective immune response necessary to neutralize such oncogenic viruses. Indeed, there is a recent report documenting the isolation of a virus belonging to the papova group (which is well known for its capacity to produce cancer in certain experimental systems) from a lymphoma invading the brain of a patient with the Wiskott-Aldrich syndrome[162]. However, this possibility must be considered an unproven hypothesis at this time.

Another somewhat related hypothesis is based on the known role of specific antibody in the elimination of antigen and feedback control of immune functions[163]. The failure to produce sufficient quantities of specific antibodies, as would be seen under most circumstances in patients with immunodeficiency diseases, could easily result in prolonged stimulation of various cells comprising the immune system. Prolonged antigenic stimulation without the usual antibody feedback control mechanisms (also, see below) might occasionally induce individual lymphocyte clones to proliferate sufficiently for an immunoglobulin end-product to be detectable by a clinical laboratory as a serum monclonal gammopathy. Indeed, as has already been mentioned, such monoclonal gammopathies are seen in patients with the Wiskott-Aldrich syndrome[157]. As an extension of this concept, prolonged stimulation of immune cells might provide a favorable environment for the activation of oncogenic viruses endogenous (but normally latent) in lymphoid cells[164]. Again, these interesting concepts must be considered subjects for further reserach.

17.3 Abnormalities of Cellular Regulatory Control

Yet another potential explanation for the association between immunodeficiency and cancer is based on the abnormalities of cellular control of lymphocyte differentiation which can be seen in such patients. On one level, the exponential burst of normal lymphocyte proliferation which may be seen following specific antigenic or polyclonal activation is reminiscent of neoplastic cellular proliferation, except that the expansion of normal lymphocyte clones is strictly limited. The critical role of suppressor T cells (and other regulatory cells) in modulating normal lymphocyte clonal expansion has already been discussed. It is likely that certain immunodeficiency diseases may have an associated abnormality of one or more classes of regulatory suppressor cells. The immune system in such patients might be characterized by the loss of a timely and effective cellular mechanism for terminating the expansion of clones, which is part of ordinary immune responses to a variety of antigens. This is not really conceptually different from the loss of humoral antibody feedback control. Such cellular control mechanisms can be antigen-specific, or they may be nonspecific. Chronic, unregulated lymphocyte proliferation *per se* may favor the emergence of neoplastic lymphocytes. Even in the subset of patients with common variable immunodeficiency who are known to have excessive suppressor T-cell function, one could still envision circumstances that favor the development of lymphoid malignancy. In a long-term microenvironment of suppressor overactivity, truly autonomous (neoplastic) clones might have a selective advantage over clones which remain sensitive to the ongoing state of negative regulation.

Other theories may be proposed to account for the interrelationship between immunodeficiency disease and cancer, and the theories discussed above should be taken only as starting points for future clinical research. It is likely that no one unifying theory to account entirely for this interrelationship can be constructed.

18. IMMUNOLOGIC STRATEGIES FOR THE FUTURE THERAPY OF CANCER

An awareness of the more recent concepts dealing with the cellular control of immune function, and especially suppressor-cell function in human neoplasia, may alter the perspective of pediatric oncologists and researchers. There is a real possibility that chemotherapy, radiotherapy, and surgical intervention might benefit certain cancer patients by an indirect effect on regulatory cells as well as the obvious direct effect on the tumor itself.

Most current chemotherapy reserach focuses on direct tumoricidal activity. Traditionally, the side-effects that any given agent may exert on the immune system have been tolerated as an unavoidable price for tumor cytotoxicity. However, data from several different laboratories imply that a variety of ordinary chemotherapeutic agents can actually augment host-immune responses in the right set of circumstances. For example, if rabbits are given antigen a few days after the completion of a seven-day course of 6-mercaptopurine, the humoral-immune response is greatly potentiated as compared to that of controls [165]. This increase may conceivably be due to the selective removal of suppressor cells. In one mouse model, tumor growth was inhibited by the administration of hydrocortisone three to five days after tumor inoculation [166]. This action seemed to occur because hydrocortisone impaired suppressor-cell function. Adrenocortical steroids, which are widely used by pediatric and medical oncologists in the treatment of lymphoproliferative malignancies, can eliminate precursors of suppressor cells. The overall deficiency of mature suppressor cells that secondarily develops might allow the host to mount an increased cytotoxic response against the neoplasm, under some circumstances. Similarly, one of the most clinically useful chemotherapeutic agents available—cyclophosphamide—has been shown to eliminate suppressor-cell activity in a variety of experimental situations, and this finding could explain situations in which this drug actually augments certain immune responses [167–173]. In many ways, one of the most intriguing situations involves mice that exhibit a genetically determined activation of specific suppressor cells that prevent immune responses to certain synthetic polymeric antigens. As discussed earlier in this chapter, this form of genetically-predetermined immunosuppression is encoded by the *I-J* region of the major histocompatibility complex [37]. The administration of cyclophosphamide actually enhances immunity in these genetically nonresponsive mice by neutralizing suppressor-cell function for the relevant antigen [168]. There are also recent data to suggest that cyclophosphamide-sensitive T cells may suppress the *in vivo* differentiation of cytotoxic effector T lymphocytes [173]. Thus, pretreatment of mice with a single dose of cyclophosphamide augments the generation of alloimmune and hapten-immune cytotoxic T-effector cells.

Another clinically useful modality of cancer therapy is ionizing irradiation. It is known that ionizing irradiation may potentiate certain *in vivo* immune responses by eliminating or inactivating suppressor cells [169, 174–176]. Moreover, the removal of suppressor cells is thought to be the reason that irradiation of the host before transplantation can retard the growth of lethal tumors in certain murine models [177]. There are recent data to indicate that in mice total body X-irradiation can neutralize suppressor T cells that would otherwise accelerate tumor growth [178, 179]. The data indicate that, at least early in tumor growth, suppressor cells are recruited from a population that is sensitive to X-irradiation. It is worth emphasizing that in many situations supressor cells may be relatively short-lived. There are data to suggest suppressor cells either lose their regulatory capacity or die promptly after extirpation of gross tumor mass. Therefore, even direct operative intervention could conceivably have the hidden benefit of tipping the immunoregulatory balance in favor of the host without eradicating every neoplastic cell.

It is extremely important to learn whether human suppressor T cells express antigenic markers comparable to the *I-J*-coded products found in mice. The serologic classification of human T-cell subsets will be among the most crucial areas of immunologic research in the immediate future. Antisera raised against so-called Th_2 antigens hold promise as tools for characterizing suppressor T-cell subsets in normal individuals and patients with certain immunologically related diseases [180]. Eventually, the use of antisera to human T-cell neoplasms that have retained suppressor-cell activity might prove very useful in the characterization, isolation, and clinical manipulation of suppressor T-cell subsets.

As discussed earlier, the administration of antisera directed against antigenic products of the *I-J* region in mice can lead to the elimination of suppressor cells and a retardation of tumor growth. If human suppressor cells (or the factors they secrete) express antigens encoded by a region analogous to the *I-J* region of mice, it might be feasible to raise heteroantibodies capable of eliminating undesirable suppressor T cells from tumor bearing patients (and thereby promoting tumor rejection). It might be possible to find alloantisera with the appropriate specificities in multiparous women, multiply transfused individuals, or patients with a tendency to form autoantibodies against lymphocytes (for example, patients with systemic lupus erythematosus). Moreover, it is very likely that therapeutically useful monoclonal (hybridoma) antibodies with selective toxicity for regulatory T-cell subsets will become available soon.

On another front, it may become possible to pharmacologically manipulate helper-cell or suppressor-cell function. For example, Sugimoto et al. have reported that a chemically defined synthetic peptidoglycan increases the generation of helper cells [181]. There are data to suggest that a relatively non-toxic agent such as colchicine can inactivate suppresor-cell activity under some conditions [182]. Highly promising, but as yet preliminary, observations of the use of indomethacin to inhibit the excessive production of immunologically inhibitory prostaglandins by suppressor cells in Hodgkin's disease have been discussed earlier [110]. In fact, indomethacin has already reported to restore *in vivo* cell-mediated immunity in a patient with acquired hypogammaglobulinemia [183].

Finally, an understanding of the cellular control of lymphocyte differentiation and suppressor-cell function may induce a re-thinking of therapeutic strategies based on nonspecific immunoadjuvants. Bacillus Calmette-Guérin (BCG) and *Corynebacterium parvum* organisms exert profound changes in the immunoregulatory system. In general, most oncologists have been disappointed with what little impact immunoadjuvant therapy has made on the practical treatment of cancer [184]. This poor showing may have resulted, in part, from the intrinsic capacity of conventional immunotherapeutic agents to activate suppressor cells, as well as host cells engaged in the destruction of tumor cells. For example, Kirchner et al. [185] have shown that injection of *C. parvum* into mice can induce a depression of specific antitumor immunity through the activation of macrophage-like suppressor cells. Klimpel and Henney [186] have also demonstrated macrophage-like suppressor cells (capable of inhibiting cytotoxic T-cell generation) after BCG injection. Immunostimulation *per se* is not always a desirable objective in treating cancer. Moreover, nonspecific immunotherapy that is effective in inhibiting local tumor growth (with the use of an agent such as BCG) will not, as a simple matter of course, result in improved systemic immunity against the same tumor. In fact, overt enhancement of a second tumor graft has been documented after inhibition of a primary tumor graft with BCG [187]. Cancer therapists must constantly bear in mind that nonselective immunostimulation may actually contribute to tumor growth under some conditions, or may worsen an existing level of generalized immunologic impairment. An urgent requirement of future research is to develop strategies that selectively activate host cells involved in tumor destruction, while nullifying suppressor cells that oppose tumoricidal immune effector mechanisms.

19. CONCLUSION

The study of immunology and, in particular, the cellular system involved in the regulation of immune function, is complex. However, this area of investigation provides the pediatric oncologist with deeper insights into immunodiagnostic and therapeutic modalities that are available now or are likely to become available for cancer patients in the future.

REFERENCES

1. Gershon RK: T cell control of antibody production. Contemp Top Immunobiol 3:1–40, 1974.
2. Waldmann TA, Broder S: Suppressor cells in the regulation of the immune response. Prog Clin Immunol 3:155–199, 1977.
3. Broder S, Waldmann TA: The suppressor-cell network in cancer. N Engl J Med 299:1281–1284, 1335–1341, 1978.
4. Gathings WE, Lawton AR, Cooper MD: Immunofluorescent studies of the development of pre-B cells, B lymphocytes and immunoglobulin isotype diversity in humans. Eur J Immunol 7:804–810, 1977.
5. Pearl ER, Vogler LB, Okos AJ, Crist WM, Lawton AR, Cooper MD: B lymphocyte precursors in human bone marrow. J Immunol 120:1169–1175, 1978.
6. Zinkernagel RM, Callahan GN, Althage A, Cooper S, Klein PA, Klein J: On the thymus in the differentiation of '*H-2* self-recognition' by T cells: evidence for dual recognition? J Exp Med 147:882–896, 1978.
7. Rajewsky K, Eichmann K: Antigen receptors of T helper cells. Contemp Top Immunobiol 7:69–112, 1977.
8. Binz H, Wigzell H: Antigen-binding, idiotypic T-lymphocyte receptors. Contemp Top Immunobiol 7:113-117, 1977.

9. Krawinkel U, Carmer M, Imanishi-Kari T, Jack RS, Rajewsky K, Mäkelä O: Isolated hapten-binding receptors of sensitized lymphocytes. I. Receptors from nylon-wool enriched mouse T-lymphocytes lack serological markers of immunoglobulin constant domains but express heavy chain variable portions. Eur J Immunol 7:566–573, 1977.
10. Cantor H, Boyse E: Regulation of the immune response by T-cell subclasses. Contemp Top Immunobiol 7:47–68, 1977.
11. Broder S, Edelson RL, Lutzner MA, Nelson DL, MacDermott RP, Durm ME, Goldman CK, Meade BD, Waldmann TA: The Sézary syndrome: a malignant proliferation of helper T cells. J Clin Invest 58:1297–1306, 1976.
12. Moretta L, Webb SR, Grossi CE, Lydyard PM, Cooper MD: Functional analysis of two human T-cell subpopulations. Help and suppression of B-cell responses by T-cell bearing receptors for IgM or IgG. J Exp Med 146:184–200, 1977.
13. Nelson DS: Nonspecific immunoregulation by macrophages and their products. In: Immunobiology of the macrophage, Nelson DS (ed.). New York: Academic Press, 1976, pp 235–253.
14. Oehler JR, Herberman RB, Holden HT: Modulation of immunity by macrophages. J Pharmacol Ther 2:551–593, 1978.
15. Zembala M, Asherson GL: T cell suppression of contact sensitivity in the mouse. II. The role of soluble suppressor factor and its interaction with macrophages. Eur J Immunol 4:799–804, 1974.
16. Asherson GL, Zembala M: T cell suppression of contact sensitivity. III. The role of macrophages and the specific triggering of nonspecific suppression. Eur J Immunol 4:804–807, 1974.
17. Ptak W, Zembala M, Gershon RK: Intermediary role of macrophages in the passage of suppressor signals between T-cell subsets. J Exp Med 148:424–434, 1978.
18. Mann RB, Jaffe ES, Berard CW: Malignant lymphomas—a conceptual understanding of morphologic diversity: a review. Am J Path 94:105–192, 1979.
19. Chessells, JM, Hardisty RM, Rapson NT, Greaves MF: Acute lymphoblastic leukaemia in children: classification and prognosis. Lancet 2:1307–1309, 1977.
20. Greaves MF, Brown G, Rapson NT, Lister TA: Antisera to acute lymphoblastic leukemia cells. Clin Immunol Immunopath 4:67–84, 1975.
21. Vogler LB, Crist WM, Bockman DE, Pearl ER, Lawton AR, Cooper MD: Pre-B-cell leukemia: a new phenotype of childhood lymphoblastic leukemia. N Engl J Med 298:872–878, 1978.
22. Borella L, Sen L: T cell surface markers on lymphoblasts from acute lymphocytic leukemia. J Immunol 111:1257–1260, 1973.
23. Kersey JH, Sabad A, Gajl-Peczalska K, Hallgren HM, Yunis EJ, Nesbit ME: Acute lymphoblastic leukemic cells with T (thymus-derived) lymphocyte markers. Science 182:1355–1356, 1973.
24. Brouet JC, Valensi F, Daniel MT, Flandrin G, Preud'homme JL, Seligmann M: Immunological classification of acute lymphoblastic leukaemias: evaluation of its clinical significance in a hundred patients. Br J Haematol 33:319–326, 1976.
25. Dow LW, Borella L, Sen L, Aur RJA, George SL, Mauer AM, Simone JV: Initial prognostic factors and lymphoblast–erythrocyte rosette formation in 109 children with acute lymphoblastic leukemia. Blood 50:671–682, 1977.
26. Tsukimoto I, Wong KY, Lampkin BC: Surface markers and prognostic factors in acute lymphoblastic leukemia. N Engl J Med 294:245–248, 1976.
27. Flandrin G, Brouet JC, Daniel MT, Preud'Homme JL: Acute leukemia with surface markers. Blood 45:183–188, 1975.
28. Brodsky FM, Parham P, Barnstable CJ, Crumpton MJ, Bodmer WF: Monoclonal antibodies for analysis of the HLA-system. Immunol Rev 47:3–61, 1979.

29. Seligmann M, Brouet JC: Antibody activity of human myeloma globulins. Semin Hematol 10:163–177, 1973.

30. Kubagawa H, Vogler L, Conrad M, Lawton A, Cooper M: The extent of clonal involvement in multiple myeloma and Waldenstrom's macroglobulinemia. Fed Proc 37:1765, 1978.

31. Rohrer JW, Vasa K, Lynch RG: Myeloma cell immunoglobulin expression during *in vivo* growth in diffusion chambers: Evidence for repetitive cycles of differentiation. J Immunol 119:861–866, 1977.

32. Rohrer JW, Lynch RG: Antigen-specific regulation of myeloma cell differentiation *in vivo* by carrier-specific T cell factors and macrophages. J Immunol 121:1066–1074, 1978.

33. Fu SM, Chiorazzi N, Kunkel HG, Halper JP, Harris SR: Induction of *in vitro* differentiation and immunoglobulin synthesis of human leukemic B lymphocytes. J Exp Med 148:1570–1578, 1978.

34. Bach FH, van Rood JJ: The major histocompatibility complex—genetics and biology. N Engl J Med 295:806–813, 872–878, 927–936, 1976.

35. Shreffer DC, David CS: The *H-2* major histocopatibility complex and the *I* immune response region: genetic variation, function, and organization. Adv Immunol 20:125–195, 1975.

36. Benacerraf B, Dorf M: The nature and function of specific H-linked immune response genes and immune suppression genes. In: The role of products of the histocompatibility gene complex in immune responses, Katz DH, Benacerraf B (eds). New York: Academic Press, 1976, pp 225–248.

37. Benacerraf B, Germain RN: The immune response genes of the major histocompatibility complex. Immunol Rev 38:70–119, 1978.

38. Metzgar RS, Bertoglio J, Anderson JK, Bonnard GD, Ruscetti FW: Detection of *HLA*-DRw (Ia-like) antigens on human T lymphocytes grown in tissue culture. J Immunol 122:949–953, 1979.

39. Taussig MJ, MunrO AJ: Antigen-specific T-cell factor in cell cooperation and genetic control of the immune response. Fed Proc 35:2061–2066, 1976.

40. Mozes E: The nature of antigen specific T cell factors involved in the genetic regulation of immune responses. In: The role of products of the histocompatibility gene complex in immune responses. Katz DH, Benacerraf B (eds). New York: Academic Press, 1976, pp 485–505.

41. Tada T, Taniguchi M, Okumura K: Regulation of antibody response by antigen specific T-cell factors bearing *I*-region determinants. Prog Immunol 3:369–377, 1977.

42. Rich SS, Rich RR: Regulatory mechanisms in cell-mediated immune responses. III. *I*-region control of suppressor cell interaction with responder cells in mixed lymphocyte reactions. J Exp Med 143:672–677, 1976.

43. Tada T, Taniguchi M, David CS: Properties of the antigen-specific suppressive T-cell factor in the regulation of antibody response of the mouse. IV. Special subregion assignment of the gene(s) that codes for the suppressive T-cell factor in the *H-2* histocompatibility complex. J Exp Med 144:713–725, 1976.

44. Theze J, Waltenbaugh C, Dorf M, Benacerraf B: Immunosuppressive factor(s) specific for *L*-glutamic acid[50]-L-tyrosine[50] (GT). II. Presence of *I-J* determinants on the GT-suppressive factor. J Exp Med 146:287–292.

45. Green MI, Pierres A, Dorf ME, Benacerraf B: The *I-J* subregion codes for determinants on suppressor factor(s) which limit the contect sensitivity response to picryl chloride. J Exp Med 146:293–296, 1977.

46. Tada T, Takemori T, Okumura K, Nonaka M, Tokuhisa T: Two distinct types of helper T cells involved in the secondary antibody response: independent and synergistic effects of Ia− and Ia+ helper T cells. J Exp Med 147:446–458, 1978.

47. Taniguchi M, Miller J: Specific suppressive factors produced by hybridomas derived from the fusion of enriched suppressor T cells and a T lymphoma cell line. J Exp Med 148:373–382, 1978.

48. Taniguchi M, Saito T, Tada T: Antigen-specific suppressive factor produced by a transplantable *I-J* bearing T-cell hybridoma. Nature 278:555–558, 1979.

49. Kapp JA: Immunosuppressive factors from lymphoid cells on nonresponder mice primed with 1-glutamic acid[60]-1-alanine[30]-1-tyrosine[10]. IV. Lack of strain restrictions among allogeneic, nonresponder donors and recipients. J Exp Med 147:997–1006, 1978.

50. Taniguchi M, Tada T, Tokuhisa T: Properties of the antigen-specific suppressive T-cell factor in the regulation of antibody response of the mouse. III. Dual gene control of the T-cell-mediated suppression of the antibody response. J Exp Med 144:20–31, 1976.

51. Pierres M, Germain RN, Dorf ME, Benacerraf B: *In vivo* effects of an anti-Ia alloantisera. I. Elimination of specific suppression by *in vivo* administration of antisera specific for *I-J* controlled determinants. J Exp Med 147:656–666, 1978.

52. Engleman EG, McDevitt HO: A suppressor T cell of the mixed lymphocyte reaction specific for the *HLA-D* region in man. J Clin Invest 61:828–838, 1978.

53. Schlossman SF, Chess L, Humphreys RE, Strominger JL: Distribution of Ia-like molecules on the surface of normal and leukemic cells. Proc Nat Acad Sci USA 73:1288–1292, 1976.

54. Broder S, Mann DL, Waldmann TA: Participation of suppressor T cells in the immunosuppressive activity of a heteroantiserum to human Ia-like antigens. J Exp Med 151:257–262, 1980.

55. Voisin GA: Immunological facilitation, a broadening of the concept of the enhancement phenomenon. Prog Allergy 15:328–484, 1971.

56. Hellstrom KE, Hellstrom I: Cellular immunity against tumor antigens. Adv Cancer Res 12:167–223, 1969.

57. Chard T: Immunological enhancement by mouse isoantibodies: the importance of complement fixation. Immunology 14:583–589, 1968.

58. Broder S, Whitehouse F Jr: Immunologic enhancement of tumor xenografts by pepsin-degraded immunoglobulin. Science 162:1494–1495, 1968.

59. Sjögren HO, Hellstrom I, Bansal SC, Hellström KE: Suggestive evidence that the 'blocking antibodies' of tumor-bearing individuals may be antigen-antibody complexes. Proc Nat Acad Sci USA 68:1372–1375, 1971.

60. Baldwin RW, Price MR, Robbins RA: Blocking of lymphocyte-mediated cytotoxicity for rat hepatoma cells by tumour-specific antigen-antidody complexes. Nature, New Biol 238:185–187, 1972.

61. Fujimoto S, Greene M, Sehon AH: Immunosuppressor T cells and their factors in tumor-bearing hosts. In: Suppressor cells in immunity, Singhal SK, Sinclair NR (eds). Toronto: University of Western Ontario Press, 1975, pp 136–148.

62. Fujimoto S, Green M, Sehon AH: Regulation of the immune response to tumor antigens. I. Immunosuppressor cells in tumor-bearing hosts. J Immunol 116:791–799, 1976.

63. Fujimoto S, Greene M, Sehon AH: Regulation of the immune response to tumor antigens. II. The nature of immunosuppressor cells in tumor-bearing hosts. J Immunol 116:800–806, 1976.

64. Greene MI, Fujimoto S, Sehon AH: Regulation of the immune response to tumor antigens. III. Characterization of thymic suppressor factor(s) produced by tumor-bearing hosts. J Immunol 119:757–764, 1977.

65. Perry L, Greene MI: Modulation of the immune response to tumor antigen in tumor-bearing hosts (TBH). Fed Prod 37:1452, 1978.

66. Greene MI, Dorf ME, Pierres M, Benacerraf B: Reduction of syngeneic tumor growth by an anti-*I-J* alloantiserum. Proc Nat Acad Sci USA 74:5118–5121, 1977.

67. Hodes RJ, Hathcock KS: *In vitro* generation of suppressor cell activity: Suppression of *in vitro* induction of cell-mediated cytotoxicity. J Immunol 116:167–177, 1976.
68. Yu A, Watts H, Jaffee N, Parkman R: Concomitant presence of tumor-specific cytotoxic and inhibitor lymphocytes in patients with osteogenic sarcoma. N Engl J Med 297:121–127, 1977.
69. Ninnemann JL: Melanoma-associated immunosuppression through B cell activation of suppressor T cells. J Immunol 120:1573–1579, 1978.
70. Gorczynski RM: Immunity to murine sarcoma virus-induced tumors. II. Suppression of T-cell mediated immunity by cells from progressor animals. J Immunol 112:1826–1838, 1974.
71. Kirchner H, Chused TM, Herberman RB, Holden HT, Lavrin DH: Evidence of suppressor cell activity in spleens of mice bearing primary tumors induced by Moloney sarcoma virus. J Exp Med 139:1473–1487, 1974.
72. Eggers AE, Wunderlich JR: Suppressor cells in tumor-bearing mice capable of nonspecific blocking of *in vitro* immunization against transplant antigens. J Immunol 114: 1554–1556, 1975.
73. Kilburn DG, Smith JB, Gorczynski RM: Nonspecific suppression of T lymphocyte responses in mice carrying progressively growing tumors. Eur J Immunol 4:784–788, 1974.
74. Fernbach BR, Kirchner H, Bonnard GD, Herberman RB: Suppression of mixed lymphocyte response in mice bearing primary tumors induced by murine sarcoma virus. Transplantation 21:381–386, 1976.
75. Pope BL, Whitney RB, Levy JG, Kilburn DG: Suppressor cells in the spleens of tumor-bearing mice: enrichment by centrifugation on Hypaque-Ficoll and characterizations of the suppressor population. J Immunol 116:1342–1346, 1976.
76. Veit BC, Feldman JD: Altered lymphocyte functions in rats bearing syngeneic Moloney sarcoma tumors. II. Suppressor cells. J Immunol 117:655–660, 1976.
77. Glaser M, Kirchner H, Herberman RB: Inhibition of *in vitro* lymphoproliferative responses to tumor-associated antigens by suppressor cells from rats bearing progressively growing gross leukemia virus-induced tumors. Int J Cancer 16:384–393, 1975.
78. Poupon MF, Kolb JP, Lespinats G: Evidence for splenic suppressor cells in C3H/He, T-cell-deprived C3H/He, and nude mice bearing a 3-methylcholanthrene-induced fibrosarcoma. J Nat Cancer Inst 57:1241–1247, 1976.
79. Kruisbeek AM, van Hees M: Role of macrophages in the tumor-induced suppression of mitogen responses in rats. J Nat Cancer Inst 58:1653–1660, 1976.
80. Good RA: Relations between immunity and malignancy. Proc Nat Acad Sci USA 69:1026–1032, 1972.
81. Jeunet FS, Good RA: Thymoma immunologic deficiencies, and hematological abnormalities. Birth Defects 4:192–206, 1968.
82. Waldmann TA, Strober W: Metabolism of immunoglobulins. Prog Allergy 13:1–110, 1969.
83. Waldmann TA, Durm M, Broder S, Blackmann M, Blaese M, Strober W: Role of suppressor T cells in pathogenesis of common variable hypogammaglobulinaemia. Lancet 2:609–613, 1974.
84. Siegal FP, Siegal M, Good RA: Suppression of B-cell differentiation by leukocytes from hypogammaglobulinemic patients. J Clin Invest 58:109–122, 1976.
85. Dosch HM, Gelfand EW: Functional differentiation of B lymphocytes in agammaglobulinemia. III. Characterization of spontaneous suppressor cell activity. J Immunol 121:2097–2105, 1978.

86. Herrod HG, Buckley RH: Use of a human plaque-forming cell assay to study peripheral blood bursa-equivalent cell activation and excessive suppressor cell activity in humoral immunodeficiency. J Clin Invest 63:868–876, 1979.

87. Stobo JD, Paul S, Van Scoy RE, Hermans PE: Suppressor thymus-derived lymphocytes in fungal infection. J Clin Invest 57:319–328, 1976.

88. Waldmann TA, Broder S, Durm M, Blackman M, Krakauer R, Meade B: Suppressor T cells in the pathogenesis of hypogammaglobulinemia associated with thymoma. Trans Assoc Am Physicians 88:120–134, 1975.

89. Fahey JL, Scoggins R, Utz JP, Szwed CF: Infection, antibody response and gamma globulin components in multiple myeloma and macroglobulinemia. Am J Med 35:698–707, 1963.

90. Cone L, Uhr JW: Immunological deficiency disorders associated with chronic lymphocytic leukemia and multiple myeloma. J Clin Invest 43:2241–2248, 1964.

91. Broder S, Humphrey R, Durm M, Blackman M, Meade B, Goldman C, Strober W, Waldmann T: Impaired synthesis of polyclonal (non-paraprotein) immunoglobulins by circulating lymphocytes from patients with multiple myeloma: role of suppressor cells. N Engl J Med 293:887–892, 1975.

92. Lindström FD, Hardy WR, Eberle BJ, Williams RC: Multiple myeloma and benign monoclonal gammopathy: differentiation by immunofluorescence of lymphocytes. Ann Intern Med 78:837–844, 1973.

93. Abdou NI, Abdou NL: The monoclonal nature of lymphocytes in multiple myeloma: effects of therapy. Ann Intern Med 83:42–45, 1975.

94. Chen Y, Bhoopalam N, Yakulis V, Heller P: Changes in lymphocytic surface immunoglobulins in myeloma and the effect of an RNA-containing plasma factor. Ann Intern Med 83:625–631, 1975.

95. Bhoopalam N, Chen Y, Yakulis V, Heller P: Surface immunoglobulins of lymphocytes in plasmacytoma. V. The effect of RNA-rich extract from mouse plasmacytoma MOPC-104E on the immune response. Clin Exp Immunol 24:357–367, 1976.

96. Bhoopalam N, Yakulis V, Costea N, Heller P: Surface immunoglobulins of circulating lymphocytes in mouse plasmacytoma. II. The influence of plasmacytoma RNA on surface immunoglobulins of lymphocytes. Blood 36:465–471, 1972.

97. Giacomoni D, Yakulis V, Wang SR, Cooke A, Dray S, Heller P: In vitro conversion of normal mouse lymphocytes by plasmacytoma RNA to express idiotypic specificities on their surface characteristic of the plasmacytoma Ig. Cell Immunol 11:389–400, 1974.

98. Heller P, Bhoopalam N, Cabana V, Costea N, Yakulis V: The role of RNA in the immunological deficiency of plasmacytoma. Ann NY Acad Sci 207:468–479, 1973.

99. Katzmann J, Giacomoni D, Yakulis V, Heller P: Characterization of two plasmacytoma fractions and their RNA capable of changing lymphocyte surface immunoglobulins (cell conversion). Cell Immunol 18:98–109, 1975.

100. Salmon SE: Immunoglobulin synthesis and tumor kinetics of multiple myeloma. Semin Hematol 10:135–147, 1973.

101. Krakauer RS, Strober W, Waldmann TA: Hypogammaglobulinemia in experimental myeloma: the role of suppressor factors from mononuclear phagocytes. J Immunol 118:1385–1390, 1977.

102. Kolb JP, Arrian S, Zolla-Pazner S: Suppression of the humoral immune response by plasmacytomas: mediation by adherent mononuclear cells. J Immunol 118:702–709, 1977.

103. Paglieroni T, MacKenzie MR: Studies on the pathogenesis of an immune defect in multiple myeloma. J Clin Invest 59:1120-1133, 1977.

104. Zembala M, Mytar B, Popiela T, Asherson GL: Depressed in vitro peripheral blood lymphocyte response to mitogens in cancer patients: the role of suppressor cells. Int J Cancer 19:605–613, 1977.

105. Lamb D, Pilney F, Kelly WD, Good RA: A comparative study of the incidence of anergy in patients with carcinoma, leukemia, Hodgkin's disease and other lymphomas. J Immunol 89:555–558, 1962.

106. Kelly WD, Lamb DI, Varco RL, Good RA: An investigation of Hodgkin's disease with respect to the problem of homotransplantation. Ann NY Acad Sci 87:187–202, 1960.

107. Twomey JJ, Laughter AH, Farrow S, Douglass CC: Hodgkin's disease: an immunodepleting and immunosuppressive disorder. J Clin Invest 56:467–475, 1975.

108. Engleman EG, Hoppe R, Kaplan H, Comminskey J, McDevitt HO: Suppressor cells of the mixed lymphocyte reaction in healthy subjects and patients with Hodgkin's disease and sarcoidosis. Clin Res 26:513A, 1978.

109. Hillinger SM, Herzig GP: Impaired cell-mediated immunity in Hodgkin's disease mediated by suppressor lymphocytes and monocytes. J. Clin Invest 61:1620–1627, 1978.

110. Goodwin JS, Messner RP, Bankhurst AD, Peake GT, Saiki JH, Williams RC: Prostaglandin-producing suppressor cells in Hodgkin's disease. N Engl J Med 297:963–968, 1977.

111. Khalifa AS, Take H, Cejka J, Zuelzer WW: Immunoglobulins in acute leukemia in children. J Pediatr 85:788–791, 1974.

112. Broder S, Poplack D, Whang-Peng J, Durm M, Goldman C, Muul L, Waldmann TA: Characterization of a suppressor-cell leukemia: evidence for the requirement of an interaction of two T cells in the development of human suppressor effector cells. N Engl J Med 298:66–72, 1978.

113. Broder S, Mann D, Waldmann TA: Pro-suppressor T-cell leukemia Clin Res 26:374A, 1978.

114. Uchiyama T, Sagawa K, Takatsuki K, Uchino H: Effect of adult T-cell leukemia cells on pokeweed mitogen-induced normal B-cell differentiation. Clin Immunol Immunopathol 10:24–34, 1978.

115. Feldmann M, Beverley PCL, Woody J, McKenzie IFC: T-T interactions in the induction of suppressor and helper T cells: analysis of membrane phenotype of precursor and amplifier cells. J Exp Med 145:793–801, 1977.

116. Basten A, Miller JFAP, Loblay R, Johnson P, Gamble J, Chia E, Pritchard-Briscoe H, Callard R, McKenzie IFC: T cell-dependent suppression of antibody production. I. Characteristics of suppressor T cells following tolerance induction. Eur J Immunol 8:360–370, 1978.

117. Broder S, Edelson RL, Lutzner MA, Nelson DL, MacDermott P, Durm ME, Goldman CK, Meade BD, Waldmann TA: The Sézary syndrome: a malignant proliferation of helper T cells. J Clin Invest 58:1297–1306, 1976.

118. Lawrence EC, Broder S, Jaffe ES, Braylan RC, Dobbins WO, Young RC, Waldmann TA: Evolution of a lymphoma with helper T cell characteristics in Sézary syndrome. Blood 52:481–492, 1978.

119. Roder JC, Tyler L, Singhal SK, Ball JK: Are T-cell lymphomas immunocompetent? Nature 273:540–541, 1978.

120. Saxon A, Stevens RH, Golde DW: Helper and suppressor T-lymphocyte leukemia in ataxia telangiectasia. N Engl J Med 300:700–704, 1979.

121. Kruger GRF, Malmgren RA, Berard CW: Malignant lymphomas and plasmacytosis in mice under prolonged immunosuppression and persistent antigenic stimulation. Transplantation 11:138–144, 1971.

122. Kersey J, Spector B, Good RA: Immunodeficiency and cancer. In: Advances in cancer research, Weinhouse S, Klein G (eds). New York: Academic Press, New York, 1973, pp 211–230, 1973.

123. Gatti RA, Good RA: Occurrence of malignancy in immunodeficiency diseases. Cancer 28:89–98, 1971.

124. Waldmann TA, Strober W, Blaese RM: Immunodeficiency disease and malignancy: various immunologic deficiencies of man and the role of immune processes in the control of malignant disease. Ann Intern Med 77:605–628, 1972.
125. Penn I: Occurrence of cancer in immune deficiencies. Cancer 34:858–866, 1974.
126. Penn I: Second malignant neoplasma associated with immunosuppressive medications. Cancer 37:1024–1032, 1976.
127. Schneck SA, Penn I: De-novo brain tumours in renal-transplant recipients. Lancet 1:983–986, 1971.
128. Spector BD, Perry GS III, Kersey JH: Genetically determined immunodeficiency diseases (GDID) and malignancy: report from the immunodeficiency-cancer registry. Clin Immunol Immunopath 11:12–29, 1978.
129. DiGeorge AM: Congenital absence of the thymus and its immunologic consequences: concurrence with congenital hypoparathyroidism. In: Immunologic deficiency disease in man, Bergsma D, Good RA (eds). The National Foundation, 1968, pp 116–123.
130. Lischner HW, DiGeorge AM: Role of the thymus in humoral immunity. Observations in complete or partial congenital absence of the thymus. Lancet 2:1044–1049, 1969.
131. Lischner HW, Huff DS: T-cell deficiency in DiGeorge syndrome. In: Immunodeficiency in man and animals, Bergsma D, Good RA, Finstad J, Paul NW (eds). Sinauer, Sunderland, 1975, pp 16–21.
132. Steele RW, Limas C, Thurman GB, Schulein M, Bauer H, Bellanti JA: Familial thymic aplasia attempted reconstitution with fetal thymus in a millipore diffusion chamber. N Engl J Med 287:787–791, 1972.
133. Gajl-Peczalska KJ, Park BH, Biggar WD, Good RA: B and T lymphocytes in primary immunodeficiency disease in man. J Clin Invest 52:919–928, 1973.
134. Kikkawa Y, Kamimura K, Hamajirna I, Sekiguchi T, Kawai T, Takeaka M, Tada T: Thymic alymphoplasia with hyper-IgE-globulinemia. Pediatrics 51:690–696, 1973.
135. Polmar SH, Waldmann TA, Terry WD: IgE in immunodeficiency. Am J Pathol 69:499–512, 1972.
136. Touraine JL, Touraine F, Dutruge J, Gilly J, Colon S, Gilly R: Immunodeficiency diseases. I. T-lymphocyte precursors and T-lymphocyte differentiation in partial DiGeorge syndrome. Clin Exp Immunol 21:39, 1975.
137. Wara DW, Goldstein AL, Doyle NE, Ammann AJ: Thymosin activity in patients with cellular immunodeficiency. N Engl J Med 292:70–74, 1975.
138. Boder E: Ataxia-telangiectasia: Some historic, clinical and pathologic observations. In: Immunodeficiency in man and animals, Bergsma D, Good RA, Finstad J, Paul NW (eds). Sinauer, Sunderland, 1975, pp 255–270.
139. Boder E, Sedgwick RP: Ataxia-telangiectasia. A familial syndrome of progressive cerebellar ataxia, oculocutaneous telangiectasia and frequent pulmonary infection. Pediatrics 21:526–554, 1958.
140. McFarlin DE, Strober W, Waldmann TA: Ataxia-telangiectasia. Medicine 51:281–314, 1972.
141. Bar RS, Levis WR, Rechler MM, Harrison LC, Siebert C, Podskalny J, Roth J, Muggeo M: Extreme insulin resistance in ataxia telangiectasia: defect in affinity of insulin receptors. N Engl J Med 298:1164–1171, 1978.
142. Waldmann TA, McIntire KR: Serum-alpha-fetoprotein levels in patients with ataxia-telangiectasia. Lancet 2:1112–1115, 1972.
143. Buckley RH: Clinical and immunologic features of selective IgA deficiency. In: Immunodeficiency in man and animals, Bergsma D, Good RA, Finstad J, Paul NW (eds). Sinauer, Sunderland, 1975, pp 133–142.
144. Polmar SH, Waldmann TA, Balestra JT, Jost MC, Terry WD: Immunoglobulin E in immunologic deficiency diseases. I. Relation of IgE and IgA to respiratory tract disease in

isolated IgE deficiency, IgA deficiency and ataxia telangiectasia. J Clin Invest 51:326–330, 1972.

145. Biggar WD, Good RA: Immunodeficiency in ataxia-telangiectasia. In: Immunodeficiency in man and animals, Bergsma D, Good RA, Finstad J, Paul NW (eds). Sinauer, Sunderland, 1975, pp 271–276.

146. Kraemer KH: Progressive degenerative diseases associated with defective DNA repair: xeroderma pigmentosum and ataxia telangiectasia. In: DNA repair processes, Nichols WW, Murphy DG (eds). Symposia Specialists Inc, 1977, p 37.

147. Taylor AMR, Harnden DG, Arlett CF, Harcourt SA, Lehmann AR, Stevens S, Bridges BA: Ataxia telangiectasia: a human mutation with abnormal radiation sensitivity. Nature 258:427–429, 1975.

148. Webb I, Harnden DG, Harding M: The chromosome analysis and susceptibility to transformation by simian virus 40 of fibroblasts from ataxia-telangiectasia. Cancer Res 37:997–1002, 1977.

149. Hecht F, McCaw BK, Koler RD: Ataxia-telangiectasia: clonal growth of lymphocytes. N Engl J Med 289:286–291, 1973.

150. Rosen FS, Janeway CA: The gamma globulins. III. The antibody deficiency syndromes. N Engl J Med 275:709–715, 1966.

151. Page AR, Hansen AE, Good RA: Occurrence of leukemia and lymphoma in patients with agammaglobulinemia. Blood 21:197–206, 1963.

152. DeVita VT Jr, Chabner B, Hubbard SP, Canellos GP, Schein P, Young RC: Advanced diffuse histiocytic lymphoma, a potentially curable disease: results with combination chemotherapy. Lancet 1:248–250, 1975.

153. Wiskott A: A familiarer, angeborener morbus werlhofli? Monatsschr Kinderheilkd 68:212–216, 1937.

154. Aldrich RA, Steinberg AG, Campbell DC: Pedigree demonstrating a sex-linked recessive condition characterized by draining ears, eczematoid dermatitis and blood diarrhea. Pediatrics 13:133–138, 1954.

155. Blaese RM, Strober W, Brown RS, Waldmann TA: The Wiskott-Aldrich syndrome: a disorder with a possible defect in antigen processing or recognition. Lancet 1:1056–1061, 1968.

156. Poplack DG, Bonnard GD, Holiman BJ, Blaese RM: Monocyte-mediated antibody-dependent cellular cytotoxicity: a clinical test of monocyte function. Blood 48:808–816, 1976.

157. Bruce RM, Blase RM: Monoclonal gammopathy in the Wiskott-Aldrich syndrome. J Pediatr 85:204-207, 1974.

158. Faraci RP, Hoffstrand HJ, Witebsky FG, Blaese RM, Beazley RM: Malignant lymphoma of the jejunum in a patient with Wiskott-Aldrich syndrome. Surgical treatment. Arch Surg 110:218–220, 1975.

159. Heidelberger KP, LeGolvan DP: Wiskott-Aldrich syndrome and cerebral neoplasia: report of a case with localized reticulum cell sarcoma. Cancer 33:280–284, 1974.

160. Thomas L: Reactions to homologous tissue antigens in relation to hypersensitivity. In: Cellular and humoral aspects of the hypersensitive states Lawrence HS (eds). Hoeber-Harper, 1959, pp 529–532.

161. Burnet FM: The concept of immunological surveillance. Prog Exp Tumor Res 13:1–27, 1970.

162. Takemoto KK, Rabson AS, Mullarkey MF, Blaese RM, Garon CF, Nelson D: Isolation of papovavirus from brain tumor and urine of a patient with Wiskott-Aldrich syndrome. J Nat Can Inst 53:1205–1207, 1974.

163. Uhr JW, Moller G: Regulatory effect of antibody on the immune response. Adv Immunol 8:81–127, 1968.

164. Schwartz RS: Immunoregulation, oncologic viruses, and malignant lymphomas. Lancet 1:1266–1269, 1972.
165. Chanmougan D, Schwartz RS: Enhancement of antibody synthesis by 6-mercaptopurine. J Exp Med 124:363–378, 1966.
166. Schecter B, Feldman M: Hydrocortisone affects tumor growth by eliminating precursors of suppressor cells. J Immunol 119:1563–1568, 1977.
167. Turk JL, Parker D, Poulter LW: Functional aspects of the selective depletion of lymphoid tissue by cyclophosphamide. Immunology 23:493–501, 1972.
168. Debre P, Waltenbaugh C, Dorf ME, Benacerraf B: Genetic control of specific immune suppression. IV. Responsiveness to the random copolymer L-glutamic acid ^{50} L-tyrosine ^{50} induced in BALB/c mice by cyclophosphamide. J Exp Med 144:277–281, 1976.
169. Chiorazzi N, Fox DA, Katz DH: Hapten-specific IgE antibody responses in mice. VI. Selective enhancement of IgE antibody production by low doses of X-irradiation and by cyclophosphamide. J Immunol 117:1629–1637, 1976.
170. Whisler RL, Stobo JD: Heterogeneity among suppressor T cells. In: Regulatory mechanisms in lymphocyte activation, Lucas DO (ed.) New York: Academic Press, 1977, pp 748–750.
171. Askenase PW, Hayden BJ, Gershon RK: Augmentation of delayed-type hypersensitivity by doses of cyclophosphamide which do not affect antibody responses. J Exp Med 141:697–702, 1975.
172. Easmon CS, Glynn AA: Effect of cyclophosphamide on delayed hypersensitivity to Staphylococcus aureus in mice. Immunology 33:767–776, 1977.
173. Rollinghoff M, Stafzinski-Powitz A, Pfizenmaier K, Wagner H: Cyclophosphamide-sensitive T lymphocytes suppress the in vivo generation of antigen-specific cytotoxic T lymphocytes. J Exp Med 145:455–459, 1977.
174. Tada T, Taniguchi M, Okumura K: Regulation of homocytotropic antibody formation in the rat. II. Effect of X-irradiation. J Immunol 106:1012–1018, 1971.
175. Anderson RE, Warner NL: Ionizing radiation and the immune response. Adv Immunol 24:215–335, 1976.
176. De Macedo MS, Catty D: Effect of X-irradiation on homocytotopic and agglutinating antibody production in mice. Immunology 33:611–619, 1977.
177. Rotter V, Trainin N: Inhibition of tumor growth in syngeneic chimeric mice mediated by a depletion of suppressor T cells. Transplantation 20:68–74, 1975.
178. Hellstrom KE, Hellstrom I: Evidence that tumor antigens enhance tumor growth in vivo by interacting with a radiosensitive (suppressor?) cell population. Proc Nat acad Sci USA 75:436–440, 1978.
179. Hellstrom KE, Hellstrom I, Kant JA, Tamerius JD: Regression and inhibition of sarcoma growth by interference with a radiosensitive T-cell population. J Exp Med 148:799–804, 1978.
180. Reinhertz EL, Parkman R, Rappeport J, Rosen FS, Schlossman SF: Aberrations of suppressor T cells in human graft-versus-host disease. N Engl J Med 300:1061–1068, 1979.
181. Sugimoto M, Germain RN, Chedid L, Benacerraf B: Enhancement of carrier-specific helper T cell function by the synthetic adjuvant, N-acetyl muramyl-L-alanyl-D-isoglutamine (MDP). J Immunol 120:980–982, 1978.
182. Shek PN, Waltenbaugh C, Coons AH: Effects of colchicine on the antibody response. II. Demonstration of the inactivation of suppressor cell activities by colchicine. J Exp Med 147:1228–1235, 1978.
183. Goodwin JS, Bankurst AD, Sellinger DS, Messner RP: Reversal of anergy with indomethacin administration in a patient with adult acquired hypogammaglobulinemia. Clin Res 26:121A, 1978.

184. Present status of trials in man. In: Immunotherapy of cancer, Terry WD, Windhorst DB (eds). New York: Raven Press, 1977.
185. Kirchner HB, Glaser M, Herberman RB: Suppression of cell-mediated tumour immunity by Corynebacterium parvum. Nature 257:396–398, 1975.
186. Klimpel GR, Henney CS: BCG-induced suppressor cells. I. Demonstration of a macrophage-like suppressor cell that inhibits cytotoxic T cell generation *in vitro*. J Immunol 120:563–569, 1978.
187. Piessens W, Campbell M, Churchill WH: Inhibition or enhancement of rat mammary tumors dependent on dose of BCG. J Nat Cancer Inst 59:207–211, 1977.

2. The Potential Use of HLA to Predict Risk of Malignant Diseases and Outcome of Therapy

RONALD T. ACTON and BRUCE O. BARGER

1. INTRODUCTION

Interest in the association of genetically determined polymorphic markers with disease states arose from the field of blood group genetics. The clinical implications of typing for blood group antigens were recognized during the late 1930s. A subsequent flurry of activity led to the discovery of hundreds of blood group markers and several new genetic systems. As the blood groups were shown to vary in frequency between various populations and ethnic groups, numerous research opportunities became apparent, one of them being the study of possible associations between the blood groups and specific diseases. In 1953, Aird et al. [1] were the first to demonstrate convincingly an association between the blood group A antigen of the ABO system on red blood cells and carcinoma of the stomach. In the extensive number of studies since then most reports of increased risk to a person carrying a particular blood group marker are rarely greater than twice that for an individual who does not carry the marker (see ref. [2] for review). The most impressive association found to date is reported in the study by Jick et al. [3]. They observed an increased risk of thromboembolism in American women on oral contraceptives who have the A blood group.

Aside from the variety of interesting associations that have been observed between blood groups and diseases, work in this field has provided a conceptual framework for extended studies with other genetic markers. At the same time as the genetics of blood group markers was being unraveled, other investigators were involved in studies leading to the discovery of other types of tissue antigens. Contributions in this area can be found as early as 1903 when Jensen [4] was able to demonstrate the continuous propagation of an alveolar carcinoma in inbred strains of white mice while transplantation of the same tumor to another strain of mice resulted in rejection. This was followed by other individuals who began to realize that tumor transplantation in mice

G. B. Humphrey et al. (eds.), Pediatric oncology 1, 47–77. All rights reserved.

was under genetic control. Gorer[5] was able to demonstrate that the successful implantation of a tumor depended on genes coding for alloantigens. This was followed by a number of other investigations which demonstrated that normal tissues also express alloantigens. These pioneering efforts provided the foundation for the immunological theory of tissue transplantation, much of which is fundamentally compatible with contemporary concepts of all types of tissue and organ transplantation. In the 1940s Medawar and collaborators[6] were able to perfect the technique of skin grafting which was a major step forward in experiments to establish the immunological basis of tissue rejection. Through the use of congenic lines of mice, Snell[7] was able to identify the antigens responsible for tissue rejection which he termed histocompatibility antigens. Our present understanding of the major histocompatibility complex (MHC) of mice is based on these early investigations and the information resulting from the explosion of research activities following them (see ref. [8] for review). The conceptual framework supplied by studies in mice served as the basis for a search for similar tissue antigens in man. Dausset[9] in 1954 was the first to demonstrate human leukocyte antigens by the observation that patients who received a large number of blood transfusions often produced antibodies that would agglutinate leukocytes. As additional histocompatibility antigens were defined in man and their frequency in various populations determined, it became possible to establish the association of these genetic markers with disease. Again, the impetus for these studies was the information available from studies of the major histocompatibility complex of mice. It was recognized very early on that various inbred strains of mice differed in their susceptibility to oncogenic viruses (see ref. [10] for review). Lilly[11] was the first to demonstrate that the susceptibility to Gross leukemic virus was an hereditary trait and, subsequently, that the gene controlling susceptibility was linked to the H-2 region in mice[12]. In addition to the genes controlling susceptibility to cancer, other genes regulating the immune response through a variety of mechanisms as well as genes coding for complement components have been defined in the region of the major histocompatibility complex in mice[13, 14]. These data have been important in allowing for a more thorough interpretation of studies on the MHC in man.

In assessing the published reports for this review, it became clear to the authors that it would be important to select only those studies that represent the state of the art. Thus, we have chosen to discuss in detail only those studies which demonstrate a statistically significant association of a given HLA marker with a malignant disease. Included in this review are numerous studies that have been conducted during the past decade as well as extracts from composite data maintained by Ryder, Anderson, and Svejgaard in the HLA and disease registry in Copenhagen[15]. The third report by these investigators provides a catalog of all studies conducted to date with regard to

HLA and numerous diseases including cancer. For investigators desiring to conduct additional studies reference to this registry is recommended as a comprehensive compilation of previous studies where the data did not reach a level of statistical significance. We will summarize the basic genetics of the major histocompatibility complex in man, describe the approach to studies of HLA and disease, summarize the significant associations that have been found, as well as take the liberty of interpreting these results and suggest areas for future studies. We would hope that, after reading this review, all can agree that while evidence for the association of HLA with malignant disease is not as impressive as for other disease states there is enough to warrant continued research.

2. GENETICS OF THE MAJOR HISTOCOMPATIBILITY COMPLES (MHC) OF MAN

The HLA system is the most complex genetic system known to exist in humans. It is a closely associated group of genetic loci coding for polymorphic cell surface components originally identified through their role in graft rejection. The system of alloantigens that has been revealed, primarily as a result of intensive efforts to circumvent their role in transplantation, appears to be a part of a common mechanism among vertebrates for effecting biological identity. The equivalent system was first recognized in mice, and later in dogs, chickens, guinea pigs and a presently expanding host of other members of the animal kingdom. The term Major Histocompatibility Complex (MHC) is used to refer to the region of chromosome 6 containing the HLA system. The MHC region contains a diverse group of associated loci that control a variety of biological functions such as immune responsiveness, immune surveillance, susceptibility to diseases and possibly, morphogenesis. A fundamental role of the HLA system within the MHC is to control the interaction of the various cells of the immune system. Our understanding of the complexity of this genetic region has been broadened by the discovery that another complex biological system related to immune capabilities is located within the MHC. This is the complement system, which acts in concert with immunoglobulins to effect the destruction of foreign organisms. There are several interesting reviews concerning the historical development of the HLA system and H-2 system that the authors recommend [13–17].

The MHC is distally located on the short arm of human chromosome 6 as diagrammatically represented in Figure 1. It is bounded on the telomeric end by the locus coding for urinary pepsinogen (Pg) and on the centromeric end by the locus coding for the isozyme, glyoxylase-1 (GLO-1) [18–20]. Within the MHC are the loci coding for the HLA linkage groups which have been assigned the designations A, B, C and D/DR. These loci, as diagrammatically

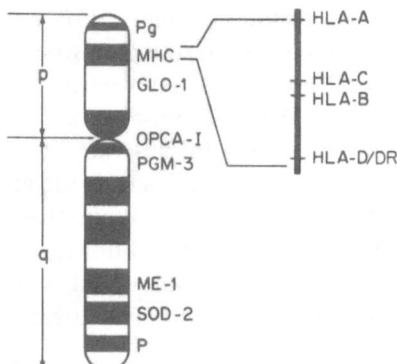

Figure 1. A synopsis of the gene map of chromosome six. The major histocompatibility complex is located on the short arm (p) between the genes for pepsinogen and glyoxalase-1.

shown in Figure 2, are from the centromere outward in the order D/DR, B, C, and A, which is reflective of the sequence of discovery of each individual loci. Also within the MHC are the loci coding for the polymorphic variants of certain complement components (C2, C4) and Properdin factor B (Bf), as well as the loci coding for the 21-Hydroxylase Deficiency gene designated AH for the disease state adrenal hyperplasia [21]. It has recently been shown that the red blood cell antigens identified as Chido and Rodgers are actually the polymorphic variants of C4 previously designated as C4S and C4F, respectively [22]. The evidence to date supports the positioning of all of these loci on the centromeric side of the HLA-B locus. It has been suggested that, in addition to these known loci, there remains within the approximately 1.8 centimorgan span between the A and D/DR loci sufficient genetic material to code for a minimum of several hundred genetic traits. Intensive research is currently devoted to identifying the products of these loci, which has led to the recent report of a new allelic system, HT (Human T), that segregates with the HLA system [23, 24]. It is thought that the human equivalent of the

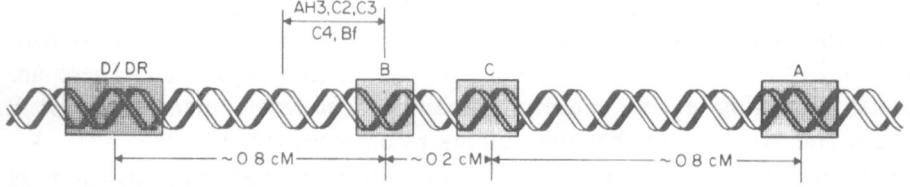

Figure 2. Diagrammatic representation of the major histocompatibility complex in man. The relative distances between the four loci, ie. D/DR, B, C and A are defined by a unit termed centimorgan (cM). A centimorgan represents a cross-over value of 1%. Other genes such as those coding for the complement components C2, C3, C4, properdin factor B and the susceptibility gene for adrenal hyperplasia (AH3) are also found at this region of chromosome 6 but their exact order or location has not been determined.

immune response loci discovered in mice will be located within this region possibly in a position near the D/DR locus.

The HLA system consists of antigens that for purposes of discussion can be separated into two unique categories based on the methods required for their detection. One group is made up of serologically-defined antigens (SD-antigens) of the A, B, C and DR loci. This group includes the majority of the antigens within the HLA system. These can be identified by two methods. The HLA-A, B and C locus antigens are found on the cells of most tissues and are easily detectable using the original microcytotoxicity technique or variants thereof [25 – 28]. These antigens were the first discovered within the HLA system. In 1973 it was reported that another group of antigens later designated HLA-DR (HLA-D related) could be detected on B-lymphocytes and macrophages using special serological methods [29]. The other category of antigens of the HLA system, HLA-D, can be detected using cellular typing methods, such as mixed lymphocyte culturing (MLC) [30] or a refinement of this method which utilizes homozygous typing cells (HTC) [29]. These are considered lymphocyte-defined antigens (LD-antigens). Included among the cellular typing methods, is primed lymphocyte typing (PLT); a technical advancement holding promise as a tool for further clarification of the genetics of the MHC region [31]. The genes coding for HLA-D antigens are very closely associated with those controlling synthesis of the HLA-DR antigens. At one time D and DR were thought to be identical but there is presently available evidence suggesting they may be two independent but closely associated loci [32]. Both the HLA-D and DR antigens are thought to correspond to the immune region associated antigens described in mice.

Although the cellular typing methods have contributed greatly to our understanding of the HLA system the recently described techniques for the generation of monoclonal antibodies may in the future provide a means for identifying D-locus markers which will circumvent a tedious and time consuming procedure.

During the last decade human geneticists and biochemists have focused attention on a detailed critical analysis of the HLA system. The need for practical information in transplantation has provided the framework for the disease association studies, which have received so much attention in the latter part of the 1970s and are continuing unabated into the 1980s. A by-product of this research has been the acquisition of an unparalleled body of evidence defining the genetics of any set of traits in humans. The HLA system is an exquisitely complex set of linked genetic loci coding for a highly polymorphic set of biochemically and biologically definable markers found on the surface of the human leucocyte. The antigens are inherited as simple codominant mendelian traits governed by the single autosomal regions (A, B, C or D/DR). At each locus multiple alleles have been identified which code

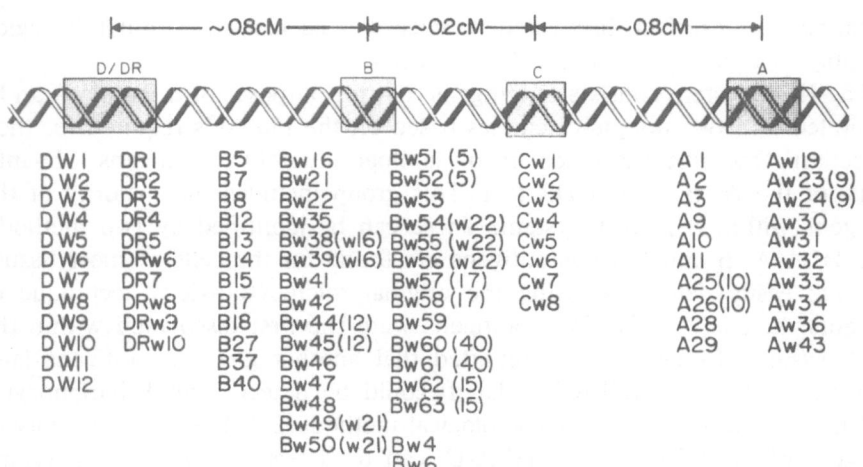

Figure 3. Nomenclature of the HLA specificities officially recognized by the 1980 World Health Organization HLA Nomenclature Committee [33].

for the histocompatibility antigens. At present there are 18 A-, 32 B-, 8 Cw-, 10 DR- and 12 D-locus antigens that have been approved by the 8th International Histocompatibility Workshop (WHO-IUIS Terminology Committee, 1980) [33]. The presently recognized antigens are listed in Figure 3.

Credit for the rapid and orderly progress made during the past two decades must be extended to those pioneers in the field of HLA studies who had the vision and wisdom to realize the tremendous potential for advancement through a continuing international collaborative endeavor. Begun in 1964 by D.B. Amos, the International Histocompatibility Workshops have been convened every two or three years to report the findings of the previous period since the last Workshop and to outline direction for the coming Workshop. The Workshops are organized around a common set of antibodies obtained from throughout the world which have been subjected to extensive testing to identify them as standard reagents. These are distributed to every participating laboratory and serve as the common measure of uniformity for the many studies of populations, transplantation outcome and disease associations. The data are then submitted to the host laboratory, which is different each time, for analysis. It has been through this complex mechanism that the segregant series have been defined, that the universality of the mode of inheritance established, as well as evidence of the general distribution of the antigens in every population examined. The Workshops in recent years have developed a considerable body of data describing the associations of HLA determinants with specific diseases, thus expanding the audience for the findings of this group. The proceedings from each of the Workshops provide an interesting chronology of the major developments leading to our present understanding of the HLA system [34–40].

Another organization instrumental in maintaining uniformity has been the international Terminology Committee sponsored by the World Health Organization (WHO) previously mentioned. This group was mandated with the responsibility for effecting suitable standards of nomenclature. Through its efforts, the term 'HLA' came into use as well as a number of other terms used throughout this chapter. Originally, H was for human, L for leucocyte and A for the designation applied to the first locus, but as our knowledge of the system expanded to include the newer segregant series, the term came to be applied to the entire series of histocompatibility antigens. It has been through the efforts of the WHO committee that the HLA nomenclature has evolved to its current form, wherein each antigen is identified by a letter for the locus which controls it, followed by a number defining the particular specificity. As you will notice in Figure 3, some of the antigens bear a 'w' designation as well. The 'w' is a provisional designation, identifying antigens that are not fully accepted specificities and must be subjected to further analysis before being accepted. The 'w' designation is removed when sufficient evidence accrues to support its acceptance as a fully-defined specificity.

A point of historical interest to which the authors would like to direct your attention is the antigen assignments for the A and B loci. There is no duplication of numbers in these two series. For example, there is an A1 but no B1. This convention of nomenclature has its roots in the early history of HLA and is a rule that is not applicable to the other segregant series, which are all sequentially numbered and thus not interdependent relative to nomenclature.

Because of intense efforts in recent years, only a relatively small fraction of the frequency of genes at the A and B loci is still unaccounted for in the caucasian population. This is in contrast to the C and D/DR loci wherein there remains a large frequency of 'blanks' as these markers are termed, i.e., more blanks where the defined antisera does not detect an antigen on the cells of a particular individual which presumably represents an undetected or undefined allele. For example, in caucasians about 96% of the antigens of the A series, 95.6% of the B series, 47% of the C series and 73.2% of the DR series have been identified. The occurrence of blanks in blacks and orientals is not appreciably different from that of the caucasians, for example, in blacks, 90.5% of the A, 93.2% of the B, 49.3% of the C and 87.3% of the DR have been identified based on the report of the latest workshop [33].

The genes of the HLA system show a markedly different distribution pattern in different ethnic groups; a factor of particular importance for disease association studies. This is sometimes true even within an ethnic group. For

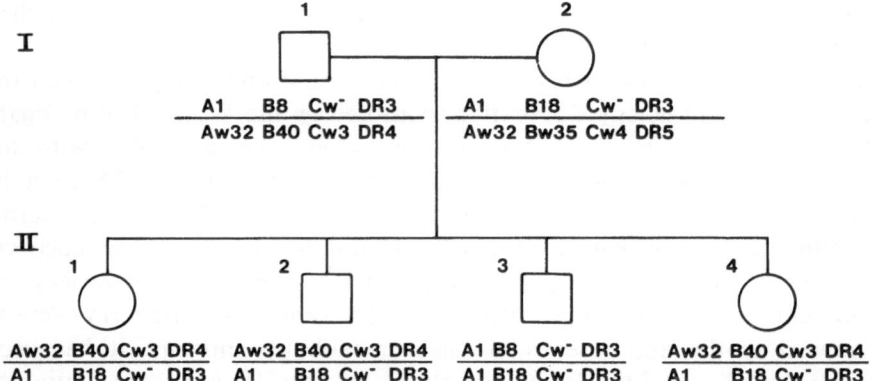

Figure 4. An example of the inheritance pattern of HLA as depicted in a two-generation family. In the first generation the father has A1, B8, Cw⁻, DR3 on one of the pairs of chromosome 6 (a haplotype) and AW3, B40, Cw3, DR4 on the other. The mother has A1, B18, Cw⁻, DR3 and Aw32, Bw35, Cw4, DR5 on each of the two pairs of chromosome 6. The children by these two individuals would therefore receive a chromosome 6 from the father and one from the mother as illustrated, which would each contain a set of A, B, C and D/DR locus antigens. In this illustration only DR antigens are shown since the Dw phenotype has not been determined. The Cw⁻ indicates that a C locus antigen was not observed in this particular haplotype.

instance, B8 occurs in only 10% of Mediterranean populations whereas it is above 30% in the population of Scotland. Moreover, among caucasians there is considerable variation within certain geographic regions such as Europe, where it has been observed that there is a decline in the frequency of A1 and B8 as well as A3 and B7 from North to South Europe. Other population groups have their own frequency of HLA components that is highly characteristic of the group. For instance, the frequency of Aw30, Bw42, Bw57 and Bw58 is greater in negroes than orientals or caucasians. In orientals, the occurrence of Aw24, and the Bw22 split, Bw54, is greater and that of the common 'caucasian' antigens, A1, A3, B8 and B18 is lower than in other population groups. This evidence makes it clear that for disease studies typing must be performed on the disease group and on a control group who, if at all possible come from the same local population [40].

Studies of the mode of inheritance of the alleles of the various segregant series have demonstrated that no person possesses more than two antigens from each series, i.e., a person has only 2 A-locus antigens, 2 B-locus antigens, etc. This can easily be seen in the example provided in Figure 4 wherein parent 1 (Father) has two A-locus antigens, A1 and Aw32; two B-locus antigens, B8 and B40, considering only these two loci, whereas parent 2 (Mother) has A1, Aw32 and B18, Bw35. For these examples the genotypes are described as being heterozygous, i.e., the two alleles inherited at each locus are different. If the genotypes are the same at any one locus, the alleles are considered homozygous. A common example of the homozygous condition among caucasians is the person with A1, A1; B8, B8. The example in Figure 4 can also be extended conceptually to demonstrate another facet of the mode of inheritance which, simply stated, is that since the loci of each segregant series are so closely linked or associated on the same chromosome, they are donated as a 'block' to each child during the meiotic association. Additionally, each parent donates only one 'block' of antigens to each child. Thus, children 1, 2 and 4 inherited the 'haplotype', as each 'block' is termed, Aw32-B40-Cw3-DR4 from the father and A1-B18-Cw(-)-DR3 from the mother. Having received the same haplotypes, these children are considered haploidentical. On the other hand, child 3 received the same haplotype as the other children from the father, while the mother donated the alternative haplotype potentially available in her set of two, i.e., A1-B8-Cw(-)-DR3. Thus, each parent contributes one-half of the genetic material received by each child in the meiotic exchange, i.e., the genetics of the HLA system is governed by simple Mendelian assortment. Recombination, another mode of inheritance which results in non-Mendelian assortment of genetic material occurs rarely.

Variations from the expected frequency of the joint occurrence of certain alleles is important in disease association studies including cancer. Genetic theory predicts that the alleles of two closely linked loci will occur together with a frequency not substantially different from that determined by the product of their two independent gene frequencies. The assumption is that equilibrium in the distribution of the HLA alleles should have been attained, given the span of time available for random assortment. However, there are several examples of the perturbation of such random associations. A common example of non-random assortment or 'linkage disequilibrium' is seen in the frequency distribution of A1 and B8 in caucasians. From Table 1, it can be seen that the individual frequencies of A1 and B8 are 0.17 and 0.11, respectively. The estimated frequency for the occurrence of these two alleles together on the same haplotype is 0.019, i.e., 0.17 times 0.11. However, the observed frequency of association of these two determinants is 0.088 which is 4.6 times more often than the occurrence predicted by random assortment. Examples of linkage disequilibrium exist for combinations of each segregant

Table 1. Example of linkage disequilibrium.

A1	0.17
B8	0.11
A1,B8	0.019 expected
A1,B8	0.088 observed

Extent of linkage disequilibrium between alleles $= 0.088 - 0.019 = 0.069$.

series, i.e. Cw3 with B15 and Dw3 with B8. However, as a general rule, the strength of such associations decreases with increasing distance between the corresponding loci. Consequently, the strongest associations are between the B and C loci, which are approximately 0.2 centimorgans apart. The impact of such non-random effects on disease associations can readily be seen. For instance, using A1, B8 as an example, when B8 is found to be associated with a particular disease, one might expect to also find that disease associated with A1. This is very often the case, and is a factor that must be considered in any interpretation of the association of HLA gene products with disease. It then becomes necessary to subject the data to analytical procedures designed to determine with which allele the disease is associated, or if it is actually associated with both and the strength of the association.

3. METHODS FOR STUDYING HLA AND DISEASE

The two approaches which have been utilized in studies of HLA and disease relationships are association and linkage analyses. These will now be discussed along with examples of each, since the studies to be reviewed of HLA and malignant disease have used both these approaches. In addition, statistical procedures assessing the significance of the data will also be briefly discussed. Hopefully, this will provide background sufficient for those individuals who do not actually work in this field to understand the data that will subsequently be presented.

3.1. Association

In an association study one looks at the frequency of occurrence of alleles among a disease population and then compares those frequencies to the frequency with which those alleles occur in a group of healthy subjects ideally, from the same geographic area. In these studies none of the subjects in either the diseased or control groups can be related to each other. If the allele is associated with the disease, then it will occur with greater frequency in the diseased population than expected by chance alone. The association between a given HLA allele and a disease may be due to the direct involvement of the gene product in the disease process, implying a causal relationship. Alternatively, the association between a gene coding for a particular HLA antigen and a disease susceptibility gene may be due to nothing more than linkage between the two where there would be no cause and effect relationship.

Once an increased or decreased frequency of occurrence of a genetic polymorphism in the diseased population has been observed the next step is to determine whether there is a statistically significant deviation between the two groups. This is accomplished by establishing a two-by-two contingency table and calculating the significance using the Chi-square test or Fisher's exact test [41]. Since there are now 80 HLA-A,-B,-C and -D/DR antigens that can be assessed in association studies there is the possibility that some of these antigens will deviate significantly at the 0.05 probability level by chance alone. One can attempt to correct for this possibility by multiplying the p-value by the number of HLA antigens that were analyzed in the study. As pointed out by Svejgaard et al. [42], this is a somewhat conservative approach that tends to obviate false associations that might appear. However, this conservative correction is only necessary in the first study. Subsequent studies which may prove or disprove the reported deviation of a specific antigen can rely on demonstrating significance at the 0.05 probability level without correction. Having computed the statistical significance of the deviation of the HLA antigen frequencies between the diseased population and healthy controls the strength of an association can be determined. This can be done by using Woolf's cross products or incidence ratio formula [43]. This statistical comparison is used as an estimate of the relative risk of an individual possessing a particular polymorphic marker developing a disease compared to an individual developing the disease who lacks the marker. An example of how this relative risk estimate is calculated is shown in Table 2. Here a two-by-two table has been constructed utilizing the data from a study of the association of HLA-DR antigens with insulin-dependent diabetes mellitus

Table 2. Method for establishing disease association.

Subjects	No. of individuals		Total
	DR4 positive	DR4 negative	
IDDM	a 18 (31.58%)	b 39 (68.42%)	57
Controls	c 9 (8.65%)	d 95 (91.35%)	104

Strength of association: relative risk $= \dfrac{a \times d}{c \times b}$ where

a is the number of patients possessing the particular HLA antigen,
b is the number of patients lacking the particular HLA antigen,
c is the number of controls possessing the particular HLA antigen,
d is the number of controls lacking the particular HLA antigen.

The relative risk of developing IDDM for a person possessing DR4 would be:
$\dfrac{18 \times 95}{9 \times 39} = 4.87$

The significance of the association as determined by the likelihood ratio asymptotic Chi square method is $p < 0.003$. The corrected p value for the number of D locus antigens compared is $p < 0.003 \times 6 = p < 0.0018$.

(IDDM) in the American black population. As can be seen, the relative risk of an American black developing IDDM with the DR4 antigen is 4.87 [44]. The significance of this observation then can be calculated by a number of statistical methods including the classic Chi-square test, Fisher's exact test, or as shown here, the likelihood ratio asymptotic Chi-square method.

It should be stressed again that in studies that aim to determine the association of a genetic polymorphism with a disease, it is important to have a large healthy local control population. Ideally, this population should be free of any major disease as well as have no family history of the disease in question.

3.2. Linkage

The other major approach to studying the relationship between a genetic trait and disease is linkage analysis. Here one may ask whether the gene for a given disease occurs on the same chromosome in close proximity to another gene whose product can be assayed. In these studies, one can determine the position of the disease susceptibility gene on the chromosome map. Ideally these studies are conducted by analyzing families in which more than one individual is affected with the given disease. HLA is a convenient marker in such studies as previously stated due to the fact that there are four closely linked loci A, B, C and D/DR each with multiple alleles. These four loci are inherited as a unit termed a haplotype. An HLA haplotype is inherited from each parent. Recombinational events or cross-overs between these four loci are very rare. This almost assures heterozygosity at the marker loci and makes it easier to identify doubly heterozygous individuals which are essential for studies of linkage between the MHC and a disease susceptibility gene. It should be stressed that the association of a genetic trait such as HLA with a disease can be due to a different phenomena from linkage of the trait to the disease. Two examples will illustrate this point. First, as already mentioned the association of the A blood group substance with thromboembolism in American women on oral contraceptives is a consistent association found in this particular population for which no measurable linkage can be detected between the susceptiblity gene(s) for the disorder and the gene for the blood group (3). Second, the association found in various racial and ethnic groups between HLA-B8, B15, B18, DR3 and DR4 and insulin dependent diabetes mellitus [44, 45] can be attributed to genetic linkage. The susceptibility gene for this disease is linked to the MHC and due to linkage disequilibrium with the aforementioned HLA types which are found more frequently in the patients. Studies assessing linkage between a genetic marker and a disease susceptibility gene are much more difficult to perform than association studies. This is because complete families where more than one individual is affected with the disease need to be studied.

The linkage of known genetic markers and disease susceptibility genes within families is measured by the frequency of crossing over events occurring in a segment of a chromosome which adjoins both the genetic marker and the gene(s) of interest. These cross over events can only be readily discerned in the offspring of individuals who are heterozygous for the genetic marker and the gene(s) of interest. For example, if we assume an individual has the following genotype linkage between two loci, A and D, AD/ad, where the *AD* chromosome is of paternal origin and the *ad* chromosome is of maternal origin, that individual can produce four types of gametes; AD, ad, Ad, and aD. The last two of these are results from single cross over events occurring between the A and D loci, and should occur at much lower frequencies in the offspring than the non-recombinant events. If, however, the frequency of these gametic types, observed in the offspring, occur at equal frequencies then these two loci are considered to be either too far apart on a chromosome for any measurable linkage or are located on entirely different chromosomes.

The measurement of the degree of linkage between two loci is determined statistically by taking the ratio of the likelihood of observing a particular frequency of recombination in the offspring of doubly heterozygous individuals, over the likelihood that there is 50% recombination, which is the frequency of recombinant types if there is no linkage. This ratio gives you the relative odds of the two loci being linked at that distance (recombination frequency) to that of their being unlinked. Odds of 1000 to 1 in favor of linkage is considered to be highly significant. The classical methodology is to take the log of this ratio, which is the difference in the two log likelihoods (lod score), and thus a difference of 3 is indicative of linkage. How close the linkage is depends on the recombination frequency at which a lod of 3.0 is detected.

4. HLA AND MALIGNANT DISEASES

Because malignant diseases were among the first in which an association with HLA was sought, there is a substantial amount of literature on this subject. We have limited ourselves to those studies in which the statistical significance is equal to or less than the 0.05 probability level after 'correcting' for the number of antigens studied, i.e., determining if the p-value remains significant after being multiplied by the number of antigens examined. This is a common mechanism for minimizing certain biases inherent in such studies. For a more detailed listing of the malignant diseases which have been investigated please refer to the third report of HLA and Disease Registry maintained in Copenhagen by Ryder *et al.* [15]. References [46–48] pertain to reviews of other studies on malignant diseases.

4.1. Association Studies

Table 3 is a compilation of those malignant diseases for which the association of HLA is statistically significance. Data for acute lymphocytic leukemia (ALL) has been combined from 15 studies for which Ryder *et al.* [15] have evaluated and calculated the statistical significance. As can be seen, in 1099 caucasoid patients studied, A2 and B12 have been shown to be increased compared to healthy controls. Thus, caucasian individuals in the population who possess A2 or B12 have a relative risk of 1.39 and 1.24 respectively for developing ALL. Some of the more impressive data has been the association of HLA with various types of carcinoma. Hammond *et al.* [49] studied 249 South African Indian cancer patients and found an increase in the frequency of the HLA-A11 and -Bw52 in patients with malignancies compared to 603 control subjects. The patient population consisted of four major Asian Indian ethnic groups. A significant association was also found between Bw52 and breast carcinoma in the Telegu Indians in South Africa. However, since only 14 patients were studied, this observation must be subjected to independent confirmation. When the data of nine separate studies on Caucasian patients with carcinoma of the breast was combined by the HLA and Disease Registry, Bw35 was found to be significantly increased when compared with healthy controls [15]. Jing *et al.* [50], in a study of 76 Chinese patients from California with nasopharyngeal carcinoma, found an increase in A2 in the patient group compared to healthy controls. However, this increase was not significant when corrected for the number of antigens examined. HLA-A11 was found to be decreased in the patient population but again this was not significant after correction. These investigators, however, observed that the combination of A2 and less than two antigens at the B locus (i.e., blanks at the B locus) occurred together more freqently in Chinese nasopharyngeal carcinoma patients than healthy controls. When corrected for the number of antigens tested this observation held up as significant. Simons *et al.* [51, 52] have also observed an increase of A2 in Chinese patients from Singapore with nasopharyngeal carcinoma. In addition, they have observed an increase of the B locus antigen originally termed Sin-2 which has now been shown to be analogous to the Bw46 specificity. These investigators also observed an increased incidence of A2 and Bw46 occurring together in the patient population. Studies by this group as well as Payne *et al.* [53] have shown that A2 and Bw46 are in genetic disequilibrium. Bertrams *et al.* [54] have shown a significant increase in B18 in a group of patients with carcinoma of the ovaries. However, because only 20 patients were studied, this observation needs further confirmation. Toomey *et al.* [55] found an increased frequency

Table 3. The association of HLA with onset of malignant diseases.

Disease	Geographic area	Racial/ethnic [1] group	HLA type	Antigen frequency				Significance	Relative risk	Ref.
				Patients		Controls				
				Total	% pos	Total	% pos			
ALL*	Combined	Cau	A2†	1099	46–68	7490	37–60	6.6×10^{-7}	1.39	15
			B12†	1099	17–75	7490	16–36	3.0×10^{-3}	1.24	
CARCINOMA										
Breast	Africa	Note 2	Bw52†	14	42.9	288	10.5	1.8×10^{-2}	6.45	49
	Combined	Cau	Bw35†	1528	13–31	6213	5–26	7.7×10^{-5}	1.35	15
Nasopharyngeal	USA	Ch	A2<2 Ag 2nd locus †	76	26.3	97	12.4	6.2×10^{-2}	3.53	50
	Singapore	Ch	A2†	153	63	91	52	4.8×10^{-2}	1.62	51.52
			Bw46†	153	39	91	25	2.3×10^{-2}	1.84	
			A2/Bw46†	130	35	73	18	2.6×10^{-3}	2.38	
Ovarium	Germany	Cau	B18†	20	35	1000	10	2.4×10^{-2}	4.85	54
Gynecologic squamous	USA	Cau	B8†	40	37.5	2550	16.4	5×10^{-2}	3.06	55
Teratocarcinoma	USA	Cau	Dw7†	26	46	150	9	1×10^{-2}	8.33	56
Stomach	Japan	Ja	B5↓	87	17.2	355	40	5×10^{-3}	0.32	58
CLL+	USA	Cau	B5, B18† Bw35†	13	69	383	30	3.6×10^{-2}	5.24	59

* ALL = Acute lymphocytic leukemia
+ CLL = Chronic lymphocytic leukemia
Note 1: Abbreviations; Cau, Caucasian; Ch, Chinese; Ja, Japanese
Note 2: Telegu Indians

Table 3. (continued).

Disease	Geographic area	Racial/ ethnic [1] group	HLA type	Antigen frequency				Significance	Relative risk	Ref.
				Patients		Controls				
				Total	% pos	Total	% pos			
CML#	England	Cau	A2 + A9†	9	67	145	5	1.1×10^{-2}	39.42	60
HODGKIN'S										
Lymphogranu-lomatosis	Combined	Cau	A1†	2669	29–62	13694	20–49	1×10^{-10}	1.38	15
			B5†	2668	0.25	13600	3–22	1.6×10^{-5}	1.33	15
			B8†	2670	11–35	13692	12–33	4.7×10^{-5}	1.23	15
			B18†	2306	3–29	11424	2–16	1.4×10^{-3}	1.30	15
	Sweden,	Cay	B12†	27	48	100	19	2.3×10^{-2}	1.58	64
	Australia	Cau	A11†	127	28.4	273	13.6	9×10^{-3}	2.52	65
			B5†	127	32.3	127	12.1	5×10^{-4}	3.54	65
Mixed cellularity	USA	Cau	B5†	39	31.0	459	6.0	2×10^{-3}	6.84	66
			B18†	39	13.0	459	2.0	2×10^{-2}	7.35	66
Lymphocyte predominance			B5†	12	33.0	459	6.0	4×10^{-2}	8.0	66
Familial	USA	Cau	Bw35†	13	54.0	629	16.0	1×10^{-2}	6.10	67
			B37†	13	23.0	629	4.0	3×10^{-2}	7.25	67
Long survival	Sweden	Cau	B18†	40	20.0	1263	5.0	3.2×10^{-2}	4.76	68
nodular sclerosis			B17↓	298	1–3	3409	7–8	1.8×10^{-3}	0.36	15
Prospective	Combined	Cau	A1†	741	33–42	3446	28–34	6.0×10^{-4}	1.37	15

Note 1: Abbreviations; Cau, Caucasian; Ch, Chinese; Ja, Japanese
CML = Chronic myelogenous leukemia

Table 3. (continued).

Disease	Geographic area	Racial/ ethnic [1] group	HLA type	Antigen frequency				Significance	Relative risk	Ref.
				Patients		Controls				
				Total	% pos	Total	% pos			
HYPERNEPHROMA	Germany	Cau	Aw30/Aw31†	44	25	300	6.6	7×10^{-3}	4.60	69
LYMPHOMA, follicular	Australia	Cau	B12†	56	62.5	273	32.3	5×10^{-3}	3.51	70
LYMPHOMA, lymphocytic	USA	Cau	B12†	39	44	383	22.0	1.8×10^{-3}	2.75	59
MULTIPLE MYELOMA	Combined	Cau	B5†	235	3–36	1792	4–22	2.2×10^{-3}	1.93	15
RETINOBLASTOMA	Germany	Cau	Bw35†	122	25.4	255	11.0	2×10^{-2}	2.76	71
			B12†	122	9.8	255	25.1	2×10^{-2}	0.33	
SARCOMA (connective tissue)	USA	Cau	B5†	63	28	389	9	4.2×10^{-2}	4.05	72
WILM'S	Czech.	Cau	A1 or A9†	46	71.7	301	44.5	1.4×10^{-2}	3.16	73

Note 1: Abbreviations; Cau, Caucasian; Ch, Chinese; Ja, Japanese

of B8 in Caucasian patients with gynecologic carcinoma. This included 43 patients of which 33 had cervical squamous carcinoma, seven had vulvar or lower vaginal squamous carcinoma, and three had uterine adenocarcinoma. No increase in HLA antigens were found for adenocarcinomas of the same organs. A report of the association of B8 with squamous cell carcinoma of the cervix and vulva was not significant for these two groups of cancers when corrected for the number of antigens tested. De Wolf et al. [56] observed a significant increase in Dw7 in 26 patients with teratocarcinoma. This is the first report of an association with a D locus antigen and a malignant disease. It is interesting that the relative risk for an individual developing teratocarcinoma carrying Dw7 is one of the highest for any of the malignant diseases summarized in Table 3. The importance of additional studies of D locus antigens will be discussed in section 5. Carr and Bach [57] found an increase in the frequency of Aw24 in patients with metastatic teratocarcinoma as compared with the frequency of this antigen in patients with non-metastatic tumor. These two studies on teratocarcinoma are of great interest but due to the small number of patients observed they need to be corroborated testing for all known A, B, C, and D/DR locus antigens.

Tsuji et al. [58] found a significant decrease in B5 in patients with carcinoma of the stomach. A significant increase in A and B locus antigens was not observed by this group. Dick et al. [59] in an early study of 154 patients with various types of lymphomas found a significant increase in the 4c antigen with chronic lymphocytic leukemia. Antisera that recognized the 4c antigen in 1972 has subsequently been shown to recognize B5, B18 and Bw35. Although this observation was statistically significant, only 13 patients were investigated and the antisera was not as clearly defined as is presently the case. Although others have not shown this same association, this study definitely needs to be repeated with a larger patient population using antisera which detects all the currently known HLA specificities. A study by Dickson [60] of 54 caucasian patients from London having various types of leukemia revealed that A2 and A9 occurred together more frequently in nine patients with chronic myelogenous leukemia than in healthy controls. Here is another study that is statistically significant but, because of the small number of patients sampled needs to be replicated before the data can be unequivocably accepted. Moreover, other investigators have shown an increased frequency of A3 [61] and B5 and Bw17 [62] in patients with chronic myelocytic leukemia. These conflicting reports will be resolved by additional studies where a larger number of patients and more defined antisera are used.

The first malignant disease in which an association with HLA antigens was sought was Hodgkin's disease by Amiel [63]. Since that time there have been more studies of Hodgkin's patients than for any other malignant disease. As can be seen in Table 3 there are 25 studies of greater than 2500 caucasian patients with lymphogranulomatosis type of Hodgkin's disease. The combined data from the HLA and Disease Registry has shown that A1, B5, B8, and B18 are significantly increased in patients with this type of Hodgkin's disease. However, the risk for an individual developing Hodgkin's who possesses these antigens is still very small due to the low strength of this association. Björkholm [64] observed an increase of B12 in caucasian individuals with Hodgkin's disease in Stockholm, Sweden. The increase was most marked in patients below 40 years of age with a favorable histopathology. Although B8 was slightly increased in patients over 40 years of age, this observation was not significant when the *p*-value was corrected. Forbes and Morris [65] observed A11 and B5 to be increased in patients with Hodgkin's disease. B5 was found to be relatively common in males with the lymphocytic predominant type of Hodgkin's disease while A11 was found to be more common in females with the nodular sclerosis type of the disease. Graff *et al.* [66] found B5 increased in the mixed cellularity and lymphocyte predominant histological subtype of Hodgkin's disease while B18 was significantly increased in the mixed cellularity type but not in the other histological types. Green *et al.* [67] observed a significant increase of Bw35 and Bw37 in the probands from 13 families prone to Hodgkin's disease. Hornmark-Stenstam *et al.* [68] in Lund, Sweden observed a significant increase in B18 in patients who had survived Hodgkin's disease for an average of 23 years. In addition, B18 was found to be significantly increased in patients with the nodular sclerosis type of Hodgkin's disease. This observation does not coincide with two combined studies from the HLA and Disease Registry where B17 was found to be decreased in 298 patients with the nodular sclerosis type of Hodgkin's disease compared to normal controls. Also from the HLA and Disease Registry the results of six combined prospective studies of Hodgkin's disease involving 741 patients revealed that A1 was significantly increased as compared with the healthy control population. The studies on Hodgkin's disease are informative because they stress the need to be aware of the possible existence of heterogeneity within a given malignant disease. The results of studies seeking an association between HLA and Hodgkin's disease as a whole have not been nearly as impressive as those from studies attempting to correlate the frequencies of a given HLA type with various histological subgroups of the disease. Thus, it appears that HLA might be important in subgrouping malignant disease in addition to predicting susceptibility based on a given HLA type.

There has been one relatively recent study where Aw30/Aw31 was found to be significantly increased in caucasian patients with hypernephroma from Munich, Germany [69]. It will be interesting to see if this observation can be repeated by other investigators. Forbes and Morris [70] found a significant association between B12 and follicular lymphoma in 56 patients studied in Melbourne, Australia. Although 154 patients were studied with various types of lymphoma a significant association was only found for the one subtype. Dick *et al.* [59] observed an increased frequency of B12 in patients with lymphocytic lymphomas. Although 154 patients with various types of lymphoid tumors were investigated, only this latter type was found to be associated with B12. Seven studies combined in the HLA and Disease Registry [15] demonstrate an increased frequency of B5 in caucasian patients with multiple myeloma. It is interesting that B5 appears to be increased in leukemia and lymphoma type of malignancies. One study of 122 German children with retinoblastoma by Bertrams [71] has demonstrated a significantly increased frequency of Bw35 and a decreased frequency of B12. Although these investigators were fortunate enough to have a large number of patients for the study and the data is statistically significant there is still the need for other studies containing an equal or greater number of patients from other parts of the world. Tarpley [72] found a 3-fold increase of B5 in patients with connective tissue sarcomas. The association was only with the occurrence of the disease itself since there was no significant deviation of the frequency of B5 relative to time of survival after treatment. In a study of 46 caucasian subjects from Czechoslavakia with Wilms tumor an increased frequency of A1 or A9 was found in these patients compared to normal controls [73]. An association with various HLA antigens and neuroblastoma was also sought in this study. Although an increased frequency of B13 and Bw21 was observed, the data was not statistically significant.

As is obvious from this review, there are few malignant diseases where large numbers of patients have been investigated in a definitive study. Only in studies on ALL, carcinoma of the breast in caucasians, nasopharyngeal carcinoma in Chinese, stomach carcinoma in Japanese, Hodgkin's disease in caucasians, multiple myeloma and retinoblastoma have the sample sizes been sufficiently large to place some confidence in the results. Of these, there are only a few in which the strength of the association is at all impressive. Among those malignancies with a large number of patients involved, it is only for nasopharyngeal carcinoma in the Chinese and subtypes of Hodgkin's disease in caucasians that the risk for individuals possessing a particular HLA-phenotype developing the disease exceed 3-fold. Another deficiency in the studies performed to date is that there is a paucity of information regarding the association of D locus antigens with malignant diseases. The only disease studied in this context so far has been teratocarcinoma for which there was only a very small number of subjects. When viewed as a whole the data are promising, however, and demonstrate that HLA-A and -B locus antigens are indeed associated with various types of malignant diseases. Perhaps one of the more intriguing aspects of studies looking for an association of HLA with malignant diseases has been the findings that HLA might be useful in predicting the outcome of therapy.

Table 4. Association of HLA with outcome of therapy.

Disease	Racial/ethnic group	HLA type	Association	References
ALL	Caucasian	A2	Survival and resistance	48, 74–77
		A9	Survival and resistance	
AML	Caucasian	A2	Survival and resistance	48, 78
		B12	Survival and resistance	79
		B17	Remission less frequently	80
Breast carcinoma	Caucasian	B7	Longer metastases-free	81
		B8	Survival	82
Nasopharyngeal carcinoma	Chinese	Bw46	Poorer survival rate	51
Bronchogenic carcinoma	Caucasian	Aw19	Resistance	83
		B5	Resistance	
Hodgkin's	Caucasian	A1	Survival	48, 84, 85
		B8	Survival	
		A28	Poor prognosis	64
		A28	Good prognosis	68
Melanoma	Caucasian	B5	Deficiency develop metastatic disease	86
Cancer	Caucasian	Hetero-zygosity	Decreased susceptibility	87

Table 4 summarizes the data suggesting that for a number of malignant diseases an individuals HLA phenotype may be useful in determining prognosis. Although many of these studies could be challenged as not being specific, the data associating HLA with survival and resistance in ALL and Hodgkin's disease has been reproduced in several laboratories and appears to be sound. There is one area of conflict. Two separate laboratories have reported opposite findings with regard to the use of A28 for establishing prognosis in Hodgkin's disease. The finding that melanoma patients who lack B5 are more likely to develop metastatic disease is interesting as is the report that geriatric patients who are more heterozygous with regard to HLA-A and -B locus have a decreased susceptibility to malignant diseases. One would suspect that further studies with geriatric subjects who are relatively disease-free would reveal an association of various HLA types with persistent health and longevity.

To date there have been no clear cut studies unequivocally linking the susceptibility gene for a given malignant disease to the major histocomptability complex in man. Although familial aggregation of select malignant diseases has been reported, breast cancer being the most obvious example, large pedigrees with multiply affected individuals have not been observed very often [88]. Lynch *et al.* [89] have investigated seven independently ascertained families which include a total of 950 members of whom 450 have been HLA typed. These investigators were unable to find a single HLA antigen or haplotype that was common to all breast cancer prone kindreds or cancer family syndrome kindreds. Until additional families are identified possessing other types of malignant diseases, the issue of linkage of a given malignant disease susceptibility gene with the major histocompatibility complex in man will remain an unanswered question.

5. EXPLANATION FOR AN ASSOCIATION OF HLA WITH MALIGNANT DISEASES

At this juncture enough is known about the major histocompatibility complex in mouse and man to speculate as to the role genes at the major histocompatibility complex play in determing ones susceptibility to disease. Table 5 summarizes some of these possibilities. The first category is the possibility that HLA is directly involved in predisposing an individual to a malignant disease. There are several mechanisms by which this could occur. The first category of possibilities would be the direct involvement of HLA in the disease process. Although viruses have not been shown unequivocably to cause cancer in man, the animal data and the data on Burkitt's lymphoma suggest that at least some types of malignant diseases may be caused by a viral agent [90]. If this was the case, HLA could serve as a receptor site whereby oncogenic viruses could attach to the cell of a host expressing a particular HLA specificity and therefore gain entry into that cell. Human and mouse histocompatibility antigens have been identified as cell surface receptors for Semliki Forest virus [91]. Therefore one could speculate that HLA plays a similar role for oncogenic virus. Another way in which HLA may be directly involved in the disease process is that it may be taken up by

Table 5. Possible explanation for association of HLA with malignant diseases.

Possibilities	Mechanism
Direct involvement of HLA	Receptor for oncogenic virus
	Uptake by oncogenic virus
	Molecular mimicry
Linkage of other genes to HLA-A, B, C, D/DR	Immune response
	Immune regulation
	Cell-cell recognition
	Complement
Other unknown linked genes	?

oncogenic viruses there by allowing the agent to escape detection by the immune system. Azocar and Essex [92] have in fact shown that HLA antigens are incorporated into the envelope of feline leukemic viruses grown in human cells. Mouse RNA tumor viruses have also been shown to incorporate host histocompatibility antigens as well as other cell surface antigens and virion envelope proteins [93]. Lastly, direct involvement of HLA in the onset of malignant diseases could be ascribed to the fact that oncogenic viruses contain genetic material which directs the cell to synthesize virion envelope proteins that are antigenically related to certain HLA specificities. This would be another mechanism to allow the agent to escape detection by the immune system and effect infection of other individuals who possess that particular HLA specificity. Another category of possibilities explaining the association of HLA with malignant diseases could be due to linkage of other genes at the major histocompatibility complex to the genes at the A, B, C and D/DR locus. As has been discussed, the phenomena of linkage disequilibrium operates at this region of chromosome 6. Therefore, genes responsible for modulating or controlling the immune response or complement components which are effector substances of the immune reaction could be in linkage disequilibrium with certain HLA specificities which are found to be associated with various malignant diseases. This latter possibility is strengthened by the knowledge that genes at the MHC do in fact govern the immune response and cell–cell interactions necessary for T as well as B cell immunity (see ref. [94] for review). Although most of these phenomena have been demonstrated by using the mouse model there has recently been numerous reports of similar genes at the MHC of man. For example, there are studies suggesting genes at the MHC of man modulate the immune response. Sasazuki *et al.* [95] have reported on the association of a particular HLA haplotype (HLA-A9 -B5 -DHO) in the Japanese population with low immune responsiveness to tetanus toxoid. The strongest association was found in individuals possessing DHO which is a new D locus specificity. Similar studies by De Vries *et al.* [96] have shown an association between low responsiveness to vaccinia virus and HLA-Cw3. Marsh *et al.* [97] in an investigation of subjects allergic to the ragweed antigen, Ra3 found A2 to be associated with response to Ra3 while A3 was associated with no response. They suggested that alleles at the A locus function as immune response and/or immune suppressor genes or that these alleles are epistatic to such genes. There are other studies worth noting that suggest an association between immune response capabilities and various HLA antigens which might be more relevant to an understanding of malignant disease. Sybesma *et al.* [98] found in a group of patients with Hodgkin's disease that 80% of those who failed to produce antibodies to influenza virus had the HLA-A12 antigen as compared to 14% of those patients who responded to the vaccine. Schacter *et al.* [99] found that the effector lymphocytes from healthy donors that carry the HLA-B7 or B27 specificity gave a significantly less spontaneous cell mediated cytotoxicity to renal cell carcinoma cell lines than donors who lacked these antigens. Lastly, Osoba and Falk [100] found that the leukocytes from healthy controls as well as untreated Hodgkin's disease patients who possessed the HLA-B8 pheno-type gave higher responses in one-way mixed leukocyte culture reactions than leukocytes from subjects who lacked B8. These investigators suggested that a gene in linkage disequilibrium with B8 which controls the proliferative response to alloantigens may explain the increased frequency of B8 in long-term survivors of carcinoma of the breast and Hodgkin's disease.

Other studies have provided evidence that cell surface components coded by genes at the MHC of man play a role in the interaction of thymus-derived (T) lymphocytes with other cells to effect an immune response. The ability of T-lymphocytes to recognize and generate a cytotoxic response to male H-Y antigen [101], dinitrophenylated cells [102], cells infected with influenza virus [103] as well as Epstein-Barr (E-B) virus infected cells [104] requires that the responder cells possess the same HLA-A and -B antigens as the stimula-tor cells. The full biological implication of the HLA restriction of cytotoxic T-cell responses has yet to be unraveled.

It is likely that the genes at the MHC of man involved in regulating the immune response are also polymorphic in nature and inheritance patterns give rise to individuals who have various degrees of susceptibility to a specific disease or diseases. There is also the possibility that there are other undefined genes which are linked to the HLA specificities shown to be associated with malignant diseases that in some way, not understood at this time, predispose an individual to that disease.

6. SUMMARY AND IMPLICATIONS FOR THE FUTURE

The early investigations aimed at determining whether HLA is associated with malignant diseases were by-and-large rather disappointing. However, as the quality of the antisera improved and more HLA specificities were defined, additional studies involving larger numbers of patients who were clinically defined in more detail have been forthcoming. Now it is known that certain HLA phenotypes are significantly associated with various malignant diseases. Although these results are promising it is disappointing that the association of malignant diseases wiht D/DR locus products have not been more extensive-ly evaluated. It is generally accepted that the D/DR locus is analogous to the I region of mouse where genes controlling immune responsiveness along with T and T as well as T and B cell interactions have been mapped. Therefore, one can anticipate that even stronger associations with certain D/DR locus products and malignant diseases will be found. In fact, many of the A and B specificities shown to be associated with malignant diseases thus far are in linkage disequilibrium with various D/DR locus genes.

The implication for the presence or absence of immune response genes is twofold. First, if indeed the immune response plays a role in warding off tumor cells or combating them once the tumor has taken hold then lack of genes directing this process in an individual would place that individual at an increased risk for developing a malignancy. Second, Purtilo[90] has presented the hypothesis that E-B virus can produce malignant lymphoma in immune deficient hosts. The X-linked lymphoproliferative syndrome is a case in point where affected individuals are immune deficient to EB virus and have an increased susceptibility to lymphoma[105]. Although the disease susceptibility gene for this particular disorder is not on chromosome 6 one can imagine how lack of the appropriate immune response genes at the MHC could predispose an individual to EB and subsequently lymphoma.

Based on the data collected thus far one can predict future experimentation will reveal HLA to be a most useful clinical test in assessing malignant diseases on a number of fronts. No doubt HLA will be a valuable aid in predicting individuals susceptible to a given type of malignancy. Determining individuals at risk early in life for a given type of malignancy offers exciting challenges to society and physicians for preventing the disease. For example, suppose an individual at birth could be determined to be genetically suscep-tible to lung cancer. One would hope that with this knowledge, the parents would be extremely aggressive in attempting to prevent the child from smok-ing while the physician(s) attending the individual throughout life would want to continuously monitor for signs of the disease. Moreover, as knowledge increases as to environmental insults which can initiate malignant diseases there will be the need to assure that exposure to these insults by individuals with a given genetic susceptibility for malignant disease(s) be minimized. The data in Table 4 suggest that HLA can be used to subgroup malignant diseases. This particularly appears to be the case for Hodgkin's disease. Additional well designed studies should extend the usefulness of HLA in this area as has been the case for other diseases such as rheumatoid arthritic disorders and autoimmune endocrinopathies[15]. However, once an individual is affected with a given malignant disease and a firm diagnosis of subgroup made HLA again will most likely be found useful in selecting treatment modality and establishing prognosis. We believe the fact that a group of affected individuals given the same course of treatment respond differently is attributed to differences in their genetic constitution. Viewed from another angle, there are other non-malignant diseases where HLA has been shown associated with response to treatment which could also be inter-preted to be due to differences in genetic constitution of the patients. For example, Perris et al. [106] have observed in 82 patients with affective disorders a significantly higher frequency of A3 in those patients on lithium therapy who did not relapse. Smeraldi et al. [107] found B5 was increased among non-relapsed Italian affective disorder patients on long term lithium therapy. It will be extremely important to continue these types of studies with malignant and other diseases. An ideal situation would be to study those patients on cooperative group protocols where the association of HLA with different modalities of treatment could be assessed. The immediate future should be quite exciting as the validity of the aforementioned possibilities are determined by additional studies using carefully defined large patient populations as well as families where more than one individual is affected. The concepts and tools that hopefully will arise from these studies should provide the clinician greater potential to predict, diagnose and treat malignant diseases.

ACKNOWLEDGEMENTS

We would like to express appreciation to Dr. Rodney Go for his advice and criticism and Ms. Susan Snead and Ms. Mary Estock for secretarial assistance. Supported in part by grants CA15338 and CA18609 from the National Cancer Institute and the Diabetes Trust Fund.

REFERENCES

1. Aird I, Bental HH, Roberts JAF: The relationship between cancer of the stomach and the ABO blood groups. Br Med J 1:799–801, 1953.
2. Mourant AE, Kopec AC, Domaniewska-Sobczak K: A study of associations of diseases with blood groups and other polymorphisms. In: Blood groups and diseases, Oxford Monographs on Medical Genetics. Oxford: Oxford University Press, 1978.
3. Jick H, Slone D, Westerholm B, Inman WHW, Vessey MP, Shapiro S, Lewis GP, Worcester J: Venous thromboembolic disease and ABO blood type. Lancet i:539–542, 1969.
4. Jensen CO: Experimentelle unterstukungen über Krebs bei Maüsen. Centralbl Bakteriol Parasiteuk Infektiouskrankg 34:28–34, 1903.
5. Gorer PA The genetic and antigenic basis of tumor transplantation. J Pathol Bacteriol 44:691–697, 1937.
6. Medawar PB: The behaviour and fate of skin autografts and skin homografts in rabbits. J Anat 78:176–200, 1944.
7. Snell GC: Methods for the study of histocompatibility genes. J Genet 49:87–108, 1948.
8. Klein J: Biology of the mouse histocompatibility-2 complex. New York: Springer-Verlag, 1975.
9. Dausset J: Leuco-agglutinins. IV Leuco-agglutinins and blood transfusion. Vox Sang 4:190-198, 1954.
10. Gross L: Oncogenic viruses, 2nd edn. Oxford: Pergamon, 1970.

11. Lilly F, Boyse EA, Old LJ: Genetic basis of susceptibility to viral leukomogenesis. Lancet II:1207–1209, 1964.
12. Lilly F: The histocompatibility-2 locus and susceptibility to tumor induction. Nat Cancer Inst Monogr 22:631–641, 1966.
13. Klein J: The major histocompatibility complex of the mouse. Science 203:516-521, 1979.
14. Snell G, Daussett J, Nathenson S: Histocompatibility, New York, Academic Press, 1976.
15. Ryder LP, Andersen E, Svejgaard A (eds): HLA and disease registry, 3rd Report. Copenhagen: Munksgaard, 1979.
16. Bach FH and van Rood JJ: The major histocompatibility complex—genetics and biology. New Engl J Med 295:806–813, 1976.
17. Bodmer W (ed): The HLA system. Br Med Bull 34:3, 1978.
18. Lamm LR, Friedrich U, Petersen GB, Jørgensen J, Nielsen J, Therkelsen AJ, Kissmeyer-Nielsen F: Assignment of the major histocompatibility complex to chromosome No. 6 in a family with a pericentric inversion. Hum Hered 24:273–284, 1974.
19. Third International Workshop on Human Gene Mapping. Birth Defects: Original Article Series, Vol XII, No. 7, 1975.
20. Bakker E, Pearson PL, Khan PM, Schreuder GMTh, Madan K: Orientation of major histocompatibility (MHC) genes relative to the centromere of human chromosome 6. Clin Genet 15:198–202, 1979.
21. Yang SY, Levine LS, Zachmann M, New MI, Prader A, Oberfield SE, O'Neill GJ, Pollack MS, Dupont B: Mapping of the 21 hydroxylase deficiency gene within the HLA linkage group. Transpl Proc X(4):753–755, 1978.
22. O'Neill GJ, Yang SY, Dupont B: Chido and Rodgers blood groups: relationship to C4 and HLA. Transpl Proc X(4):749–751, 1978.
23. Gazit E, Terhorst C, Mahoney R, Yunis E: Alloantigens of the human T (HT) genetic region of the HLA linkage group. Human Immunol 2:97–108, 1980.
24. Gazit E, Terhorst C, Yunis E: The human 'T' genetic region of the HLA linkage group is a polymorphism detected on lectin-activated lymphocytes. Nature 284:275–277, 1980.
25. Terasaki PI, McClelland JD: Microdroplet assay of human serum cytotoxins. Nature 204:998–1000, 1964.
26. Terasaki PI, Bernoco D, Park MS, Ozturk G, Iwaki Y: Microdroplet testing for HLA-A, -B, -C and -D antigens, The Philip Levine Award Lecture. Am J Clin Histopath 69:103–120, 1978.
27. Mittal KK: Standardization of the HLA typing method and reagents. Vox Sang 34:58-63, 1978.
28. Amos DB, Bashir H, Boyle W, MacQueen M, Tiïlikainen: A simple microcytotoxicity test. Transpl 7:220–222, 1970.
29. Leeuwen AV, Schuit HRE, Rood JJV: Typing for MLC (LD) II. The selection of non-stimulator cells by MLC inhibition tests using SD identical stimulator cells (MISTS) and fluorescent antibody studies. Transpl Proc 5:1539–1542, 1973.
30. Bach FH, Hirschhorn K: Lymphocyte interaction: a potential histocompatibility test *in vitro*. Science 143:813–814, 1964.
31. Sheehy MJ, Sondel PM, Bach ML, Wank R, Bach FH: HL-A LD (lymphocyte defined) typing: a rapid assay with primed lymphocytes. Science 188:1308–1310, 1975.
32. Balner H: Are D and DR antigens identical? A review of available data for man and the rhesus monkey. Transpl Proc 11:657–664, 1979.
33. Terasaki PI (ed): Predata Report of the World Health Organization Terminology Committee. 8th Int. Histocompatibility Workshop, 1980.
34. Rood JJV (ed): Histocompatibility testing. Copenhagen: Munksgaard, 1965.
35. Curtoni ES, Mattiuz PL, Tosi RM (eds): Histocompatibility testing. Copenhagen: Munksgaard, 1967.

36. Terasaki PI (ed): Histocompatibility testing. Copenhagen: Munksgaard, 1970.
37. Dausset J, Colombani J (eds): Histocompatibility testing: Copenhagen: Munksgaard, 1973.
38. Kissmeyer-Nielsen E (ed): Histocompatibility testing. Copenhagen: Munksgaard, 1975.
39. Bodmer WF, Batchelor JR, Bodmer JG, Festenstein H, Morris PJ (eds): Histocompatibility testing. Copenhagen: Munksgaard, 1978.
40. Terasaki PI (ed): Predata analysis. 8th Int Histocompatibility Workshop, 1980.
41. Armitage P: Statistical methods in medical research. New York: John Wiley, 1971.
42. Svejgaard A, Jersild C, Nielsen L, Stuab, Bodmer WF: HL-A antigens and disease. Statistical and genetical considerations. Tissue Antigens 4:95–105, 1974.
43. Woolf B: On estimating the relationship between blood group and disease. Ann Hum Genet 19:251–253, 1955.
44. Reitnauer PJ, Roseman JM, Barger BO, Murphy CC, Kirk KK, Acton RT: HLA associations with insulin-dependent diabetes mellitus in a sample of the American black population. Tissue Antigens (in press).
45. Murphy CC, Acton RT, Barger BO, Roseman JM, Go RCP: Genetics of diabetes mellitus: I. Evidence from linkage analysis of IDDM to HLA within multiply affected families suggests a dominant mode of inheritance of susceptibility. J Clin Invest (submitted for publication).
46. Murphy GP, Cohen E, Fitzpatrick JE, Pressman D (eds): HLA and malignancy. Progress in Clinical and Biological Research, Vol 16. New York: Alan R Liss, 1977.
47. Terasaki PI, Perdue ST, Mickey MR: HLA frequencies in cancer: a second study. In: Genetics of human cancer, Mulvihill JJ, Miller RW, Fraumeni JF, Jr. (eds). New York: Raven Press, 1977, pp 321–327.
48. Harris R, Lawler SD, Oliver RTD: The HLA system in acute leukaemia and Hodgkin's disease. Br Med Bull 34:301–304, 1978.
49. Hammond MG, Appadoo B, Brain P: HLA and cancer in South African Indians. Tissue Antigens 14:296–302, 1979.
50. Jing J, Louie E, Henderson BE, Terasaki P: Histocompatibility leukocyte antigen patterns in nasopharyngeal carcinoma cases. Natl Cancer Inst Monogr 47:153–156, 1977.
51. Simons MJ, Wee GB, Goh EH, Chan SH, Shanmugaratnam K, Day NE, de-Thé GB: Immunogenetic aspects of nasopharyngeal carcinoma. IV. Increased risk in Chinese of nasopharyngeal carcinoma associated with Chinese-related HLA profile (A2, Singapore 2). J Natl Cancer Inst 57:977–980, 1976.
52. Simons MJ, Wee GB, Day NE, Morris PJ, Shanmugaratnam K, de-Thé GB: Immunogenetic aspects of nasopharyngeal carcinoma: I. Differences in HL-A antigen profiles between patients and control groups. Int J Cancer 13:122–134, 1974.
53. Payne R, Radvany R, Grumet C: A new second locus HL-A antigen in linkage disequilibrium with HL-A2 in Cantonese Chinese. Tissue Antigens 5:69–71, 1975.
54. Bertrams J, Thraenhart O, Feldmann U, Kuwert E: HL-A antigens in carcinoma of the breast, ovarium, cervix and endometrium: possible association of haplotype HL-A10-W18 with carcinoma of the breast. Z Krebsforsch 83:219–222, 1975.
55. Twomey PL, Rogentine GN, Chretien PB: Lymphocyte function and HL-A antigen frequency in gynecologic squamous cancer. Int Surg 59:468–472, 1974.
56. De Wolf WC, Lange PH, Einarson ME, Yunis EJ: HLA and testicular cancer. Nature 277:216–217, 1979.
57. Carr BI, Bach FH: Possible association between HLA-AW24 and metastatic testicular germ-cell tumours. Lancet i:1346–1347, 1979.
58. Tsuji K, Ito M, Inouye H, Nose Y, Hoshino K, Shibuya K, Tajima T, Mitomi T: HLA antigens and Ia antibody in the gastric cancer patient. In: HLA and malignancy, Murphy GP, Chan E, Fitzpatrick JE, Pressman D (eds). New York: Alan R Liss, 1977, pp 29–37.

59. Dick FR, Fortuny I, Theologides A, Greally J, Wood N, Yunis EJ: HL-A and lymphoid tumors. Cancer Res 32: 2608–2611, 1972.
60. Dickson A: A raised incidence of HL-A2 plus HL-A9 and other anomalies of the HL-A antigens of patients with leukaemia. Acta Haemat 54:143–151, 1975.
61. Degos L, Drolet Y, Dausset J: HL-A antigens in chronic myeloid leukemia (CML) and chronic lymphoid leukemia (CLL). Transpl Proc 3:1309–1310, 1971.
62. Hester JP, Rossen R, Trujillo J, McCrodie KB, Freireich EJ: Frequency of HLA antigens in chronic myelocytic leukemia. South Med J 70:691–693, 1977.
63. Amiel JL: Study of the leukocyte phenotypes in Hodgkin's disease. In: Histocompatibility testing 1967, Curtoni ES, Mattiuz PL, Tosi RM (eds). Baltimore: Williams & Wilkins, 1967, pp 79–81.
64. Björkholm M, Holm G, Johansson B, Millstedt H, Möller E: A prospective study of HL-A antigen phenotype and lymphocyte abnormalities in Hodgkin's disease. Tissue Antigens 6:247–256, 1975.
65. Forbes JF, Morris PJ: Analysis of HL-A antigens in patients with Hodgkin's disease and their families. J Clin Invest 51:1156–1162, 1972.
66. Graff KS, Simon RM, Yankee RA, DeVita VT, Rogentine GN: HL-A antigens in Hodgkin's disease: histopathalogic and clinical correlations. J Natl Cancer Inst 52:1087–1090, 1974.
67. Greene MH, McKeen EA, Li FP, Blattner WA, Fraumeni JF, Jr: HLA antigens in familial Hodgkin's disease. Int J Cancer 23:777–780, 1979.
68. Hornmark-Stenstam B, Landberg T, Löw B: HLA antigens in Hodgkin's disease of very long survival. Oncology 17:283–288, 1978.
69. Kuntz BME, Schmidt GD, Scholz S, Albert ED: HLA-antigens and hypernephroma. Tissue Antigens 12:407–408, 1978.
70. Forbes JF, Morris PJ: Transplantation antigens and malignant lymphomas in man: follicular lymphoma, reticulum cell sarcoma and lymphosarcoma. Tissue Antigens 1:265–269, 1971.
71. Bertrams J, Schildberg P, Höpping W, Böhme U, Albert E: HL-A antigens in retinoblastoma. Tissue Antigens 3:78–87, 1973.
72. Tarpley L, Chretien PB, Rogentine GN, Jr, Twomey PL, Dellon AL: Histocompatibility antigens and solid malignant neoplasms. Arch Surg 110:269–271, 1975.
73. Abrahámová J, Májský A, Koutecký J: HLA systém u Wilmsova nádoru a nauroblastomu. Cesk Pediat 34:268–270, 1979.
74. Rogentine GN, Trapani RJ, Yankee RA, Henderson ES: HL-A antigens and acute lymphocytic leukemia. The nature of the HL-A2 association. Tissue Antigens 3:470–476, 1973.
75. Lawler SD, Klouda PT, Smith PG, Till MM, Hardisty RM: Survival and the HL-A system in acute lymphoblastic leukaemia. Br Med J 1:547–548, 1974.
76. Klouda PT, Lawler SD, Till MM, Hardisty RM: Acute lymphoblastic leukaemia and HL-A: a prospective study. Tissue Antigens 4:262–265, 1974.
77. Cohen E, Singal DP, Khurana U, Gregory SG, Cox C, Sinks L, Henderson E, Fitzpatrick JE, Higby D: HLA-A9 and survival in acute lymphocytic leukemia and myelocytic leukemia. In: HLA and malignancy, Vol 16, Murphy GP (ed.). New York. Alan R Liss, 1977, pp 65–70.
78. Parrish EJ, Heise ER, Cooper MR: HLA association with acute myelogenous leukemia. In: HLA and malignancy, Murphy GP, Cohen E, Fitzpatrick JE, Pressman D (eds). New York: Alan R Liss 1977, pp 81–89.
79. Harris R, Zuhrie SR, Taylor GM, Freeman CB, Wentzel J, Geary C, MacIver JE: Influence of HLA, ABO and RH(D) on survival after remission in acute myelogenous leukaemia. Lancet i:653, 1977.

80. Heise E, Parrish E, Cooper R: HLA-B17 and the HLA-A1, B17 Haplotype in acute myelogenous leukemia. Tissue Antigens 14:98–104, 1979.
81. Patel R, Habal MB, Wilson RE, Birtch AG, Moore FD: Histocompatibility (HL-A) antigens and cancer of the breast. Am J Surg 124:31–34, 1972.
82. Falk J, Osoba D: The HLA system and survival in malignant disease: Hodgkin's disease and carcinoma of the breast. In: HLA and malignancy, Murphy GP, Cohen E, Fitzpatrick JE, Pressman D (eds). New York: Alan R Liss, 1977, pp 205–216.
83. Dellon AL, Rogentine GN, Jr, Chretien PB: Prolonged survival in bronchogenic carcinoma associated with HL-A antigens W-19 and HL-A5: a preliminary report. J Natl Cancer Inst 54:1283–1286, 1975.
84. Falk JA, Osoba D: The association of the human histocompatibility system with Hodgkin's disease. J Immunogenet 1:53–61, 1974.
85. Hansen JA, Young CW, Whitsett C, Case DC, Jersild C, Good RA, Dupont B: HLA and MLC typing in patients with Hodgkin's disease. In: HLA and malignancy, Murphy GP, Cohen E, Fitzpatrick JE, Pressman D (eds). New York: Alan R Liss, 1977, pp 217–227.
86. Clark DA, Necheles T, Nathanson L: Apparent HL-A5 deficiency in malignant melanoma. Transplantation 15:326–328, 1973.
87. Gerkins VR, Ting A, Menck HT, Casagrande JT, Terasaki PI, Pike MC, Henderson BE: Brief communication: HL-A heterozygosity as a genetic marker of long-term survival. J Natl Cancer Inst 52:1909–1011, 1974.
88. Miller AB: Familial risk of cancer. CMA J 121:505–507, 1979.
89. Lynch HT, Terasaki PI, Guirgio HA, Sherard BD, Androsh KL, Harris RE, King MC, Petrakis N, Lynch J, Maloney K, Rankin K, Lynch PM, Elston R, Mulcahy G, Platt R: In: HLA and malignancy, Murphy GP, Cohen E, Fitzpatrick JE, Pressman D (eds). New York: Alan R Liss, 1977, pp 149–162.
90. Purtillo DT: Epstein-Barr virus-induced oncogenesis in immune deficient individuals. Lancet ii:300–303, 1980.
91. Helenius A, Morein B, Fries E, Senious K, Robinson, VS, Terhorst C, Strominger JL: Human (HLA-A and HLA-B) and murine (H-2K and H-2D) histocompatibility antigens are cell surface receptors for Semliki Forest virus. Proc Nat Acad Sci 75:3846–3850, 1980.
92. Azocar J, Essex M: Incorporation of HLA antigens into the envelope of RNA tumor viruses grown in human cells. Cancer Res 39:3388–3391, 1979.
93. Henley S, Acton RT, Wise KS: Effect of productive murine leukemia virus (MuLV) infection on antigen expression of EL4 lymphoblastoid cells. Unpublished observation.
94. Zinkernagel RM: Associations between major histocompatibility antigens and susceptibility to disease. Ann Rev Microbiol 33:201–213, 1979.
95. Sasazuki T, Kohno Y, Iwamotos I, Tanimura M, Nato S: Association between an HLA haplotype and low responsiveness to tetanus toxoid in man. Nature 272:359–361, 1978.
96. deVries RRP, Kreftenberg HG, Loggen HG, van Rood JJ: In vitro immune responsiveness to vaccinia virus and HLA. New Engl J Med 297:692–696, 1977.
97. Marsh DG, Chase GA, Freidhoff LR, Meyers DA, Bias WB: Association of HLA antigens and total serum immunoglobulin E level with allergic response and failure to respond to ragweed allergen Ra3. Proc Natl Acad Sci 76:2903–2907, 1979.
98. Sybesma JPHB, Holtzer JD, Borst-Eilers E, Moes M, Zeger BJM: Antibody response in Hodgkin's disease and other lymphomas related to HLA antigens, Immunoglobulin levels and therapy. Vox Sang 25:254–262, 1973.
99. Schacter B, Braun WE, Bukowski R, Deodhor S: HLA-B7 association with low spontaneous cell-mediated cytotoxicity (Sp-CMC) to renal cell carcinoma cell lines. Transpl Proc 9:1849–1851, 1977.
100. Osoba D, Falk J: HLA-B8 phenotype associated with an increased mixed leukocyte reaction. Immunogenetics 6:425–432, 1978.

101. Goulmy E, Termijtelan BA, Bradley BA, van Rood JJ: Y-antigen killing by T-cells of women is restricted by HLA. Nature 266:544–545, 1977.
102. Dickmeiss E, Soeberg B, Svejgaard A: Human cell-mediated cytotoxicity against modified target cells is restricted by HLA. Nature 270:526–528, 1977.
103. McMichael, AJ, Ting A, Zweerink HJ, Aakones BA: HLA restriction of cell-mediated lysis of influenza virus-infected human cells. Nature 270:524–526, 1977.
104. Rickinson AB, Wallace LE, Epstein MA: HLA-restricted T-cell recognition of Epstein-Barr virus-infected B cells. Nature 283:865–868, 1980.
105. Hamilton JK, Paquin LA, Sullivan JL, Maurer HS, Cruzi FG, Provisor Aj, Steuber CP, Hawkins E, Yawn D, Coonet JA, Clausen K, Finkelstein GZ, Landing B, Grunnet M, Purtilo DT: X-linked lymphoproliferative syndrome registry report. J Pediat 96:669–673, 1980.
106. Perris C, Strandman E, Wahlby L: HLA antigens and the response to prophylatic lithium. Neuropsychobiology 5:114–118, 1979.
107. Smeraldi E, Negri F, Melica AM, Scorza-Smeraldi R, Fabio G, Bonara P, Bellodi L, Sacchetti E, Sabbadini-Villa MG, Cazzullo CL and Zanussi C: HLA typing and effective disorders: a study in the Italian population. Neuropsychobiology 4:344–352, 1978.

3. Interferon and Cancer

W. ROBERT FLEISCHMANN JR. and SAMUEL BARON

In 1957, Isaacs and Lindenmann found that pieces of chick chorioallantoic membranes infected with heat inactivated influenza virus released a substance into the surrounding medium which could make other pieces of chick membrane resistant to virus[1]. They called this unique substance interferon. Similar antiviral activities were rapidly discovered in a great many vertebrates, including man[2]. These substances have been classified as interferons because they all are cellular proteins which act by inducing antiviral resistance in responding vertebrate cells. Now, we know that interferon, even within a single species, is not limited to a single molecular type but that several disparate molecules exhibit antiviral activity. For a number of years, the emphasis of interferon reserach was directed primarily toward its antiviral functions and it is only relatively recently that the immunoregulatory and antitumor activities of the interferons have come under intensive study. This paper will review some of the salient features of the antiviral and antitumor activities of the interferon system and will draw attention to the exciting prospects of employing interferons as agents for tumor management.

1. MULTIPLE TYPES OF INTERFERON

Three antigenically distinct molecular species of interferon have been recognized in the human system. These interferons can be identified as fibroblast, leukocyte, and immune interferons. They all share several important biological properties. They are normally in a repressed state and *de novo* RNA and protein synthesis are required for their production [3–11]. The interferons have antiviral activity against a broad spectrum of viruses[2]. The interferons do not directly inactivate viruses, rather their effect is a cell-mediated process involving the activation of responding cells to an antiviral state. This activation requires *de novo* RNA and protein synthesis[12–15]. So far as is known,

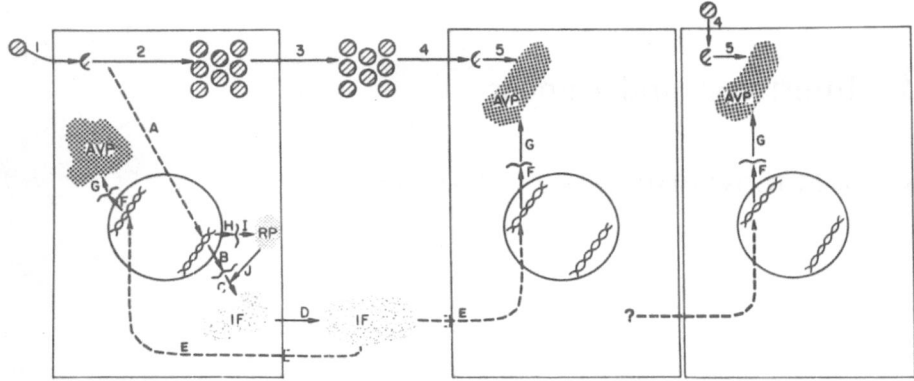

Figure 1. Cellular events of the induction and action of interferon (IF). Virus comes in contact with cell (1) and penetrates the cell membrane. The virus then releases its genetic material and replication of the virus occurs (2). The new virus leaves the cell (3) and enters the fluid around the first cell, and some of the replicated virus infects a second cell (4) where the release of the genetic material again takes place (5). During the early stages of infection of the first cell, some event (viral nucleic acid?) stimulates a gene in the DNA which contains the stored genetic information for interferon (A). This leads to the production of mRNA for interferon (IF), which leaves (B) the nucleus and is translated by the cell's ribosomes (C) into the interferon protein. Several events now occur more or less simultaneously. Some interferon is secreted by the first cell (D) and enters the surrounding fluid where it comes into contact with and stimulates the second cell (E). The second cell is thereby induced to produce a new mRNA (F), which is translated to a new protein(s) (G), the antiviral protein (AVP). This in turn modifies the cell's protein-synthesizing machinery, such that cell mRNA can be translated into protein, but viral RNA is poorly bound or translated or both. In the first cell, processes E, F, and G may also operate to form AVP and thereby reduce the virus yield in the first cell. Shortly after interferon is synthesized in the first cell, another mRNA (H) is believed to be synthesized from the cell's DNA and is translated (I) into a regulatory protein (RP) (hypothesized). This RP combines with the mRNA for IF, thereby preventing the further synthesis of more IF (J). There is recent evidence that the antiviral state may be directly transferred between adjacent cells (from second to third cell at right) by the passage of an unknown (?) inducer of the AVP (from Baron S, *ASM News* 45:358–366, 1979, with permission).

all interferons possess antiviral activity, immunoregulatory activity, and anti-tumor activity, though there are degrees of difference. For example, immune interferon has been shown to more slowly activate the antiviral response than fibroblast and leukocyte interferons, possibly by a unique mechanism involv-ing the synthesis of an intermediary protein before the antiviral state is induced [16, 17]. Immune interferon is a more potent immunosuppressive agent [18] and a more potent antitumor agent than fibroblast or leukocyte interferon [19–21]. Further, it appears that there is no cross resistance of cells to the cell growth inhibitory ability of immune interferon and fibroblast interferon [22].

Each of these interferons can be induced both *in vitro* and *in vivo*. Fibroblast interferon is the predominant interferon species produced when fibroblasts

and epithelial cells are exposed to viruses, viral RNAs, or synthetic polyribo-
nucleotides such as poly (rI:rC) (Figure 1, left panel)[23–28]. Leukocyte
interferon is the predominant species produced by leukocytes and lymphoblastoid cells upon exposure to viruses and foreign or tumor cells[29–35].
Immune interferon is produced along with other lymphokines by lymphocytes
exposed to T-cell mitogens such as phytohemagglutinin-P, concanavalin A,
and staphylococcal enterotoxin A; it is also produced by lymphocytes which
have been sensitized and then challenged with specific antigens such as old
tuberculin[36–40]. Immune interferon can also be induced *in vitro* with the
enzyme galactose oxidase[41].

Fibroblast and leukocyte interferons share several biochemical properties as
well as some common inducers. However, they have been shown to be coded
by different genes and possess different N-terminal amino acids[42–45].
Immune interferon differs from fibroblast and leukocyte interferon in several
important biochemical properties (for example pH and heat stability)[46–48].
Further, antibodies against each species of interferon have been raised and the
three interferons have been shown not to cross react immunologically[49–54].

2. THE ANTIVIRAL ACTION OF INTERFERON

One of the easiest changes to quantitate and one of the most accurate in
reflecting the establishment of antiviral resistance is still that of a reduction in
virus yield by cells treated with interferon and challenged with virus (Figure 1, center panel). Exposure of cells to fibroblast interferon for 1–2 minutes
is sufficient to initiate the events involved in the establishment of the antiviral state[55, 56]. Cells possessing this antiviral state can be characterized by
both a reduced virus yield per cell and a lengthened or delayed viral infectious cycle[57–67]. Virtually all viruses are sensitive to interferon though
they each have their unique position in a spectrum extending from highly
sensitive to relatively resistant to interferon[68]. Similarly, virtually all body
cells can be protected by interferon. Tissue culture studies demonstrate that
the exposure of cells to interferon initiates a number of molecular changes
ranging from membrane effects to the synthesis of enzymes involved in
regulating host cell protein synthesis[69–88]. None of these changes has been
unambiguously correlated with the antiviral properties of the host, but some
of these molecular changes may relate to the antiviral, immunoregulatory, or
anticellular effects of interferon.

Establishment of the antiviral state does not always insure survival of the
cell, however. Some cytotoxic viruses still kill protected cells despite being
unable to replicate. Thus, the term protective is a relative term which some-

times relates more to the inhibition of viral replication and subsequent dampening of an infection than it does to individual cell survival.

Interferon has been suggested to play a major role in the normal recovery of patients from many viral infections [2, 89–93]. This suggestion is supported by *in vivo* experimental studies. Interferon and its inducers have been shown to be protective against influenza and the common cold when it is administered prophylatically [94–96]. Further, recent clinical trials have demonstrated that interferon is useful therapeutically in the treatment of hepatitis and herpesviruses [97–108]. In addition, studies in monkeys and other animals show that interferon treatment potentiates the efficacy of rabies vaccine in the prevention of rabies [109].

3. MODIFIERS OF THE ANTIVIRAL ACTION OF INTERFERON

Three features of the interferon system extend the antiviral protective effect beyond that which would normally be expected. First, pretreatment of cells with a low level of interferon establishes a condition which allows a more rapid and quantitatively greater level of protection to develop after addition of a second higher level of interferon than if the higher level of interferon was administered without interferon pretreatment (Figure 2) [110, 111]. This feature of the interferon system (priming of interferon action) might play a role

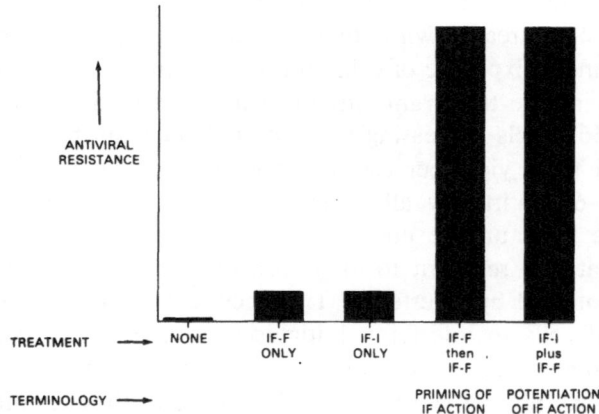

Figure 2. Enhancers of the antiviral action of interferon. Cells treated with identical amounts of fibroblast interferon (IF-F) or immune interferon (IF-I) develop approximately equal amounts of antiviral resistance. Priming of interferon action: sequential treatments of cells with either immune interferon or fibroblast interferon (shown here as IF-F then IF-F) cause a markedly greater level of antiviral resistance to develop. Potentiation of interferon action: combined treatment of cells with both immune interferon and fibroblast interferon (IF-I plus IF-F) also causes a markedly greater level of antiviral resistance to develop.

early in the infectious process when localized virus production and localized interferon production may be cyclic. Outlying cells surrounding a focus of infection might be 'primed' to respond more strongly to additional interferon by their repeated exposure to ever more concentrated interferon as virus replication spreads from the initial focus. Primed, hyperresponsive cells might then play an important role in limiting the infection.

Second, cells can transfer viral resistance from cell to cell (Figure 1, right panel)[112, 113]. In this process, cells which respond to interferon treatment transfer their ability to develop the antiviral state to adjacent non-responding cells. This was originally demonstrated as a cross species transfer of viral resistance from mouse to human cells. However, a more important biological ramification of the initial observation is that individual cells in a population vary in their sensitivities to interferon and the transfer process raises the level of viral resistance to that of the most interferon sensitive cells in the population [114]. Consequently, the transfer process greatly enhances the viral resistance of a tissue as a whole.

Third, a mixed preparation of immune and fibroblast interferon can potentiate the antiviral response of cells to interferon (Figure 2)[115]. The increased level of protection is 5- to 20-fold greater than that expected on the basis of the additive effects of the two interferons. Whatever the mechanism of potentiation, the local production of multiple types of interferon may also play a significant role in increasing the viral resistance of a tissue.

4. THE ANTITUMOR ACTIVITY OF INTERFERON

The discovery of the antitumor activity of interferon was a natural outgrowth of the interferon antiviral studies. In 1960, Atanasiu and Chany observed that interferon pretreatment of hamsters inhibited the development of polyoma virus tumors [116]. These studies were extended to show a general ability of interferon to inhibit tumor growth when a considerable number of other oncogenic virus tumors, chemically-induced tumors, radiation-induced tumors and spontaneous tumors were also shown to be sensitive to interferon treatment *in vivo* and *in vitro* in a variety of different animal systems (for recent review, see [117]).

The *in vivo* mechanism of the antitumor activity of interferon is not well understood, however, three components of the mechanism may have been identified by *in vitro* studies. First, interferon may have a direct anticellular effect. The anticellular effect is seen as an inhibition of the growth of many proliferating cells and has been demonstrated for transformed cells, normal cells, and primary cultures *in vitro* [118–124]. As is the case with many antitumor drugs, it is unclear to what extent the anticellular activity of interferon differentiates between normal and tumor cells. The susceptibility of cell growth to inhibition by interferon varies substantially. For example, the growth of normal mouse embryo cells in culture is inhibited modestly and only after 7 days exposure to interferon; some transformed cells are inhibited strongly and rapidly by interferon; other transformed cells are resistant to interferon; and, interferon-resistant cell clones can be selected from susceptible cell populations [125, 126]. Interestingly, cells resistant to fibroblast interferon may still be sensitive to immune interferon [22].

The first interferon preparations were crude preparations and there was considerable debate as to whether the anticellular activity resided with the interferon molecule or in a separate molecule contaminating the interferon preparation. The use of highly purified interferon preparations demonstrated that the anticellular component of the antitumor activity copurifies with interferon and presumably is interferon [127–129].

Available evidence suggests that the primary site of interferon action on cell growth may be on events which occur early in the cell cycle [130–132]. The *in vivo* observation that some patients under treatment with interferon suffer some reversible bone marrow depression confirms the *in vitro* suggestion that the discriminatin of the anticellular effects of interferon against normal and tumor cells is not absolute [133, 134]. However, these effects are observed only with high dosages of interferon.

The second component of interferon's antitumor mechanism involves the activation of a number of elements in the host's system. Interferon, particularly immune interferon, has been shown to be a potent regulator of the humoral immune response (Figure 3) [18, 38, 135–140]. Treatment of mouse spleen cells with interferon suppresses the *in vitro* antibody response and is believed to play a central role in immunoregulation of antibody synthesis. *In vitro* studies show that macrophages treated with interferon show an increased level of phagocytic activity [141–145]. Similarly, the *in vitro* specific cytotoxicity of sensitized lymphocytes increases with interferon treatment [87, 146, 147]. The activation of natural killer cells has also been demonstrated [148–151]. Further, interferon treatment protects normal cells but not tumor cells from natural killer cell activity [152]. These *in vitro* effects of interferon have been difficult to reconcile with some *in vivo* studies in the mouse which show that at least one presumed function of cell-mediated immunity, allograph rejection, is inhibited by interferon treatment [153–157]. On the other hand, Gresser and his colleagues inoculated mice with a clone of L1210 cells which were resistant to the anticellular and antiviral effects of interferon and found that interferon treatment still increased survival though not to the level observed when mice inoculated with interferon sensitive L1210 cells were treated with interferon [158]. Since interferon treatment was protective in the absence of a direct anticellular effect, the antitumor effect of

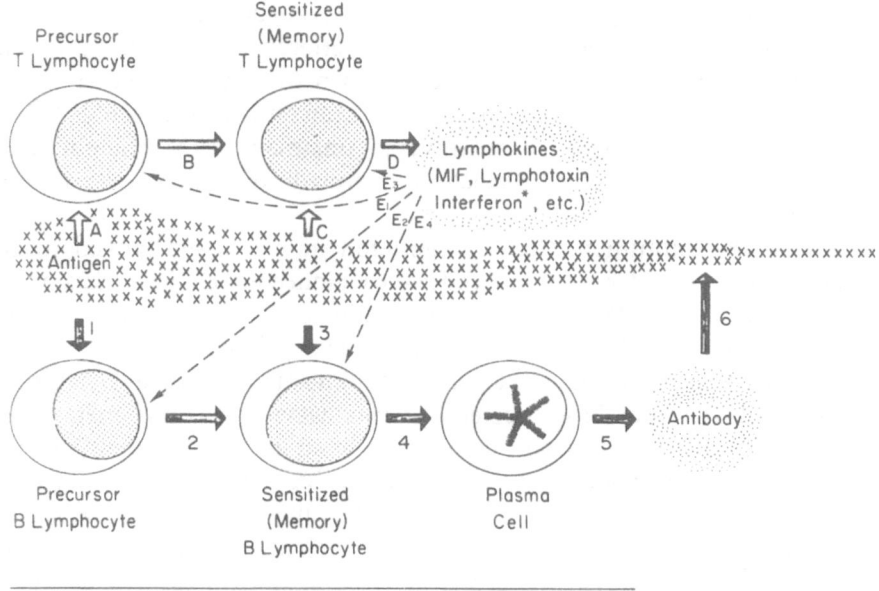

Time →

Figure 3. Cellular events in the induction and immunosuppressive action of immune interferons. Antigen comes into contact with a precursor T lymphocyte (A), which undergoes differentiation to a sensitized T lymphocyte (B). This cell, driven by antigen (C), may become a memory cell or it may release mediators known as lymphokines (D). Among the mediators produced by the T lymphocyte is antigen-type interferon. Antigen also reacts with a precursor B lymphocyte (1), which undergoes differentiation to a sensitized B lymphocyte (and memory B cell) (2). The sensitized B cell is further driven by antigen (3) to become a plasma cell (4), which is reponsible for most of the antibody (5) that is produced. This antibody reacts with the specific antigen (6). Both antigen- and virus-induced interferons are capable of suppressing precursor and sensitized T lymphocytes (E_1) and B lymphocytes (E_2). As differentiation progresses, in part as a result of continued antigen presence, it becomes progressively more difficult to inhibit lymphocyte function by interferons. Plasma cell production of antibody is resistant to inhibition by interferon. The macrophage is not included in the figure, but interferons may exert their immunosuppressive effects via a required macrophage function in the immune response. The diagrammatic scheme does not necessarily imply, therefore, a direct effect of the interferons on the lymphocytes (from Baron S, Dianzani F, Texas Rep Biol Med 35:1–10, 1977, with permission).

interferon must have been mediated by an enhancement of a host antitumor function, possibly through the stimulation of one or more elements of the host's cell-mediated immune system or through the modulation of the host's humoral immune system, described above. Thus, whatever the nature of the contribution of the host immune response to the interferon antitumor effect, interferon does enhance the host's ability to reject tumors probably by both a direct anticellular action on the tumor cells and by an indirect action mediated by the host.

Third, interferon strongly resembles certain polypeptide hormones. Thyrotropic hormone, chorionic gonadotropin, and interferon bind to the same cell receptor and interferon treatment has been shown to mimic hormone action in two other hormone systems which have been studied [159-163]. Some tumors have been shown to be sensitive to treatment with different hormones. Thus, interferon may regulate the growth of tumor cells by its hormone-like action.

Studies on the antitumor effect of interferon in man have proven to be most promising. Strander and his colleagues pioneered clinical trials with interferon. Beginning in 1971, osteosarcoma patients were treated with 3×10^6 units of partially purified leukocyte interferon daily for one month and three times weekly for one and one half years as adjuvant therapy [164]. After $2\frac{1}{2}$ years, 64% of the interferon treated patients were free from metastases compared to 30% in a concurrent, non-double blind control group of patients at other Swedish hospitals which did not receive interferon as adjuvant therapy [164]. Also, after $2\frac{1}{2}$ years, 73% of the interferon group were still living compared to 35% of the control group. They also observed the regression of juvenile laryngeal papilloma with interferon therapy. Following these and other promising clinical trials in Europe, clinical trials were begun in the United States [108]. Tumor regression has been reported in patients treated with leukocyte interferon who had advanced breast cancer, multiple myeloma, and non-Hodgkin's lymphoma [133, 134, 165, 166]. Leukocyte interferon therapy has been reported to have antileukemia effects in patients with three types of leukemia (ALL, AGL, and CGL) and to induce bone marrow remission in one patient with ALL [167, 168]. Further, fibroblast interferon treatment of individuals with malignant melanoma causes regression of the malignant melanoma lesions [169]. While these studies are in their preliminary and uncontrolled stages, the early results show promise for the future. Preliminary studies are also underway to evaluate and compare the potential antitumor efficacy of exogenous interferon therapy versus that of endogenous induction of interferon by a nuclease-resistant form of poly (rI : rC) and other inducers [170-172].

Several side effects of interferon therapy have been noted but most of the side effects are probably due to contaminating proteins in the interferon preparations [100, 133, 134, 173, 174]. Some of the initial trials employed interferon which was not highly purified. The most common side effects observed with these interferon preparations were temperature rise, myalgia, and chills. Less common side effects included malaise and lassitude. These side effects were shown to diminish in frequency and severity when more purified interferon preparations were employed. Some bone marrow suppression has been observed even with highly purified leukocyte interferon preparations and may reflect an activity attributable to the interferon molecule. The bone marrow suppression is reflected by decreases in leukocyte, platelet, and reticulocyte levels. It is readily reversible with the discontinuation of therapy, though it has been reported that this side effect has never caused complications and has never required the termination of therapy. Thus, while side effects do occur with highly purified interferon therapy, they appear to be mild and not contraindicating.

5. INTERFERON AND CANCER—PROSPECTS FOR THE FUTURE

Large scale controlled studies are underway or planned with malignant melanoma, non-Hodgkin's lymphoma, multiple myeloma, breast cancer, and leukemia. Presumeably these studies will also be expanded to include clinical trials with other types of cancers. Hopefully, these expanded studies will bring the promise of interferon as a potent antitumor substance to fruition.

Clinical trials and routine employment of interferon for tumor therapy are currently limited by the high cost and the availability of interferon. There are several principle reasons why interferon has been expensive to produce and difficult to purify. First, interferon is species specific and antigenic. Thus, interferon for human use must be produced by human cells employing expensive tissue culture methods. Second, the current method for the production of leukocyte interferon which has so far shown the most clinical promise, is dependent on blood donations. The blood cells which produce this leukocyte interferon do not readily grow *in vitro*, cannot be clonally expanded by tissue culture, and are exhausted in the interferon induction process. About 10^7 units of purified interferon can be produced for each blood donation. Since interferon therapy requires 0.5–3 million units per day, a blood donation ultimately provides only 3–20 days of therapy for a single patient.

Purification problems center on the low concentration of interferon molecules in even highly potent interferon preparations. Thus, it is difficult and costly to purify the interferon through the multistep procedures required to reduce contaminating proteins to acceptable levels.

There are several prospects for increasing the production of interferon in the future. Permanent tissue culture cell lines may be employed for the production of interferon. More streamlined methods of interferon purification may be developed and implemented. Further, exciting reports on the production of human proteins, including interferon, by bacterial cells through the use of genetic engineering techniques, raise the prospect of inexpensive, large scale production of interferons by this means [175, 176].

The clinical trials currently underway have employed only two types of interferon: leukocyte and fibroblast interferons. On the basis of *in vitro* evidence, it has been suggested that different types of cancer might respond best to different types of interferon [177]. Preliminary *in vivo* evidence with mice suggest that immune interferon is more effective an antitumor agent than fibroblast interferon against sarcoma MC-36 and osteogenic sarcoma [19, 20]. *In vitro* studies with human cells demonstrate that immune interferon has a 10–50 fold greater anticellular effect against WISH and HEp-2 cells than either fibroblast or leukocyte interferon [21]. Large scale methods for the production and purification of immune interferon have recently been described [178] and clinical trials employing immune interferon are expected to begin shortly. There is hope that the addition of immune interferon to the therapeutic armamentarium may increase either the level of the antitumor response or the number of tumors which respond to interferon therapy.

Another exciting possibility for the future is that one or more of the three mechanisms which increase the tissue antiviral activity (priming of interferon action, transfer of antiviral resistance, and potentiation of interferon action) may also play a role in increasing the antitumor activity of interferon. The contributions which priming of interferon action and the transfer of interferon's effects from one cell to another may make to the antitumor activity of interferon have not yet been evaluated. However, the possible potentiation of the antitumor activity of interferon by employing mixed preparations of interferon in antitumor therapy has been studied in the mouse system. *In vitro* studies with mouse melanoma tumor cells show that the direct anticellular activity of interferon can be potentiated by mixed fibroblast and immune interferon preparations [179]. Further, mouse studies employing the P388 tumor demonstrate that treatment with immune interferon preparations that were too dilute to be protective by themselves, potentiate the antitumor activity of fibroblast interferon when the two interferons are employed in combined therapy (Figure 4) [180]. Clinical trials to determine whether combined therapy with immune and leukocyte interferons can potentiate the antitumor activity of interferon in man are planned for the near future. It is hoped that these clinical trials will demonstrate an increase in the efficacy of interferon therapy so that interferon dosage levels and/or toxicity may be reduced, thereby conserving the interferons for broader patient application and possibly diminishing the side effects of interferon therapy.

In summary, clinical trials show that leukocyte and fibroblast interferons may be effective therapeutic agents for the management of several malignancies. These preliminary studies represent only the beginning stages of the investigation of interferon as an antitumor agent. Future experiments to determine ideal treatment dosages and schedules will maximize the antitumor activity of the interferons. The use of immune interferon, alone and in combination with leukocyte and/or fibroblast interferons holds the promise of increasing the antitumor activity still further. Finally, though the interferons are currently difficult to obtain in large quantity and expensive to produce

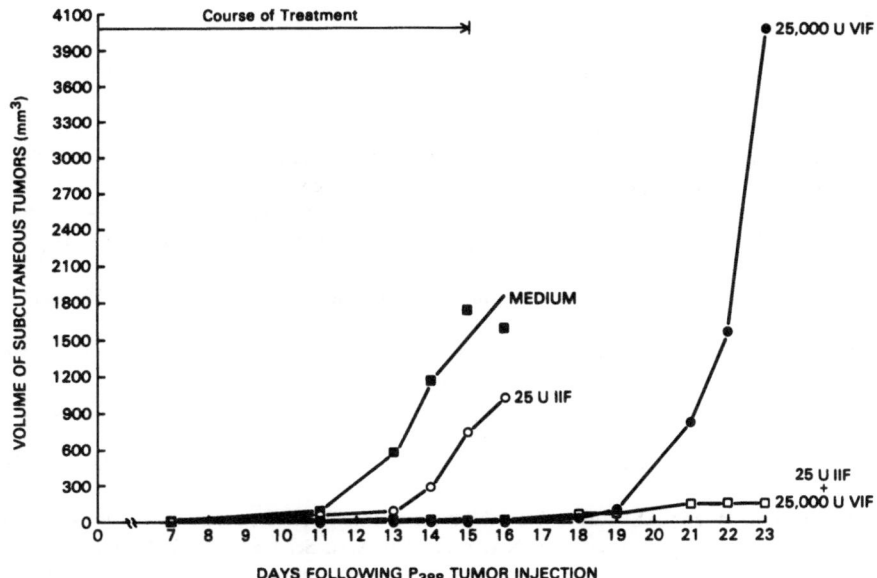

Figure 4. Potentiation of the antitumor effect of interferon. Four week old female DBA-2 mice were injected subcutaneously with 10^5 P388 cells. Interferon and mock interferon were injected at the approximate site of the tumor, beginning on the day of tumor injection and continuing for 15 days. Tumor volume was calculated by employing the standard formula for a cylinder ($r^2 1$). Mice were injected with mock interferon (medium, ■), immune interferon (IIF, ○), virus-type interferon (VIF, ●), or a combination of immune and virus-type interferon (IIF & VIF, ■).

and purify, the prospects are bright for the bulk production of virtually unlimited quantities of cheaper, more highly purified interferon within the next five to ten years. If the preliminary clinical trials can be confirmed and extended to other malignancies, and if the antitumor activity of interferon can be increased as suggested above, interferon may fulfill what is now its promise to be a broad spectrum, high therapeutic index, highly efficacious agent for the management of malignancies.

ACKNOWLEDGEMENTS

The authors wish to thank Ms Sue Ellen Gerchman, Mrs. Sophie Kozlek, Mr. Elliot Lefkowitz, and Dr. Thomas Albrecht for their assistance in assembling this manuscript.

REFERENCES

1. Isaacs A, Lindenmann, J: Virus interference. I. The interferon. Proc Roy Soc Lond B 147:258–267, 1957.
2. Isaacs A: Interferon. Adv Virus Res 10:1–35, 1963.
3. Heller E: Enhancement of Chickungunya virus replication and inhibition of interferon production by actinomycin D. Virology 21:652–656, 1963.
4. Wagner RR: Inhibition of interferon biosynthesis by actinomycin D. Nature 204:49–51.
5. Levy HB, Axelrod D, Baron S: Messenger RNA for interferon production. Proc Soc Exp Biol Med 118:384–385, 1965.
6. Burke DC, Walters S: A search for an interferon messenger RNA. Biochem J 101:25P–26P, 1966.
7. Buchan A, Burke DC: Inhibition of interferon production by puromycin and p-fluorophe-nylalanine. Abstr 6th Int Congr Biochem New York: 46, 1964.
8. Buchan A, Burke DC: Interferon production in chick-embryo cells. The effect of puromycin and p-fluorophenylalanine. Biochem J 98:530–536, 1966.
9. Ho M, Breinig MK: Metabolic determinants of interferon formation. Virology 25:331–339, 1965.
10. Wagner RR, Huang AS: Reversible inhibition of interferon synthesis by puromycin: evidence for an interferon-specific mRNA. Proc Natl Acad Sci USA 54:1112–1118, 1965.
11. Friedman RM: Interferon production and protein synthesis in chick cells. J Bacteriol 91:1224–1229, 1966.
12. Taylor J: Inhibition of interferon action by actinomycin D. Biochem Biophys Res Commun 14:447–451, 1964.
13. Lockart RZ Jr: The necessity for cellular RNA and protein synthesis for viral inhibition resulting from interferon. Biochem Biophys Res Commun 15:513–518, 1964.
14. Levine S: Effect of actinomycin D and puromycin dihydrochloride on action of interferon. Virology 24:586–588, 1964.
15. Friedman RM, Sonnabend JA: Inhibition of interferon action by p-fluorophenylalanine. Nature 203:366–367, 1964.
16. Dianzani F, Salter L, Fleischmann WR Jr, Zucca M: Immune interferon activates cells more slowly than does virus-induced interferon. Proc Soc Exp Biol Med 159:94–97, 1978.
17. Dianzani F, Zucca M, Scupham A, Georgiades JA: Immune and virus-induced interferons may activate cells by different derepressional mechanisms. Nature 283:400–402, 1980.
18. Sonnenfeld G, Mandel AD, Merigan TC: The immunosuppressive effect of Type II mouse interferon preparations on antibody production. Cell Immunol 34:193–206, 1977.
19. Crane JL Jr, Glasgow LA, Kern ER, Youngner JS: Inhibition of murine osteogenic sarcomas by treatment with Type I or Type II interferon. J Natl Cancer Inst 61:871–874, 1978.
20. Salvin SB, Youngner JS, Nishio J, Neta R: Tumor suppression by a lymphokine released into the circulation of mice with delayed hypersensitivity. J Natl Cancer Inst 55:1233–1236, 1975.
21. Blalock JE, Georgiades JA, Langford MP, Johnson HM: Purified human immune interferon has more potent anticellular activity than fibroblast or leukocyte interferon. Cell Immunol 49:390–394, 1980.
22. Falcoff E: Properties of mouse immune T interferon. In: Regulatory functions of interferon. Ann NY Acad Sci (in press).
23. Rotem Z, Cox RA, Isaacs A: Inhibition of virus multiplication by foreign nucleic acid. Nature 197:564-566, 1963.

24. Isaacs A, Cox RA, Rotem Z: Foreign nucleic acids as the stimulus to make interferon. Lancet 2:113–116, 1963.
25. Kleinschmidt WJ, Cline JC, Murphy EB: Interferon production induced by statolon. Proc Natl Acad Sci USA 52:741–744, 1964.
26. Field AK, Lampson GP, Tytell AA, Nemes MM, Hilleman MR: Inducers of interferon and host resistance. IV. Double stranded replicative form RNA (MS2-RF-RNA) from *E. coli* infected with MS2 coliphage. Proc Natl Acad Sci USA 58:2101–2108, 1967.
27. Field AK, Tytell AA, Lampson GP, Hilleman MR: Inducers of interferon and host resistance. II. Multistranded synthetic polynucleotide complexes. Proc Natl Acad Sci USA 58:1004–1010, 1967.
28. Havell EA, Hayes TG, Vilcek J: Synthesis of two distinct interferons by human fibroblasts. Virology 89:330–334, 1978.
29. Lakovic V, Borecky L: Interferon-like and antibody-like substances in mouse peritoneal cells stimulated by myxoviruses *in vivo*. Acta Virol 9:382, 1965.
30. Glasgow LA: Leukocytes and interferon in the host response to viral infections. I. Mouse leukocytes and leukocyte-produced interferon in vaccinia virus infection *in vitro*. J Exp Med 121:1001–1018, 1965.
31. Ash RJ, Bubel HC: Temporal relationship of interferon production and resistance to experimentally induced virus infection. J Infect Dis 116:1–7, 1966.
32. Lee SHS, van Rooyen CE, Ozere RL: Additional studies of interferon production by human leukemia leukocytes *in vitro*. Cancer Res 29:645–652, 1969.
33. Falcoff E, Fournier F, Chany C: Etude comparative des poids moleculaires de deux interferons humains produits *in vitro*. Ann Inst Pasteur (Paris) 111:241–248, 1966.
34. Strander H, Cantell K: Production of interferon by human leukocytes *in vitro*. Ann Med Exp Biol Fenn 44:265–273, 1966.
35. Havell EA, Yip YK, Vilcek J: Characteristics of human lymphoblastoid (Namalva) interferon. J Gen Virol 38:51–59, 1977.
36. Wheelock EF: Interferon-like virus-inhibitor induced in human leukocytes by phytohemagglutinin. Science 149:310–311, 1965.
37. Green JA, Cooperband SR, Kibrick S: Immune specific induction of interferon production in cultures of human blood lymphocytes. Science 164:1415–1417, 1969.
38. Johnson HM, Stanton GJ, Baron S: Relative ability of mitogens to stimulate production of interferon by lymphoid cells and to induce suppression of the *in vitro* immune response. Proc Soc Exp Biol Med 154:138–141, 1977.
39. Salvin SB, Youngner JS, Lederer WH: Migration inhibitory factor and interferon in the circulation of mice with delayed hypersensitivity. Infect Immun 7:68–75, 1973.
40. Stobo J, Green I, Jackson L, Baron S: Identification of a subpopulation of mouse lymphoid cells required for interferon production after stimulation with mitogens. J Immunol 112:1589–1593, 1974.
41. Dianzani F, Monohan TM, Scupham A, Zucca M: Enzymatic induction of interferon production by galactose oxidase treatment of human lymphoid cells. Infect Immun 26:879–882, 1979.
42. Cavalieri RL, Havell EA, Vilcek J, Pestka S: Synthesis of human interferon by *Xenopus laevis* oocytes: two structural genes for interferons in human cells. Proc Natl Acad Sci USA 74:3287–3291, 1977.
43. Knight E Jr, Hunkapiller MW, Korant BD, Hardy RWF, Hood LE: Human fibroblast interferon: amino acid analysis and amino terminal amino acid sequence. Science 207:525–526, 1980.
44. Zoon KC, Smith ME, Bridgen PJ, Anfinsen CB, Hunkapiller MW, Hood LE: Amino terminal sequence of the major component of human lymphoblastoid interferon. Science 207:527–528, 1980.

45. Taira H, Broeze RJ, Jayaram BM, Lengyel P, Hunkapiller MW, Hood LE: Mouse interferons: amino terminal amino acid sequences of various species. Science 207:528–530, 1980.

46. Falcoff R: Some properties of virus and immune-induced human lymphocyte interferons. J Gen Virol 16:251–253, 1972.

47. Valle MJ, Jordan GW, Haahr S, Merigan TC: Characteristics of immune interferon produced by human lymphocyte cultures compared to other human interferon. J Immunol 115:230–233, 1975.

48. Youngner JS, Salvin SB: Production and properties of migration inhibitory factor and interferon in the circulation of mice with delayed hypersensitivity. J Immunol 111:1914–1922, 1973.

49. Berg K, Ogburn CA, Paucker K, Mogensen EK, Cantell K: Affinity chromotography of human leukocyte and diploid cell interferons on Sepharose-bound antibodies. J Immunol 114:640–644, 1975.

50. Havell EA, Berman B, Ogburn CA, Berg K, Paucker K, Vilcek J: Two antigenically distinct species of human interferon. Proc Natl Acad Sci USA 72:2185–2187, 1975.

51. Paucker K, Dalton BJ, Ogburn CA, Torma E: Multiple active sites on human interferons. Proc Natl Acad Sci USA 72:4587–4591, 1975.

52. Sonnenfeld G, Mandel AD, Merigan TC: The immunosuppressive effect of Type II mouse interferon preparations on antibody production. Cell Immunol 34:193–206, 1977.

53. Maehara N, Ho M, Armstrong JA: Differences in mouse interferons according to cell source and mode of induction. Infect Immun 17:572–579, 1977.

54. Osborne LC, Georgiades JA, Johnson HM: Antibody to mouse immune interferon. IRCS Med Sci 8:212, 1980.

55. Dianzani F, Baron S: Unexpectedly rapid action of human interferon in physiological conditions. Nature 257:682–684, 1975.

56. Dianzani F, Levy HB, Berg S, Baron S: Kinetics of the rapid action of interferon. Proc Soc Exp Biol Med 152:593–597, 1976.

57. Fleischmann WR Jr, Simon EH: Effect of interferon on virus production from isolated single cells. J Gen Virol 20:127–137, 1973.

58. Cooper PD, Bellett AJD: A transmissible interfering component of vesicular stomatitis virus preparations. J Gen Microbiol 21:485–497, 1959.

59. Levine S: Some characteristics of an interferon derived from embryonated eggs infected with Newcastle disease virus. Virology 17:593–595, 1962.

60. Ho M: Kinetic considerations of the inhibitory action of an interferon produced in chick cultures infected with sindbis virus. Virology 17:262–275, 1962.

61. Lockart RZ Jr, Horn B: Interaction of an interferon with L cells. J Bacteriol 85:996–1002, 1963.

62. Levine S, Magee WE, Hamilton RD, Miller OV. Effect of interferon on early enzyme and viral DNA synthesis in vaccinia virus infection. Virology 32:33–40, 1967.

63. Gandhi SS, Stewart RB: The production and effect of interferon on influenza virus growth in chick embryo lung epithelial and fibroblast cell cultures. Can J Microbiol 15:273-277, 1969.

64. Wagner RR: Biological studies of interferon. I. Suppression of cellular infection with Eastern equine encephalomyelitis virus. Virology 13:323–337, 1961.

65. Mayer V, Sokol F, Vilcek J: Effect of interferon on the infection with Eastern equine encephalomyelitis virus and its ribonucleic acid. Acta Virol 5:264–278, 1961.

66. Taylor J: Studies on the mechanism of action of interferon. I. Interferon action and RNA synthesis in chick embryo fibroblasts infected with Semliki Forest virus. Virology 25:340–349, 1965.

67. Takemoto KK, Baron S: Non-heritable interferon resistance in a fraction of virus populations. Proc Soc Exp Biol Med 121:670–675, 1966.
68. Stewart WEII, Scott WD, Sulkin SE: Relative sensitivities of viruses to different species of interferon. J Virol 4:147–153, 1969.
69. Marcus PI, Terry TM, Levine S: Interferon action. II. Membrane-bound alkaline ribonuclease activity in chick embryo cells manifesting interferon-mediated interference. Proc Natl Acad Sci USA 72:182–186, 1975.
70. Maenner H, Bradner G: Interferon action may not be effected by induction of a cellular ribonuclease. Nature 260:637–638, 1976.
71. Meldolesi MF, Friedman RM, Kohn LD: An interferon-induced increase in cyclic AMP levels precedes the establishment of the antiviral state. Biochem Biophys Res Commun 79:239–246, 1977.
72. Eppstein DA, Samuel CE: Mechanism of interferon action. Partial purification and characterization of a low-molecular-weight interferon-mediated inhibitor of translation with nucleolytic activity. Biochem Biophys Res Commun 79:145–153, 1977.
73. Lebleu B, Sen GC, Shaila S, Cabrer B., Lengyel P: Interferon, double-stranded RNA, and protein phosphorylation. Proc Natl Acad Sci USA 73:3107–3111, 1976.
74. Roberts WK, Hovanessian A, Brown RE, Clemens MJ, Kerr IM: Interferon-mediated protein kinase and low-molecular-weight inhibitor of protein synthesis. Nature 264:477–480, 1976.
75. Hovanessian AG, Brown RE, Kerr IM: Synthesis of low molecular weight inhibitor of protein synthesis with enzyme from interferon-treated cells. Nature 268:537–540, 1977.
76. Kerr IM, Brown RE, Hovanessian AG: Nature of inhibitor of cell-free protein synthesis formed in reponse to interferon and double-stranded RNA. Nature 268:540–542, 1977.
77. Kerr IM, Brown RE: pppA2′p5′A2′p5′A: an inhibitor of protein synthesis synthesized with an enzyme fraction from interferon-treated cells. Proc Natl Acad Sci USA 75:256-260, 1978.
78. Kimchi A, Shulman L, Schmidt A, Chernajovsky Y, Fradin A, Revel M: Kinetics of the induction of three translation-regulatory enzymes by interferon. Proc Natl Acad Sci USA 76:3208–3212, 1979.
79. Zilberstein A, Federman P, Shulman L, Revel M: Specific phosphorylation in vitro af a protein associated with ribosomes of interferon-treated mouse L-cells. FEBS Lett 68:119–124, 1976.
80. Cooper JA, Farrell PJ: Extracts of interferon-treated cells can inhibit reticulocyte lysate protein synthesis. Biochem Biophys Res Commun 77:124–131, 1977.
81. Zilberstein A, Kimchi A, Schmidt A, Revel M: Isolation of two interferon-induced translational inhibitors: a protein kinase and an oligo-isoadenylate synthetase. Proc Natl Acad Sci USA 75:4734–4738, 1978.
82. Schmidt A, Zilberstein A, Shulman L, Federman P, Berissi H, Revel M: Interferon action: isolation of Nuclease F a translation inhibitor activated by interferon-induced (2′-5′) oligoisoadenylate. FEBS Lett 95:257–264, 1978.
83. Schmidt A, Chernajovsky Y, Shulman L, Federman P, Berissi H, Revel M: An interferon-induced phosphodiesterase degrading (2′-5′) oligoisoadenylate and the C-C-A terminus of tRNA. Proc Natl Acad Sci USA 76:4788–4792, 1979.
84. Ohtsuki K, Dianzani F, Baron S: Decreased initiation factor activity in mouse L cells treated with interferon. Nature 269:536–538, 1977.
85. Kohn LD, Friedman RM, Holmes JM, Lee G: Use of thyrotropin and cholera toxin to probe the mechanism by which interferon initiates its antiviral activity. Proc Natl Acad Sci USA 73:3695–3699, 1976.
86. Knight E Jr, Korant BD: A cell surface alteration in mouse L cells induced by interferon. Biochem Biophys Res Commun 74:707–713, 1977.

87. Lindahl P, Leary P, Gresser I: Enhancement by interferon of the specific cytotoxicity of sensitized lymphocytes. Proc Natl Acad Sci USA 69:721–725, 1972.

88. Lindahl P, Leary P, Gresser I: Enhancement by interferon of the expression of surface antigens on murine leukemia L_{1210} cells. Proc Natl Acad Sci USA 70:2785–2788, 1973.

89. Baron S: The biological significance of the interferon system. Arch Intern Med 126:84–93, 1970.

90. Baron S: Mechanism of recovery from viral infection. Adv Virus Res 10:39–64, 1963.

91. Merigan TC: Symposium on interferon and host response to virus infection. Arch Intern Med 126:49–50, 1970.

92. Vilcek J: Interferon. In: Virology monographs, Gard S, Hallaver C, Meyer KF (eds). New York: Springer-Verlag, 1969, Vol 6.

93. Grossberg SE: The interferons and their inducers: molecular and therapeutic considerations. New Engl J Med 287:13–19, 79–85, 122–128, 1972.

94. Merigan TC, Reed SE, Hall TS, Tyrrell DAJ: Inhibition of respiratory virus infection by locally applied interferon. Lancet 1:563–567, 1973.

95. Solov'ev VD: The results of controlled observations on the prophylaxis of influenza with interferon. Bull Wld Hlth Org 41:683–688, 1969.

96. Panusarn C, Stanley ED, Dirda V, Rubenis M, Jackson GG: Prevention of illness from rhinovirus infection by a topical interferon inducer. New Engl J Med 291:57–61, 1974.

97. Merigan TC, Rand KH, Pollard RB, Abdallah PS, Jordan GW, Fried RP: Human leukocyte interferon for the treatment of herpes zoster in patients with cancer. New Engl J Med 298:981–987, 1978.

98. Desmyter J, De Groote J, Desmet VJ, Billiau A, Ray MB, Bradburne AF, Edy VG, DeSomer P, Mortelmans J: Administration of human fibroblast interferon in chronic hepatitis B infection. Lancet 2:645–647, 1976.

99. Greenberg HB, Pollard RB, Lutwick LI, Gregory PB, Robinson WS, Merigan TC: Effect of human leukocyte interferon on hepatitis B virus infection in patients with chronic active hepatitis. New Engl J Med 295:517–522, 1976.

100. Jordan GW, Fried RP, Merigan TC: Administration of human leukocyte interferon in herpes zoster. I. Safety, circulating antiviral activity, and host responses to interferon. J Infect Dis 130:56–62, 1974.

101. Sundmacher R, Neumann-Haefelin D, Cantell K: Successful treatment of dendritic keratitis with human leukocyte interferon. A controlled clinical study. Albrecht von Graefes Arch Klin Exp Ophthal 201:39–45, 1976.

102. Jones BR, Coster DJ, Falcon MG, Cantell K: Topical therapy of ulcerative herpetic keratitis with human interferon. Lancet 2:128, 1976.

103. Arvin AM, Yeager AS, Merigan TC: Effect of leukocyte interferon on urinary excretion of cytomegalovirus by infants. J Infect Dis 133 (Suppl): A 205–210, 1976.

104. Larsson A, Forsgren M, Hard af Segerstad S, Strander H, Cantell K: Administration of interferon to an infant with congenital rubella syndrome involving persistent viremia and cutaneous vasculitis. Acta Paediatr Scand 65:105–110, 1976.

105. O'Reilly RJ, Everson LK, Emodi G, Hansen J, Smithwick EM, Grimes E, Pahwa S, Pahwa R, Schwartz S, Armstrong D, Siegal FP, Gupta S, DuPont B, Good RA: Effects of exogenous interferon in cytomegalovirus infections complicating bone marrow transplanatation. Clin Imm Immunopathol 6:51–61, 1976.

106. Emodi G, Rufli T: Antiviral action of interferon in man: use of interferon in varicella-zoster infections in man. Tex Rep Biol Med 35:511–515, 1977.

107. Desmyter J: The use of interferon in viral hepatitis B. Tex Rep Biol Med 35:516–522, 1977.

108. Dunnick JK, Galasso GJ: Clinical trials with exogenous interferon: summary of a meeting. J Infect Dis 139:109–123, 1979.

109. Baer GM, Shaddock JH, Moore SA, Yager PA, Baron S, Levy HB: Successful prophylaxis against rabies in mice and rhesus monkeys: the interferon system and vaccine. J Infect Dis 136:286–291, 1977.

110. Sheaff ET, Stewart RB: Interaction of interferon with cells: induction of antiviral activity. Can J Microbiol 15:941–953, 1969.

111. Fleischmann WR Jr: Priming of interferon action. Tex Rep Biol Med 35:316–325, 1977.

112. Blalock JE, Baron S: Interferon-induced transfer of viral resistance between animal cells. Nature 269:422–425, 1977.

113. Blalock JE, Baron S: Mechanism of interferon induced transfer of viral resistance between animal cells. J Gen Virol 42:363–372, 1979.

114. Blalock JE: A small fraction of cells communicates the maximal interferon sensitivity to a population. Proc Soc Exp Biol Med 162:80–84, 1979.

115. Fleischmann WR Jr, Georgiades JA, Osborne LC, Johnson HM: Potentiation of interferon activity by mixed preparations of fibroblast and immune interferon. Infect Immun 26:248–253, 1979.

116. Atanasiu P, Chany C: Action d'un interferon provenant de cellules malignes sur l'infection experimentale du hamster nouveau—ne par le virus du polyome. CR Acad Sci (Paris) 251:1687–1689, 1960.

117. Gresser I, Tovey MG: Antitumor effects of interferon. Biochem Biophys Acta 516:231–247, 1978.

118. Gresser I, Brouty-Boye D, Thomas MT, Macieira-Coelho A: Interferon and cell division. I. Inhibition of the multiplication of mouse leukemia L 1210 cells in vitro by interferon preparations. Proc Natl Acad Sci USA 66:1052–1058, 1970.

119. Paucker K, Cantell K, Henle W: Quantitative studies on viral interference in suspended L-cells. III. Effect of interfering viruses and interferon on the growth rate of cells. Virology 17:324–334, 1962.

120. Collyn d'Hooghe M, Brouty-Boye D, Malaise EP, Gresser I: Interferon and cell division. XII. Prolongation by interferon of the intermitotic time of mouse mammary tumor cells in vitro. Microcinematographic analysis. Exp Cell Res 105:73–77, 1977.

121. Tovey M, Brouty-Boye D, Gresser I: Early effect of interferon on mouse leukemia cells cultivated in a chemostat. Proc Natl Acad Sci USA 72:2265–2269, 1975.

122. Lindahl-Magnusson P, Leary P, Gresser I: Interferon and cell division. VI. Inhibitory effect of interferon on the multiplication of mouse embryo and mouse kidney cells in primary culture. Proc Soc EXp Biol Med 138:1044–1050, 1071.

123. Knight E Jr: Interferon: effect on the saturation density to which mouse cells will grow in vitro. J Cell Biol 56:846–849, 1973.

124. Lee SHS, O'Shaughnessy MV, Rozee KR, Kind LS: Interferon induced growth depression in diploid and heteroploid human cells. Proc Soc Exp Biol Med 139:1438–1440, 1972.

125. Baron S, Merigan TC, McKerlie ML: Effect of crude and purified interferon on the growth of uninfected cells in culture. Proc Soc Exp Biol Med 121:50–52, 1966.

126. Lindahl-Magnusson P, Leary P, Gresser I: Interferon and cell division. VI. Inhibitory effect of interferon on the multiplication of mouse embryo and mouse kidney cells in primary cultures. Proc Soc Exp Biol Med 138:1044–1050, 1971.

127. Knight E Jr: Antiviral and cell growth inhibitory activities reside in the same glycoprotein of human fibroblast interferon. Nature 262:302-303, 1976.

128. Stewart WE II, Gresser I, Tovey MG, Bandu MT, Le Goff S: Identification of the cell-multiplication inhibitory factors in interferon preparations as interferons. Nature 262:300–302, 1976.

129. Iwakura Y, Yonehara S, Kawade Y: Purification of mouse L-cell interferon. Essentially pure preparations with associated cell growth inhibitory activity. J Biol Chem 253:5074–5079, 1978.

130. Lundgren E, Larsson I, Miorner H, Strannegard O: Effects of leukocyte and fibroblast interferon on events in the fibroblast cell cycle. J Gen Virol 42:589–595, 1979.

131. Fuse A, Kuwata T: Effects of interferon on the human clonal cell line, RSa: inhibition of macromolecular synthesis. J Gen Virol 33:17–24, 1976.

132. O'Shaughnessy MV, Lee SHS, Rozee KR: Interferon inhibition of DNA synthesis and cell division. Can J Microbiol 18:145–151, 1972.

133. Gutterman J, Yap Y, Buzdar A, Alexanian R, Hersh E, Cabanillas F, Geenberg S: Leukocyte interferon induced tumor regression in patients with breast cancer and B cell neoplasms. Proc Am Assoc Cancer Res 20:167, 1979.

134. Merigan TC, Sikora K, Breeden JH, Levy R, Rosenberg SA: Preliminary observations on the effect of human leukocyte interferon in non-Hodgkins's lymphoma. New Engl J Med 299:1449–1453, 1978.

135. Braun W, Levy HB: Interferon preparations as modifiers of immune responses. Proc Soc Exp Biol Med 141:769–773, 1972.

136. Chester TJ, Paucker K, Merigan TC: Suppression of mouse antibody producing spleen cells by various interferon preparations. Nature 246:92–94, 1973.

137. Gisler RH, Lindahl P, Gresser I: Effects of interferon on antibody synthesis in vitro. J Immunol 113:438–444, 1974.

138. Johnson HM, Smith BG, Baron S. Inhibition of the primary in vitro antibody response of mouse spleen cells by interferon preparations. IRCS (Med Sci) 2:1616, 1974.

139. Johnson HM, Smith BG, Baron S: Inhibition of the primary in vitro antibody response by interferon preparations. J Immunol 114: 403–409, 1975.

140. Johnson HM: Cyclic AMP regulation of mitogen-induced interferon production and mitogen suppression of immune response. Nature 265:154–155, 1977.

141. Schultz RM, Chirigos MA, Heine UI: Functional and morphologic characteristics of interferon-treated macrophages. Cell Immunol 35:84–91, 1978.

142. Schultz RM, Papamatheakis JD, Chirigos MA: Interferon: an inducer of macrophage activation by polyanions. Science 197:674–676, 1977.

143. Huang KY, Donahoe RM, Gordon FB, Dressler HR: Enhancement of phagocytosis by interferon-containing preparations. Infect Immun 4:581–588, 1971.

144. Imanishi J, Yokota Y, Kishida T, Mukainaka T, Matsuo A: Phagocytosis-enhancing effect of human leukocyte interferon preparation on human peripheral monocytes in vitro. Acta Virol 19:52–58, 1975.

145. Kishida T, Morikawa K, Ito H, Yokota Y: Influence de l'interferon sur l'inhibition par les macrophages, de la multiplication in vitro de la cellule maligne murine (FM$_3$A). Cr Soc Biol (Paris) 167:1502–1505, 1973.

146. Zarling JM, Sosman J, Eskra L, Borden EC, Horoszewicz JS, Carter WA: Enhancement of T cell cytotoxic responses by purified human fibroblast interferon. J Immunol 121:2002–2004, 1978.

147. Heron I, Berg K, Cantell K: Regulatory effect of interferon on T-cells in vitro. J Immunol 117:1370–1377, 1976.

148. Trinchieri G, Santoli D, Dee RR, Knowles BB: Anti-viral activity induced by culturing lymphocytes with tumor-derived virus-transformed cells. Identification of the antiviral activity as interferon and characterization of the human effector lymphocyte subpopulation. J Exp Med 147:1299–1313, 1978.

149. Gidlund M, Orn A, Wigzell H, Senik A, Gresser I: Enhanced NK cell activity in mice injected with interferon and interferon inducers. Nature 273:759–761, 1978.

150. Svet-Moldavsky GJ, Chernyakhovskaya IJ: Interferon and the interaction of allogeneic normal and immune lymphocytes with L-cells. Nature 215:1299–1300, 1967.

151. Chernyakhovskaya IY, Slavina EG, Svet-Moldavsky GJ: Antitumor effect of lymphoid cells activated by interferon. Nature 288:71–72, 1970.

152. Trinchieri G, Santoli D: Antiviral activity induced by culturing lymphocytes with tumor-derived or virus-transformed cells. Enhancement of human natural killer cell activity by interferon and antagonistic inhibition of susceptibility of target cells to lysis. J Exp Med 147:1314–1333, 1978.

153. Hirsch MS, Ellis DA, Black PH, Monaco AP, Wood ML: Immunosuppressive effects of an interferon preparation *in vivo*. Transplantation 17:234–236, 1974.

154. Imanishi J, Oishi K, Kishida T, Negoro Y, Iizuka M: Effects of interferon preparations on rabbit corneal xenograft. Arch Virol 53:157–161, 1977.

155. Mobraaten LE, DeMaeyer E, DeMaeyer-Guignard J: Prolongation of allograft survival in mice by inducers of interferon. Transplantation 16:415–420, 1973.

156. DeMaeyer E, Mobraaten L, DeMaeyer-Guignard J: Prolongation par l'interferon de la survie des greffes de peau chez la souris. C R Acad Sci 277:2101–2103, 1973.

157. DeMaeyer E, Mobraaten LE, DeMaeyer-Guignard J: Prolongation of allograph survical in mice by interferon inducers and interferon preparations. In: Effects of interferon on cells, viruses, and the immune system, Geraldes A (ed.). New York: Academic Press, 1975, pp 367–379.

158. Gresser I, Maury C, Brouty-Boye D: Mechanism of the antitumor effect of interferon in mice. Nature 239:167–168, 1972.

159. Baron S: The biological significance of the interferon system. In: Interferon, Finter NB (ed.). Philadelphia: WB Saunders, 1966, pp 268–293.

160. Kohn LD, Friedman RM, Holmes JM, Lee G: Use of thyrotropin and cholera toxin to probe the mechanism by which interferon initiates its antiviral activity. Proc Natl Acad Sci USA 73:3695–3699, 1976.

161. Besancon F, Ankel H: Inhibition de l'action de l'interferon par des hormones glycoproteiques. C R Acad Sci 283: 1807–1810, 1976.

162. Blalock JE, Stanton JD: Common pathways of interferon and hormonal action. Nature 283:406–408, 1980.

163. Blalock JE, personal communication.

164. Einhorn S, Strander H: Interferon therapy for neoplastic diseases in man *in vitro* and *in vivo* studies. In: Human interferon: production and clinical use, Stinebring WR, Chapple PJ (eds). New York: Plenum Press, 1978, pp 159–174.

165. Blomgren H, Cantell K, Johansson B, Lagergren C, Ringborg V, Strander H: Interferon therapy in Hodgkin's disease. Acta Med Scand 199:527–532, 1976.

166. Mellstedt H, Ahre A, Bjorkholm M, Holm G, Johansson B, Strander H: Interferon therapy in myelomatosis. Lancet 1:245–247, 1979.

167. Hill NO, Loeb E, Pardue AS, Dorn GL, Khan A, Hill JM: Response of acute leukemia to leukocyte interferon. J Clin Hematol Oncol 9:137–149, 1979.

168. Hill NO, Khan A, Loeb E, Pardue A, Aleman C, Dorn G, Hill JM: Clinical trials of high dose human leukocyte interferon. In: Interferon: properties and clinical uses, Khan A, Hill NO, Dorn G (eds). Dallas: Leland Fikes Foundation Press, 1980, pp 667–677.

169. Horoszewicz JS, Leong SS, Ito M, Buffett RF, Karakovsis C, Holyoke E, Job L, Dolen JG, Carter WA: Human fibroblast interferon in human neoplasia: clinical and laboratory study. Cancer Treat Rep 62:1899–1906, 1978.

170. Borecky L, Buchvald J, Alderova E, Stodola I, Obrucnikova E, Gruntova Z, Lackovic V, Doskocil J: Results of a five year study of the curative effect of double stranded ribonucleic acid in viral dematoses and eye diseases. In: Human interferon: production and clinical use, Stirling WR, Chapple PJ (eds). New York: Plenum Press, 1978, pp 175–191.

171. Levy HB, Law LW, Rabson AS: Inhibition of tumor growth by polyinosinic-polycytidylic acid. Proc Natl Acad Sci USA 62:357–359, 1969.

172. Levine A, Krown S: Poly ICLC in cancer therapy, current status and future prospects. In: Augmenting agents in cancer therapy. Current status and future prospects, Hersh E, Mastrangelo M. (eds). New York: Raven Press, 1980 (in press).
173. Merigan TC: Pharmokinetics and side effects of interferon in man. Tex Rep Biol Med 35:541–547, 1977.
174. Billiau A, De Somer P, Edy VG, DeClercq E, Heremans H: Human fibroblast interferon for clinical trials: pharmacokinetics and tolerability in human experimental animals and humans. Antimicrob Agents Chemother 16:56–63, 1979.
175. Gilbert W, Villa-Komaroff L: Useful proteins from recombinant bacteria. Sci Am 242:74–94, 1980.
176. Nagata S, Taira H, Hall A, Johnsrud L, Streuli M, Escodi J, Boll W, Cantell K, Weissman C: Synthesis in *E. coli* of a polypeptide with human leukocyte interferon activity. Nature 284:316–320, 1980.
177. Eihorn S, Strander H: Is interferon tissue specific?—Effect of human leukocyte and fibroblast interferons on the growth of lymphoblastoid and osteosarcoma cell lines. J Gen Virol 35:573–577, 1977.
178. Georgiades JA, Langford MP, Stanton GJ, Johnson HM: Purification and potentiation of human immune interferon activity. IRCS Med Sci 7:559, 1979.
179. Fleischmann WR Jr: personal communication.
180. Fleischmann WR Jr, Kleyn K, Baron S: Potentiation of the antitumor effect of virus induced interferon by mouse immune interferon preparations. J Natl Cancer Inst 1980 (in press).

4. Tumor Heterogeneity

GLORIA H. HEPPNER, WILLIAM R. SHAPIRO and JOAN K. RANKIN

The heterogeneous nature of cancer as it appears in different patients or animals is one of the reasons for our primitive understanding and ability to control neoplastic diseases. However, inter-tumor heterogeneity is only one level of tumor variability. A second level, intra-tumor heterogeneity also contributes to the difficulties of understanding cancer. Although the idea that solid tumors are composed of mixtures of malignant cells, heterogeneous in regard to many characteristics, has long been accepted by clinical oncologists and pathologists, the majority of cancer researchers have sought to eliminate such heterogeneity from their experimental systems in order to obtain reproducible, unambiguous results. That tumor heterogeneity itself is an area suitable for experimental and clinical investigation has not been widely appreciated. The purpose of this chapter is to review the experimental and clinical basis for intra-tumor heterogeneity and to speculate on its possible significance to cancer therapeutics.

1. HETEROGENEITY OF EXPERIMENTAL TUMORS

1.1. Heterogeneous Characteristics of Animal Tumors

One of the most obvious characteristics by which tumor cells may differ is morphology. An extreme example of intra-tumor structural variability is teratocarcinoma[1]. In this neoplasm representatives of any type of adult somatic tissue, as well as 'embryonal' malignant cells, may be found. Extensive, although not as dramatic, morphological heterogeneity can be seen in other tumors as well. Kobori and Oota[2] have demonstrated the simultaneous presence of tumor cells with characteristics of gastric, intestinal, and neuroendocrine differentiation in gastric carcinomas induced in rats with N-methyl-N-nitro-N-nitrosoguanidine. Histological evaluation of spontaneous mouse mammary tumors reveals extensive inter- and intra-tumor variation in cellu-

G. B. Humphrey et al. (eds.), Pediatric oncology 1, 99–116. All rights reserved.

larity, cellular ultrastructure, and differentiation [1, 3]. Henderson and Rous [4] examined morphological heterogeneity by 'plating' various neoplastic components of epidermal and mammary carcinomas in the subcutaneous connective tissue of mice. By an ingenious technique these investigators were able to separate benign papillomas from epidermal carcinomas, as well as to propagate individual subtypes of mammary tumors previously hidden within single neoplasms. More recently, subpopulations of tumor cells with a variety of distinct morphological · features *in vitro* have been isolated from a single, mouse mammary tumor virus (MMTV)-associated, mammary tumor [5], and from a single ethylnitrosourea-induced rat neurotumor [6]. Most of these subpopulations have maintained their distinctive cellular morphology through many passages *in vitro*, suggesting that morphological variations among tumor cells are not necessarily due to pleomorphism of a single cell type, but rather reflect stable differences. Further evidence for this comes from the karyotypic diversity exhibited among tumor cells from a single tumor. The karyotypes of the isolated mammary tumor populations mentioned above vary from diploid to tetraploid to highly aneuploid. The original tumor from which they were obtained contained cells with karyotypes of the entire range seen in the subpopulations. The literature contains numerous other examples of experimental tumors which contain cells exhibiting a 'stem line' karyotype as well as other sidelines [7–12]. These observations suggest a genetic basis for at least part of the heterogeneity of solid tumors.

Tumor heterogeneity is not limited to morphological and karyotypic differences. Gray and Pierce [13] demonstrated heterogeneity in melanin production by subpopulations of a hamster melanoma. Hormone responsive mouse mammary tumors are mixed populations of high estrogen and progesterone receptor positive, hormone-dependent cells and low or negative receptor, autonomous cells [14]. Subpopulations of the MMTV-associated mammary tumor differentially express MMTV-coded, cell surface antigens [5]. Thus, tumor cell heterogeneity is also evident in production of various cell products or 'markers.'

Another manifestation of intra-tumor variability is heterogeneity in behavior. Subpopulations have been shown to grow at different rates [5, 13] when passaged, either *in vivo* or *in vitro*, as isolated clones. Klein and Klein [15] demonstrated that many solid mouse tumors contain variants able to grow as an ascites, and Ishidate *et al.* [11] found that cells within a 1-butyl-1-nitrosourea-induced, rat myeloblastic leukemia differed in ability to proliferate in bone marrow. Variani *et al.* [16], presented evidence that methylcholanthrene-induced sarcomas of mice contain subpopulations heterogeneous in migratory ability *in vitro*, a characteristic which may be related to invasiveness *in vivo*. Perhaps the most significant demonstration of behavorial heterogeneity is that of Fidler and Kripke [17], as well as others [18, 19], showing that tumors can be composed of subpopulations of cells with diverse metastatic potential. The existence of tumor subpopulations differing in such fundamental neoplastic properties as invasiveness and metastasis provides a framework for the well-known capacity of cancer behavior to change during the course of disease, a phenomenon called 'progression' [15]. It further provides an explanation for some of the 'laws of progression' as defined by Foulds [20]. This is particularly so for the concepts of independent assortability and progression of different characteristics within the same tumor, since these characteristics at a single point in time depend upon the relative 'mix' of the variable tumor subpopulations [21].

1.2. Mechanisms of Tumor Heterogeneity

The fact that many tumors consist of distinct neoplastic subpopulations raises questions about the origin and maintenance of this variability. Current thinking assigns a monoclonal origin to most cancers [22], although exceptions such as methylcholanthrene-induced sarcomas in mice do occur [23]. Clearly, a tumor of multiclonal origin would be heterogeneous from its beginning. A tumor of monoclonal origin, however, could become heterogeneous through a process involving either mutation or differentiation of a stem cell population [24, 25]. One of the mammary tumor subpopulations mentioned above produces new, morphologically distinct, tumorigenic variants following passage in vivo [26]. Candidate stem cells have also been isolated from a dimethylbenzanthracene-induced rat mammary tumor [27] and from the ethylnitrosourea-induced rat neurotumor studied by Imada and Sueoka [6]. The karyotypic instability of many tumors could also contribute to the production of variants [7], even in a precise, ordered way [28]. Furthermore, both the stem cell and the genetic mechanisms allow for a continual production of variants throughout tumor growth, thus confounding the efforts of selection pressures to produce homogeneous tumors.

Another class of mechanisms which could help maintain the heterogeneity of tumors is growth interaction between subpopulations; that is, individual subpopulations may not display as wide a range in growth capacity when growing together as they do when growing apart [29]. Recent experiments with tumor subpopulations isolated from a single mammary tumor have demonstrated such growth interactions both in vivo and in vitro [30]. In the in vivo experiments growth of selected subpopulations of cells injected on opposite flanks of host mice was compared with the growth of the individual sublines injected opposite themselves. Depending upon the particular sublines used, the presence of another subpopulation growing on the other side could either increase or decrease the growth of these specific sublines. Four-hundred rads X-irradiation of the host animal 2 days before injection of the subpopulations abolished the interaction. Comparison of the direction of the

interaction with the ability of the isolated subpopulations to immunize syngeneic mice against these various sublines [31] suggests that the mechanism of
the phenomenon is dependent upon the ability of some subpopulations to
induce effective immunity against themselves and against cells of other sublines, even though the other sublines may be nonimmunogenic.

In vitro experiments have suggested another mechanism to maintain tumor
heterogeneity. Two of the mammary tumor subpopulations have been found
to produce a factor that can inhibit growth of the other subpopulations.
Cocultivation of mixed subpopulations *in vitro* results in similar inhibition of
growth. Thus, the evidence to date is that both host and tumor factors can
regulate tumor growth in such a way as to keep the growth of tumor cell
subpopulations in balance. This suggests that the level of cancer organization
is beyond the cellular, rather akin to that of an organ.

2. HETEROGENEITY OF HUMAN CANCER

Identifying heterogeneity in human cancers requires consideration of factors
similar to those in animal systems. Heterogeneity may be functionally present
in three different circumstances. Individual patients' tumors may behave
differently despite similar pathology, especially in response to therapy. Further, a specific tumor may change over time, that is, it may undergo progression. Thirdly, the subject of this review, a patient's tumor at any one time
may be heterogeneous, that is, it may be composed of cell populations
identifiably distinct by one or several specific criteria. The criteria may be
phenotypic in nature or may be genotypic. Heterogeneity must be defined
operationally with respect to some specific circumstance. Clinically, heterogeneity may be defined in terms of whether or not the same treatment should
be applied to all patients harboring tumors with the same pathology, or must
be tailored to an individual patient's tumor or even to individual cell populations within a patient's tumor. A different operational definition may be
applicable if one is dealing with immunological parameters or is using long-
term cell lines.

2.1. Heterogeneity within a Patient's Tumor

Hints that human cancers are composed of different cell populations have
been supplied by studies of metastases. Tumors removed from metastatic
sites frequently bear little morphologic resemblance to the primary tumor.
Metastatic tumors may grow at different rates and may be more or less
malignant than the primary tumor. A formal attempt to ascertain differences
between metastatic and primary tumors was recently reported by Baylin *et
al.* [32]. They examined levels of histaminase activity, L-DOPA decarboxylase

activity, and calcitonin in multiple autopsy tissues from patients with lung cancer. Such markers may be found in cell lines in small cell carcinomas of the lung that bear characteristics of the APUD (APU = amine precursor uptake, D = L-aromatic amino acid decarboxylase) system of endocrine cells. Whereas the marker levels in mediastinal metastases were similar to those in the primary tumors, histaminase activity in hepatic metastases from four of six patients was much lower than that in the primary tumor or in mediastinal tumor nodules. Similarly, in four patients in whom L-DOPA decarboxylase activity was high in primary lung tumor or in mediastinal metastases, the enzyme activity in hepatic metastases was much lower than in the surrounding normal liver or in pulmonary metastases. In the other two patients, although the hepatic metastases had higher histaminase and L-DOPA decarboxylase activity than did the surrounding liver, the levels were in the same range found in either the primary lung tumor or in the mediastinal lesions. Sometimes the L-DOPA decarboxylase varied between hepatic tumor lesions. Calcitonin levels generally did not vary from one metastasis to another, suggesting lack of concordance among the three markers. Immunohistochemical studies of histaminase in both the primary and hepatic metastases suggested variable amounts of activity in clusters of tumor cells within each of the sites. Siracký [33] has also presented evidence of divergence in characteristics between primaries and their metastases and between different metastatic nodules from the same patient. Cell suspensions of primary and metastatic ovarian carcinoma were found to be differentially sensitive *in vitro* to a variety of commonly used drugs.

The work of Fidler and associates (see above) has indicated that, in animal tumors, metastases are derived from differing cells within the primary tumor. Proving the existence of mixed cell populations in primary human cancers is more difficult. It requires that the primary tumor be examined at one point in time (hence ignoring progression) or after periods in tissue culture (imposing potentially obfuscating artifacts—see below). Furthermore, although phenotypic behavior is most easily examined, cell population differences are more specifically proven by genotypic differences.

Pertschuk et al. [34] measured estrogen receptor in 74 primary breast cancers, 12 recurrences, 12 metastases, and eight specimens in which no tumor could be identified. Fifty-nine of the specimens were positive by fluorescence, dextran-coated charcoal and sucrose gradient centrifugation assays. Most of the positive tumors were heterogeneous for estrogen receptor in that they were composed of varying proportions of both positive and negative cells. Lee [35] also examined estrogen receptor in human mammary carcinomas. Among 19 breast cancer cases studied, only two carcinomas (one primary, one metastatic) demonstrated homogeneous populations of strongly estrogen receptorpositive cancer cells and two primaries were negative. The other fifteen mammary carcinomas were composed of cancer cells showing varying degrees of fluorescence ranging from completely negative to strongly positive cells. Such results indicate different hormone binding capacities among tumors, as well as among individual cells of the same tumor. Thus, human breast cancers should not be classified simply as estrogen receptor-positive or estrogen receptor-negative, because the majority are composed of heterogeneous populations of cancer cells of varying estrogen receptor content.

While these studies examined whole tissue specimens, others have looked for regional differences within a tumor. Byers and Johnston [36] examined antigenic differences among human osteogenic sarcoma cell suspensions taken from different locations in tumors removed at operation. The antigenic characteristics were examined by immunofluorescence using autologous or homologous anti-osteogenic sarcoma antiserum. The density of tumor associated antigen on cells from the center of the five tumor masses was low. Cells from the midzone had intermediate levels of tumor antigen density and cells at the margin contained the highest levels. Such regional differences suggest that the location of the cell within the tumor may influence its immunologic characteristics.

It is in the examination of individual cells that heterogeneity must ultimately be proven. Most studies have utilized long-term human cell lines. These experiments sometimes suggested variations between patients' tumors but similarity within the same tumor line over an extended period of time. Thus, Rogan et al. [37] used high resolution SDS-polyacrylamide slab gel electrophoresis with labelled methionine and autoradiography to demonstrate a variety of cell surface membrane proteins among 6 human lymphoid cell lines. Whereas the lines appeared to differ considerably one from the other, within each line there was a remarkable degree of consistency in the protein patterns over extended periods, in one case over two years. On the other hand, Sorg et al. [38] showed that membrane associated antigens of human malignant melanomas changed as the tumors remained in culture, and this change was associated with the appearance of subclones of cell populations differing in antigenic reactivity. Such changes are consistent with a developmental concept of cancer which suggests that tumors undergo changes as they grow, changes associated with the development of varying clonal subpopulations. Barranco and his colleagues [39] showed that four permanent cell lines of human malignant melanoma derived from a single melanoma nodule in one patient exhibited different survival responses to cytosine arabinoside as measured by colony forming assay. One strain was quite sensitive to the drug while the other three were very resistant. In part, the differences appeared to be related to variable deoxycytidine kinase activity in the four cell strains. These cell lines were also found to vary in their sensitivities to BCNU but not to bleomycin [40]. Chu [41] also demonstrated subpopulations of a human lung carcinoma that responded differently to three chemotherapeutic agents and Calabresi *et al.* [42] have reported a similar situation with a human colon carcinoma. Siracký [33] has shown differential drug sensitivity among cell suspensions taken from different regions of primary ovarian and colon carcinomas.

Such studies have emphasized phenotypic markers of heterogeneity. Ultimately, it is the genotypic pattern of individual cell populations that most specifically defines them. Unfortunately, this aspect of human cancer heterogeneity has been the least well studied. Woods *et al.* [43] established four permanent human tumor cell lines from 4 patients with ovarian adenocarcinoma. One line was derived from primary tumor tissue while the other three were from cells in malignant effusions. While the cells differed somewhat morphologically, they all had chromosomal abnormalities; several were common to all the lines, but some chromosomal defects were unique to individual lines. One problem with this kind of study is that long-term tissue culture lines tend to increase chromosomal abnormalities with increasing passage number and it is difficult to draw conclusions about the original tumor as such evolution occurs. For example, Hagemeijer *et al.* [44] performed cytogenetic analysis on three clonal cell lines derived from a human renal cell carcinoma and its lymph node metastasis. Although the primary tumor was not karyotyped, there were similar chromosomal markers in the three lines, suggesting that they were derived from a common tumor. However, there were a number of differences between the three lines indicating either that there had been evolution in tissue culture or that divergent cell populations were contained within the initial tumors.

2.2. Progression and Tumor Heterogeneity

Even though the cellular composition of a tumor may be homogeneous (by one or several criteria) at one time, it may evolve over weeks or months into a tumor with diverse characteristics. An example of this was given in a recent paper by Andreef *et al.* [45] who reported two patients whose acute leukemia changed over a year. A child with acute lymphoblastic leukemia had relapsed one year after chemotherapy. At the time of relapse, an analysis of cellular morphology revealed the presence of both lymphoid and myeloid blasts. The cells were positive for deoxynucleotidyl transferase activity and 56% of the cells expressed Fc receptors. Sedimentation techniques separated the population into myeloid cells with high RNA content and lymphoid cells with low RNA content. The DNA stemline was found to be diploid. A second patient, an adult, initially presented with deoxynucleotidyl transferase positive acute leukemia. Morphologically and cytochemically the cell line was a primitive monocytic leukemia with high RNA content and a diploid DNA stemline. After one year in remission, subsequent marrow relapse indicated the presence of cells with a triploid DNA stemline, high RNA content and negative Philadelphia chromosome. Bovine serum albumin sedimentation of these cells separated them into diploid and triploid cell populations. These two cases provide some evidence for the possibility of phenotypic and genotypic evolution in the development of acute leukemia.

Another example of tumor evolution was presented by Testa *et al.* [46] who followed the karyotypes of a series of patients with acute nonlymphocytic leukemia. The karyotypes were examined in 17 of these patients, seven of whose chromosomes were initially normal and 10 whose chromosomes were initially abnormal. Structural rearrangements and gain, or occasionally loss, of chromosomes were found in patients followed over a one- to two-year period. Some relationship between karyotypic evolution and prognosis was also found. In no instance was a full clone of chromosomally abnormal cells detected when the bone marrow was morphologically normal, but single abnormal cells of clonal origin were occasionally observed.

Morse *et al.* [47] found a high incidence of clonal abnormalities in cytogenetic studies of children with acute nonlymphoblastic leukemia. Seven patients were found to have at least two abnormalities and/or clones and five patients had one abnormality. These observations suggested multiple events leading to the initial malignant transformation, although another interpretation would be that the investigators sampled diverse marrow cell populations.

Cancers other than leukemias can also exhibit heterogeneous characteristics over the course of time. Siracký [33] sampled cancer cells from ascites fluid in 12 patients undergoing palliative chemotherapy for ovarian carcinomas. Distinct changes in ploidy were seen in sequential samples, including decreases in the number of polyploid cells. Siracký [33] also found a heterogeneity in the characteristic changes in nuclear morphology subsequent to progesterone therapy in sequential samples of cancer cells from patients with endometrial cancer. These findings suggest an intra-tumor heterogeneity in response to progesterone.

2.3. Heterogeneity of Human Brain Tumors

Recently, two of us (W.S. and J.R.) have initiated studies on the heterogeneity of human brain tumors. The most distinctive feature of the most malignant human brain tumor, the glioblastoma multiforme or astrocytoma grade IV, is the pleomorphic nature of the cell types in the tumor. Histologically one may see small darkly stained nuclei that appear to divide rapidly alongside large multinucleate cells whose rate of division is slower [48]. Rubinstein [49] has pointed out that diffuse malignant gliomas not infrequently disclose fields that suggest a proliferation of separate clones of anaplastic cells. In fact, the very term glioblastoma multiforme emphasizes the remarkable diversity of cells which comprise that tumor. Many gliomas contain fields of benign tumor reflecting the frequent clinical progression from a slowly to a rapidly growing cancer and suggesting that the cells within a glioma have variable growth rates. Many gliomas are formed not of one glial cell type but rather are a mixture of several neoplastic glial elements. One common mixed glioma is the oligodendrogliomaastrocytoma, a tumor in which fields of neoplastic oligodendroglial cells alternate or interdigitate with areas of astrocytoma [50]. Occasionally a malignant glial tumor may acquire either early, or more often late in its course, a sarcomatous element apparently through the malignant transformation of its reactive vascular stroma. The resulting gliosarcoma is a complex of malignant neural and mesenchymal cells pursuing very divergent patterns and rates of growth [51].

Recent studies in human brain tumors carried in nude mice suggested varying chemosensitivities for tumors derived from individual patients [52, 53]. One possible explanation for this differential chemosensitivity was that contained within each paient's tumor were cells that grew readily in the nude mouse and were incidentally sensitive to different drugs. There are at present some 70 established human glioma lines [54–67]. As discussed previously, tumor cell lines can generate new variant or mutant cells during the course of their evolution. This implies that cells of some established tumor cell lines may bear little resemblance to the stem or substem population of cells [68] at the time of resection. Therefore, established lines do not adequately provide information on the heterogeneity of the brain tumors from which they were derived.

To study early passage tumor cells and their clones, methods were developed to determine the extent of variability actually existing among cell types within the same tumor and among cell types from different tumors. The protocol had three objectives: (1) to identify the tumors' stem and substem cell populations; (2) to isolate single cells from these populations to generate pure clones, and (3) to identify the clones in a manner permitting us to trace their evolution *in vitro*.

Tumor tissue was obtained from patients undergoing resection and immediately dissociated mechanically into single cells which were then karyotyped and dilution plated *in vitro* [69]. The immediate karyotyping of dissociated tumor cells permitted a determination of the chromosomal complement for that tumor. Further, clones established from the single dissociated cells could be identified as cellular representatives of the brain tumor based on their karyotype. Karyotyping thus characterizes the clonal populations permitting a determination of: (1) the extent of cellular heterogeneity; (2) the evolution of each cell type; and (3) the cell behaviour of individual clones vs. mixed populations of clones.

Six tumors were analyzed in this manner; each tumor had a number of stem and substem cell populations [70]. The chromosomal complement of each cell type ranged from near-diploid (2n) to hypo- or hyper-tetraploid (4n) in chromosome numbers. This cellular heterogeneity confirmed the cytogenetic studies of Mark[71] who reported more than one cell type in each of the 50 astrocytomas analyzed. Since the study included only Giemsa stained karyotypes, Mark[71] could not determine the extent of heterogeneity in cells with the same modal numbers. Analysis of cells with the same modal number using G-banding techniques can, however, reveal two or more subpopulations, implying extensive variability in the cells' chromosomal complements[72]. Furthermore, the distribution of cell types varied with each tumor. Some tumors were predominately aneuploid; other were predominately hypodiploid and the remaining tumors were some combination of both. These observations indicate that human gliomas are not only heterogeneous in their cell populations but are different from each other. Cells with so many combinations of chromosomes will most certainly show altered gene expression and should demonstrate marked phenotypic variability. Indeed, considerable variability has been observed in these clonal populations when analyzed for cell kinetics, glial fibrillary acidic protein (GFAP), S-100 protein or chemosensitivity.

Clonal evolution was also evaluated, by observing each clone for 3–4 months, karyotyping, and recloning at even passage numbers until passage 12. Both stable and unstable clonal behavior was observed. Stable clones were those in which 80% or more of the karyotyped cells showed the parental karyotype and continued to do so for 8–12 passages. Unstable clones rapidly produced new cell types which were karyotypically different from the parent clone. All six tumors displayed stable and unstable clonal behavior. In general, near-diploid clones were stable whereas aneuploid clones were unstable[72]. If such cellular stability and instability also characterize *in vivo* clonal behavior, it might account for the tremendous diversity in cell types seen in human gliomas.

Tumor cells are well know for their often bizarre chromosomes and such marker chromosomes can be used to trace the cells' karyotypic evolution. Several mechanisms can be proposed by which tumor cells undergo karyotypic change. Tetraploid cells may arise by a process called endoreduplication in which the chromosomes replicate but the cell fails to divide, hence producing a cell with 4n chromosomes. Subsequent division may produce unequal chromosome distribution in the two daughter cells, thus yielding aneuploid cells. With time any number of cells of various chromosomal complements may form, thus explaining the heterogeneity observed in this study.

3. CLINICAL SIGNIFICANCE OF TUMOR HETEROGENEITY

The term 'heterogeneity' has yet to be defined operationally and may encompass several aspects of tumor biology. For example, heterogeneity may imply differences in tumors from one patient to another and may also imply the evolution of an individual patient's tumor over time. A more important issue relates to cellular heterogeneity within the patient's tumor. Here the definition of heterogeneity depends on the biological problem under study. For example, do we consider cellular differences at the level of cell surface markers, growth patterns, or chemosensitivity? That is, do we deal with heterogeneity of phenotypic behavior, or rather, should we approach heterogeneity at the cytogenetic level and consider chromosomal analysis to be the ultimate marker for differences between cell populations? Must we also quantitate such differences? Is it enough to consider that 1% of the cell population in a given patient's tumor may differ from the other 99%. Is this 'heterogeneity' or do we need to have larger differences that are more evenly divided among cell types? Finally, what is the clinical significance of the finding that a patient's tumor contains diverse cell populations if they are all equally sensitive to chemotherapeutic agents or radiation therapy? While it is likely that variations between individual tumors, tumor progression, cellular heterogeneity within individual tumors, and individual cellular differences all contribute to the concept of tumor heterogeneity, it seems to us that such heterogeneity is most relevant when it affects the clinical state of the patient; that is when cell populations are sufficiently different that therapy must be directed at all of the stemlines likely to yield populations resistant to the various forms of therapy. We believe this should be the operational definition of heterogeneity, at least with respect to the clinical care of patients. Other definitions apply to such aspects as cell surface markers, biochemical receptors, and of course to problems of identifying immunologically diverse cells and the reactions they induce within the patients. It is on the clinically important aspects of heterogeneity, however, that we shall now focus.

The fact that many cancers are composed of mixed populations of tumor cells with different growth properties is clearly of importance to the clinical investigation and management of neoplastic disease. Differential sensitivity of tumor subpopulations, already present before therapy, to different therapeutic modalities is undoubtedly a factor in resistance to therapy and recurrent disease. Non-curative therapy of any kind, including surgery, could be expected to affect the kinetics, and sensitivity to subsequent treatment, of the remaining tumor by changing the 'mix' and by upsetting the interactive balance (see above) among the subpopulations [73]. The simultaneous presence of drug sensitive and relatively drug insensitive subpopulations, prior to any selective pressure due to drug treatment, has been demonstrated in a number of tumors, including L1210 leukemia [74], human melanoma [39, 40], mouse methylcholanthrene-induce sarcoma [75, 76] rat hepatoma [77], mouse mammary carcinoma [78], mouse B16 melanoma [79], human colon carcinoma [42], human ovarian carcinoma [33], human lung cancer [41], and human glioma [70]. It is important to realize, however, that much of this work has been performed with cell lines, which especially in the case of the human studies, have been long removed from the patient.

The consequences of tumor heterogeneity to drug therapy may be multiple. Differential drug sensitivity, coupled with heterogeneous metastatic behavior, may be one explanation of the observed variation in drug sensitivity between primary tumors and their metastases, and vice versa [78, 80, 81]. Metastatic subpopulations of a single tumor line have also been shown to be differentially affected by drugs [33]. Lotan and Nicolson [79] found that B16 melanoma sublines which vary in metastatic capacity also vary in sensitivity *in vitro* to inhibition by retinoic acid. No correlations between metastatic behavior and drug sensitivity were seen. Thus, pharmacologic heterogeneity occurs between different metastases, as well as between metastases and their primaries.

Administration parameters of combination chemotherapy might also be affected by drug heterogeneity. Concurrent combination chemotherapy has been found to increase response frequency and remission duration over that seen with sequential chemotherapy in patients with metastatic breast cancer [82]. The fact that no difference in ultimate survival was seen between the two groups of patients [82] attests, in part, to the presence of cancer cells, both pre-existent and subsequent to therapy, resistant to drug therapy.

Response to therapeutic modalities other than cytoreductive drugs can also be affected by tumor heterogeneity. Leith *et al.* [83] have shown that mouse mammary tumor subpopulations are differentially sensitive to X-irradiation. The basis for this observation is due, in part, to a decreased ability of the cells to repair the radiation damage. The efficacy of immunotherapy is likewise subject to the heterogeneity of tumors. Heterogeneity in expression of tumor-associated antigens has been found among subpopulations of human osteogenic sarcoma [36], human melanoma [38] and mouse mammary cancer [5]. Differential ability of cells isolated from single tumors to immunize syngeneic hosts has been reported with methylocholanthrene-induced mouse and rat sarcomas [84, 85] and lymphomas [86], L1210 leukemia [87, 88], and mouse mammary tumors [31]. In the latter case, analysis of the patterns of cross-reactive immunogenicity among the subpopulations revealed both qualitative and quantitative differences in the effective expression of MMTV associated and 'unique' immunogens. Furthermore, immunization with one subpopulation can affect the response to another [30]. Thus, the immune response to tumors is complicated by their heterogeneity, and it is likely that efforts to modulate that immunity will be similarly complicated.

In addition to therapy, tumor heterogeneity poses a problem to other aspects of cancer treatment. For example, the development of *in vitro* or xenograft systems to predict drug sensitivity of individual patient's cancers can be expected to falter unless techniques are found to ensure a complete sampling of the entire tumor. Requiring the tumor cells to grow in dilute agar on in a nude mouse, thereby selecting for subpopulations capable to perform these feats, automatically introduces a bias in the test procedure in the direction of false positives since the tumor cells unable to grow under those conditions may also be insensitive to any given drug. Thus, one could predict that assays, such as that described by Salmon and co-workers [89], would be much better at predicting drug insensitivity rather than drug sensitivity. Similar considerations apply to attempts to detect cancer cells by assays for antigen or other marker production. This is particularly true in a 'monitoring' situation in which serial measurments are made during the course of therapy. A differential sensitivity of either marker positive or negative cells to therapy could greatly complicate the interpretation of results. The cophenomena of tumor heterogeneity and progression result in an unstable baseline upon which to chart neoplastic disease.

The above discussion has concentrated on the problems presented by tumor heterogeneity to clinical oncology. Understanding tumor heterogeneity, however, offers the possibility of developing new methods and strategies for ultimately more effective therapy than is currently available. It may someday be feasible to control tumor heterogeneity itself so that more homogeneous, hence predictable, targets will be available to treatment. To do this, more knowledge about the origin and maintenance of heterogeneity is necessary. If stem cell differentiation is an important mechanism in the origin of diversity, it may be possible to control the process with inducers of differentiation [42]. If growth interactions between tumor subpopulations are involved in the maintenance of heterogeneity, interruption of these interactions may disrupt the organization of the tumor and allow the therapist to dissect out the components with the various modalities available to him. Recognition of the unique characteristics of the invasive and metastatic subpopulations may allow for therapy to be focussed on the life threatening elements of the disease rather than on the more easily controlled, less malignant populations. Thus, the concept of tumor heterogeneity may not only be necessary to understanding the biology of cancer, but also lead to better ways to control neoplastic disease.

ACKNOWLEDGEMENTS

The authors' studies described in this review were supported by United States Public Health Service grants CA 27419, CA 08748, CA 25956, and by a grant from Concern Foundation.

REFERENCES

1. Pierce GB: Cellular heterogeneity of cancers. In: World symposium on model studies in chemical carcinogenesis, T'so POP, DiPaolo JA (eds), 1972, Vol B, pp 463–472.
2. Kobori O, Oota K: Neuroendocrine cells in serially passaged rat stomach cancers induced by MNNG. Int J Cancer 23:536–541, 1979.
3. Dunn T: Morphology of mammary tumors in mice. In: Pathophysiology of cancer (2nd edn), Homburger F, Fishman NH (eds). Paul B Hoeber, 1959, pp 32–84.
4. Henderson JS, Rous P: The plating of tumor components on the subcutaneous expanses of young mice. J Exp Med 115:1211–1229, 1962.
5. Dexter DL, Kowalski HM, Blazar BA, Fligiel Z, Vogel R, Heppner GH: Heterogeneity of tumor cells from a single mouse mammary tumor. Cancer Res 38:3174–3181, 1978.
6. Imada M, Sueoka N: Clonal sublines of rat neurotumor RT4 and cell differentiation. I. Isolation and characterization of cell lines and cell type conversion. Devel Biol 66:97–108, 1978.
7. Levan A, Hauschka TS: Endomitotic reduplication mechanisms in ascites tumors of the mouse. J Natl Cancer Inst 14:1–21, 1953.
8. Makino S: Further evidence favoring the concept of the stem cell in ascites tumors of rats. Ann NY Acad Sci 63:818–830, 1956.
9. Mitelman F: The chromosomes of fifty primary Rous rat sarcomas. Hereditas 69:155–186, 1971.
10. Becker FF, Klein KM, Wolman SR, Asofsky R, Sell S: Characterization of primary hepato-cellular carcinomas and initial transplant generations. Cancer Res 33:3330–3338, 1973.
11. Ishidate M, Aoshima M, Sakurai Y: Population changes of a rat leukemia by different routes of transplantation. J Natl Cancer Inst 53:773–781, 1974.
12. Nowell PC: The clonal evolution of tumor cell populations. Science 194:23–28, 1976.
13. Gray JM, Pierce GB: Relationship between growth rate and differentiation of melanoma *in vivo*. J Natl Cancer Inst 32:1201–1211, 1964.
14. Sluyser M, Evers SG, DeGoeij CCJ: Sex hormone receptors in mammary tumors of GR mice. Nature 263:386–389, 1976.
15. Klein G, Klein E: Conversion of solid neoplasms into ascites tumors. Ann NY Acad Sci 63:640–661, 1956.
16. Variani J, Orr W, Ward PA: A comparison of the migration patterns of normal and malignant cells in assay systems. Am J Pathol 90:159–171, 1978.
17. Fidler IJ, Kripke ML: Metastasis results from preexisting variant cells within a malignant tumor. Science 197:893–895, 1977.
18. Tao TW, Burger MM: Non-metastasizing variants selected from metastasizing melanoma cells. Nature 270:437–438, 1977.
19. Suzuki N, Withers HR, Koehler MW: Heterogeneity and variability of artificial lung colony forming ability among clones from mouse fibrosarcoma. Cancer Res 38:3349–3351, 1978.

20. Foulds L: Neoplastic development. New York: Academic Press, 1969, 1975, Vols 1 and 2.

21. Hager JC, Miller FR, Heppner GH: Influence of serial transplantation on the immunological-clinical correlates of BALB/cfC$_3$H mouse mammary tumors. Cancer Res 38:2492–2500, 1978.

22. Fialkow PJ: Clonal origin of human tumors. Biochim Biophys Acta 458:283–321, 1976.

23. Reddy AL, Fialkow PJ: Multicellular origin of fibrosarcomas in mice induced by the chemical carcinogen 3-methylcholanthrene. J Exp Med 150:878–887, 1979.

24. Pierce GB, Cox WJ: Neoplasms as caricatures of tissue renewal. In: Cell Differentiation and neopalsia, Saunders GF (ed.). New York: Raven Press, 1978, pp 57–66.

25. Mintz B: Genetic mosaicism and *in vivo* analyses of neoplasia and differentiation. In: Cell differentiation and neoplasia, Saunders GF (ed.). New York: Raven Press, 1978, pp 27–53.

26. Heppner GH: The challenge of tumor heterogeneity. In: Commentaries on research in breast disease, Bulbrook RD, Taylor DJ (eds). New York: Alan R Liss, 1979, pp 177–191.

27. Bennett DC, Peachey LA, Durbin H, Rudland PS: A possible mammary stem cell line. Cell 15:283–298, 1978.

28. Jansson B, Révész L: A deductive approach to the analysis of the growth of ascites tumor cell populations. In: Methods in cancer research, Busch H (ed.). New York: Academic Press, 1976, Vol XIII, pp 227–290.

29. Hauschka TS: Methods of conditioning the graft in tumor transplantation. J Natl Cancer Inst 14:723–736, 1953.

30. Heppner G, Miller B, Cooper DN, Miller FR: Growth interactions between mammary tumor cells. In: Systematics of mammary cell transformation. New York: Academic Press (in press).

31. Miller FR, Heppner GH: Immunologic heterogeneity of tumor cell subpopulations from a single mouse mammary tumor. J Natl Cancer Inst 63:1457–1464, 1979.

32. Baylin SB, Weisburger WR, Eggleston JC, Mendelsohn G, Beaven MA, Abeloff MD, Ettinger DS: Variable content of histaminase, L-DOPA decarboxylase and calcitonin in small-cell carcinoma of the lung. New Engl J Med 299:105–110, 1978.

33. Siracký J: An approach to the problem of heterogeneity of human tumour-cell populations. Br J Cancer 39:570–577, 1979.

34. Pertschuk LP, Tobin EH, Brigati DJ, Kin DS, Bloom ND, Gaetjens E, Berman PJ, Carter AC, Degenshein GA: Immunofluorescent detection of estrogen receptors in breast cancer. Cancer 41:907–911, 1978.

35. Lee SH: Cytochemical study of estrogen receptor in human mammary cancer. Am J Clin Pathol 70:197–203, 1978.

36. Byers VS, Johnston JO: Antigenic differences among osteogenic sarcoma tumor cells taken from different locations in human tumors. Cancer Res 37:3173–3183, 1977.

37. Rogan KM, Faldetta TJ, Boto W, Aiken JJ, DeMartino JL, Howe RC, Spiro RC, Humphreys RE: Heterogeneity in the membrane proteins of human lymphoid cell lines as seen in sodium dodecyl sulfate-polyacrylamide electrophoresis slab gels. Cancer Res 38:3604–3610, 1978.

38. Sorg C, Brügger J, Seibert E, Macher E: Membrane-associated antigens of human malignant melanoma IV: changes in expression of antigens on cultured melanoma cells. Cancer Immunol Immunother 3:259–271, 1978.

39. Barranco SC, Ho DHW, Drewinko B, Romsdahl MM, Humphrey RM: Differential sensitivities of human melanoma cells grown *in vitro* to arabinosylcytosine. Cancer Res 32:2733–2736, 1972.

40. Barranco SC, Drewinko B, Humphrey RM: Differential response by human melanoma cells to 1,3-bis-(2-chloroethyl)-1-nitrosourea and bleomycin. Mutation Res 19:277–280, 1973.

41. Chu MY: Tumor cell heterogeneity in human lung carcinoma. Proc AACR 20:151, 1979.
42. Calabresi P, Dexter DL, Heppner GH: Clinical and pharmacological implications of cancer cell differentiation and heterogeneity. Biochem Pharmacol 28:1933–1941, 1979.
43. Woods LK, Morgan RT, Quinn LA, Moore GE, Semple TU, Stedman KE: Comparison of four new cell lines from patients with adenocarcinoma of the ovary. Cancer Res 39:4449–4459, 1979.
44. Hagemeijer A, Hoehn W, Smit EME: Cytogenetic analysis of human renal carcinoma cell lines of common origin (NC 65). Cancer Res 29:4662–4667, 1979.
45. Andreeff M, Beck JD, Kapoor N, Steinmetz J, Melamed MR, Gee T, Miller D, Clarkson B: Clonal evolution in acute leukemia: analysis of subpopulations by velocity sedimentation and multiple markers. Proc AACR 20:112, 1979.
46. Testa JR, Mintz U, Rowley JD, Vardiman JW, Golomb HM: Evolution of karyotypes in acute nonlymphocytic leukemia. Cancer Res 39:3619–3627, 1979.
47. Morse H, Hays T, Peakman D, Rose B, Robinson A: Acute nonlymphoblastic leukemia in childhood. Cancer 44:164–170, 1979.
48. Hoshino T, Wilson CB: Cell kinetic analyses of human malignant brain tumors (gliomas). Cancer 44:956–962, 1979.
49. Rubinstein LJ: Current concepts in neuro-oncology. In: Advances in neurology, Thompson RA, Green JR (eds). New York: Raven Press, 1976, Vol 15, pp 1–25.
50. Russell DS, Rubinstein LJ: Pathology of tumors of the nervous system (4th ed). Baltimore: Williams & Wilkins, 1977.
51. Feigin I, Arlen LB, Lipkin L, Gross SW: The endothelial hyperplasia of the cerebral blood vessels with brain tumors, and its sarcomatous transformation. Cancer 11:264–277, 1958.
52. Shapiro WR, Basler GA: Chemotherapy of human brain tumors transplanted into nude mice, International symposium on multidisciplinary aspects of brain tumor therapy. Brescia, Italy, June, 1979.
53. Shapiro WR, Basler GA, Chernik NL, Posner JB: Human brain tumor transplantation into nude mice. J Natl Cancer Inst 62:447–453, 1979.
54. Chen TT, Mealey J: Effect of corticosteroid on protein and nucleotide synthesis in human glial tumors cells. Cancer Res 33:1721–1723, 1973.
55. Manuelidis EE: Long-term tissue culture lines of intracranal tumors. J Neurosurg 22:368–373, 1965.
56. Manuelidis EE: Experiments with tissue culture and heterologous transplantation of tumors. Ann NY Acad Sci 159:409–431, 1969.
57. Manuelidis L, Manuelidis EE: Cholera toxin-peroxidase: changes in surface labeling of glioblastoma cells with increased time in tissue culture. Science 193:588-590, 1976.
58. Ponten J, MacIntyre EH: Long term culture of normal and neoplastic human glia. Acta Pathol Microbiol Scand 74: 465–486, 1968.
59. Ponten J, Westermark B, Hugosson R: Regulation of proliferation and movement of human glia-like cells in culture. Exp Cell Res 58:393–400, 1969.
60. Ponten J: Neoplastic human glia cells in culture. In: Human tumor cells in vitro, Fogh J (ed.). New York: Plenum Press, 1975, pp 175–206.
61. MacIntyre EH, Grimes RA, Vatter AE: Cytology and growth characteristics of human astrocytes transformed by Rous sarcoma virus. J Cell Sci 5:583–602, 1969.
62. MacIntyre EH, Ponten J, Vatter AE: Fine structure of human glial cells in tissue culture. Fed Proc 28:754, 1969.
63. Perkins J, MacIntyre EH, Riley WD, Clark RB: Adenyl cyclase, phosphodiesterase and cyclic AMP-dependent protein kinase of malignant glial cells in culture. Life Sci 10:1069–1080, 1971.

64. Westermark B, Ponten J, Hugosson R: Determinants for the establishment of permanent tissue culture lines from human gliomas. Acta Pathol Scand Sect A 81:791–805, 1973.

65. Westermark B: The deficient density-dependent growth control of human malignant glioma cells and virus-transformed glia-like cells in culture. Int J Cancer 12:438–451, 1973.

66. Lindgren A, Westermark B, Ponten J: Serum stimulation of stationary human glia and glioma cells in culture. Exp Cell Res 95:311–319, 1975.

67. Maunoury R, Delpech A, Delpech B, Virard MN, Vedrenne C: Presence of neurospecific antigen NSA 1 in fetal human astrocytes in long-term cultures. Brain Res 112:383–387, 1976.

68. Levan A, Fredga K, Sandberg A: Nomenclature for centromeric position on chromosomes. Hereditas 55:28–38, 1966.

69. Rankin JK: In preparation.

70. Shapiro WR, Rankin JK, Yung WA, Basler GA: Heterogeneity of chemotherapy in nude mice and *in vitro* clones of human gliomas. Cancer Treatment Rep (in press).

71. Mark J: Chromosomal characteristics of neurogenic tumours in adults. Hereditas 68:61–100, 1971.

72. Rankin JK: In preparation.

73. Schiffer LM, Braunschweiger PG, Stragand JJ: Tumor cell population kinetics following noncurative treatment. In: Antibiotics and chemotherapy, Schonfeld H (ed.). Basle: S Karger, 1978, pp 148–156.

74. Law L: Origin of the resistance of leukemic cells to folic acid antagonists. Nature 169:628–629, 1952.

75. Hakansson L, Tropé C: On the presence within tumors of clones that differ in sensitivity to cytostatic drugs. Acta Path Microbiol Scand Section A, 82:35–40, 1974.

76. Hakansson L, Tropé C: Cell clones with different sensitivity to cytostatic drugs in methyl-cholanthrene-induced mouse sarcomas. Acta Path Microbiol Scand Sect A, 82:41–47, 1974.

77. Barranco SC, Haenelt BR, Gee EL: Differential sensitivities of five rat hepatoma cell lines to anticancer drugs. Cancer Res 38:656–660, 1978.

78. Heppner GH, Dexter DL, DeNucci T, Miller FR, Calabresi P: Heterogeneity in drug sensitivity among tumor cell subpopulations of a single mammary tumor. Cancer Res 38:3758–3763, 1978.

79. Lotan R, Nicolson GL: Heterogeneity in growth inhibition by β-trans-retinoic acid of metastatic B16 melanoma clones and *in vivo*-selected cell variant lines. Cancer Res 39:4767–4771, 1979.

80. Schabel FM, Jr: Concepts for systemic treatment of micrometastases. Cancer 35:15–24, 1975.

81. Fugmann RA, Anderson JC, Stolfi RL, Martin DS: Comparison of adjuvant chemotherapeutic activity against primary and metastatic spontaneous murine tumors. Cancer Res 37:496–500, 1977.

82. Chlebowski RT, Irwin LE, Pugh RP, Sadoff L, Hestorff R, Wienes JM, Bateman JR: Survival of patients with metastatic breast cancer treated with either combination or sequential chemotherapy. Cancer Res 39:4503–4506, 1979.

83. Leith JT, Zeman EM, Glicksman AS, Heppner GH: Differential response of tumor cell populations to ionizing radiation. Radiat Res, (In Press).

84. Prehn RT: Analysis of antigenic heterogeneity within individual 3-methylcholanthrene-induced mouse sarcomas. J Natl Cancer Inst 45:1039–1045, 1970.

85. Pimm MV, Baldwin RW: Antigenic differences between primary methylcholanthrene-induced rat sarcomas and post-surgical recurrences. Int J Cancer 20:37–43, 1977.

86. Schirrmacher V, Bosslet K, Shantz G, Clauer K, Hubsch D: Tumor metastases and cell-mediated immunity in a model system in DBA/2 mice. IV. Antigenic differences between a metastasizing variant and the parental tumor line revealed by cytotoxic T lymphocytes. Int J Cancer 23:245–252, 1979.
87. Fuji H, Mihich E, Pressman D: Differential tumor immunogenicity of L1210 and its sublines. J Immunol 119:983–986, 1977.
88. Killion JJ:Immunotherapy with tumor cell subpopulations. Cancer Immunol Immunother 4:115–119, 1978.
89. Salmon SE, Hamburger AW, Soehnlen B, Durie BG, Alberts DS, Moon TE: Quantitation of differential sensitivity of human-tumor stem cells to anticancer drugs. N Engl J Med 298:1321–1327, 1978.

5. Biological Markers of the Tumors of the Central Nervous System

JEROME SEIDENFELD and LAURENCE J. MARTON

1. INTRODUCTION

The concept of biochemical tumor markers began with Warburg's research on the differences in enzymatic activities between normal and neoplastic tissues from the same organ [1]. His observation that rates of aerobic glycolysis were higher for tumor tissue than for normal, nongrowing tissue was subsequently shown to depend on the degree of differentiation of the tumor [2]. Other enzymatic differences between cancer and normal cells have been reported and were reviewed recently by Weber [2]. Such intracellular differences might be reflected in alterations of the activities of specific enzymes or concentrations of specific biomolecules in physiological fluids. Because the cerebrospinal fluid (CSF) is most directly in contact with central nervous system (CNS) tissue, and because the existence of a blood–brain barrier has long been known, metabolic changes associated with neoplasms of the CNS may be observed earlier and to a greater degree in CSF than in other physiological fluids such as urine or serum. Nevertheless, several published studies on CNS tumor markers in serum and/or urine will be included in this review.

Biochemical markers of tumors have been defined [3, 4] as any substance whose presence or elevation above normal concentrations correlates with the presence of a tumor. A perfect tumor marker would be present or elevated in all tumor patients and would be absent or within the normal range of concentrations in all patients without tumor. No such ideal marker exists, but we can assess which, if any, of several less-than-perfect markers of brain tumors can be used to aid in the diagnosis and management of patients harboring CNS neoplasia. We will first describe an approach to the evaluation of the clinical utility of laboratory tests suggested by Galen and Gambino [5], and then discuss the potential uses for markers of CNS tumors. The extensive literature on clinical studies. of biochemical markers of CNS tumors and

G. B. Humphrey et al. (eds.), Pediatric oncology 1, 117–163. All rights reserved.
Copyright © 1981 Martinus Nijhoff Publishers bv, The Hague/Boston/London.

some of the methods used for their measurement will then be reviewed. Markers have been subdivided into three groups: enzymes, small biomole- cules, and immunological markers.

2. AN APPROACH TO EVALUATING THE CLINICAL UTILITY
OF LABORATORY TESTS

Galen and Gambino have published criteria for evaluating clinical laborato- ry tests used for diagnosis and screening [5]. They define four parameters: *Sensitivity,* a measure of positivity in disease, is the fraction of patients with the disease giving positive test results. *Specificity,* a measure of positivity in health, is the fraction of individuals free of the disease giving negative test results. The *predictive value* of a positive result—the major determinant of clinical utility—is the fraction of all positive results obtained that are correct. *Efficiency* is the fraction of all results that are correct. One can also calculate a predictive value for a negative result from the fraction of all negative results obtained that are correct, but this parameter is generally in a more acceptible range than the predictive value of a positive result, and is thus of less critical importance.

The first two of the parameters can be calculated directly from results obtained in a clinical study. In practice, preliminary studies are used to establish a cut-off value for a positive test result, which is set usually at greater than two standard deviations above the mean for a reference group. Measurements are then made in a substantially larger population of individ- uals. Data can then be divided into four categories: true positives, true negatives, false positives, and false negatives. Sensitivity is the ratio of true positives to the sum of true positives plus false negatives, and specificity is the ratio of true negatives to the sum of true negatives plus false positives.

The second two parameters cannot be calculated directly from the results of a clinical study because they depend on the prevalence of the disease in the population being tested. When a clinical laboratory test is applied to a large segment of the population, many more healthy individuals will be tested than usually found in the average preliminary clinical study; while the percentage of false positives may remain the same, the absolute number certainly will increase greatly when a test is applied to a broad population. The predictive value of a positive result must be calculated from the numbers obtained in actual use of the test, rather than from the more limited data provided by preliminary clinical studies. The same is true for efficiency. In practice, some arbitrary, large number of subjects to be tested is chosen. The product of the disease's prevalence and the total number of subjects gives the number of patients suffering from the disease, while the remainder of those tested will

Table 1. Methods for calculating the four parameters of Galen and Gambino.

From the data of a clinical study:

Sensitivity = true positives/(true positives + false negatives)
Specificity = true negatives/(true negatives + false positives)

From prevalence and an assumed total subject population:

	No. of subjects Giving positive test results	No. of subjects Giving negative test results	Totals
No. of subjects with disease	True positives (sensitivity × all subjects with disease)	False negatives (all subjects with disease − true positives)	All subjects with disease (prevalence × all subjects tested)
No. of subjects without disease	False positives (all subjects without disease − true negatives)	True negatives (specificity × all subjects without disease)	All subjects without disease (all subjects tested − all subjects with disease)
Totals	All positives (true positives + false positives)	All negatives (false negatives + true positives)	All subjects tested

Predictive value = true positives/all positives.
Efficiency = (true positives + true negatives)/all subjects tested.

be free of the disease. To find the number of true positives in actual use of the test, sensitivity is multiplied by the number of patients with the disease. The difference between this product and the total number of patients with the disease is equal to the number of false negative results that would be obtained in actual use of the test. Similarly, the product of specificity times the total number of disease-free patients gives the number of true negatives, and the difference between all disease-free patients and true negatives gives the total number of false positives. Predictive value is then calculated as the ratio of true positives to the sum of true positives plus false positives, while efficiency is the ratio of the sum of true positives plus true negatives to the total number of subjects tested. Table 1 summarizes the methods used to calculate these parameters. When sufficient data are available, we will apply this predictive value model to evaluate the potential clinical utility of the CNS tumor markers reviewed here.

The sensitivity and specificity of a given test depends on a chosen cut-off point or referent value [6]. Raising the cut-off improves the specificity at the expense of decreased sensitivity, while lowering the referent value will have the opposite effect. Thus for a given test, sensitivity and specificity must be balanced to maximize predictive value. As Galen has pointed out [6], many tests show improved specificity if a series of referent values that are related to the age, sex, or other factors of the subject being tested are used in place of a single cut-off point. For instance, a marker whose concentration in serum increases with the age of the subject will provide more false positives among older test subjects unless a set of age-related referent values are used.

The predictive value of a positive result strongly depends on the prevalence of the disease being tested in the population. Consider the predictive value of a test with 95% sensitivity and 95% specificity used 1) to screen for a disease with a prevalence of 10,000 cases per 100,000 individuals and 2) for a disease with a prevalence of only 1000 cases per 100,000 subjects. In the first case, the test would has a predictive value of 68% for a positive result, while in the second case the predictive value declines to 16%. More dramatically, the predictive value for the same test drops to 2% if used to test for a disease with a prevalence of 100 in 100,000 individuals: there would be 98 false positives for every two patients found suffering from the disease.

If there are a number of markers available to test for a given disease, multiple marker tests that will have better predictive value than the individual markers used may be designed. If two markers were measured simultaneously on all subjects, the criterion for a positive test could be set as either an elevation of one marker or elevations for both markers. The first approach would result in a very sensitive test that has a large number of false positives; the second would lead to an increased specificity but would carry with it a loss of sensitivity. Measurement of the two markers in sequence, with the second determation made only for those subjects giving positive results with the first marker, is a better approach. A preliminary screen with a very sensitive test would eliminate the majority of disease-free individuals without missing many of those harboring the disease. A second test that was fairly specific would eliminate most of the false positives obtained with the first screen, but only if the second test were used for individuals who gave positive results with the preliminary screen. If the second test were applied to all patients, almost as many new false positives would be added as were eliminated.

3. POTENTIAL USES FOR CNS TUMOR MARKERS

We have previously proposed four uses for CSF markers of brain tumors [7, 8]: 1) screening, 2) diagnosis, 3) long-term evaluation of tumor growth, and 4) short-term evaluation of the efficacy of a specific mode of therapy. For the purpose of this review, we would like to further subdivide diagnosis into two separate categories. The first is the determination of whether or not a patient with a given set of symptoms has a CNS tumor, and the second is the classification and grading of a tumor already known to be present. We will examine each of the five areas in turn to establish criteria with which the potential utility of individual biochemical markers can be judged.

3.1. Screening for Brain Tumors

It is assumed that a screening test for a particular disease would be used for the whole of the general population, and would be performed for each person whether or not they exhibited symptoms of the disease. It is obvious that a diagnostic test based on CSF markers could never be used in this way. Lumbar puncture, which is necessary for obtaining CSF, would not be routinely submitted to by individuals who felt themselves to be in good health. Moreover, lumbar puncture of a patient who may harbor brain tumor risks herniation if a tumor is present. Lumbar puncture should only be undertaken by neurologists or neurosurgeons trained to expect and capable of dealing with all eventualities.

Let us assume, however, that obtaining CSF from a normal population was not a problem, or that we could develop a screening test for CNS tumors using markers in serum or urine. If the predictive value model of Galen and Gambino[5] is applied to such a screening test, the test is of no value. Calculation of the predictive value of a test with an assumed sensitivity of 90%, an assumed specificity of 90%, and an estimated prevalence of brain tumors in the general population of 4.5 cases per 100,000 individuals would be 0.04%. Only four out of every 10,000 subjects with positive results would really have a CNS tumor. For a next-to-perfect test with sensitivity and specificity both equal to 99%, the predictive value would only rise to 0.44% for a disease with an incidence of only 4.5 cases per 100,000 individuals. The only direct effect of instituting a mass screening program for CNS tumors would be to overload the diagnostic facilities of neurology and neurosurgery departments. Screening for brain tumors in CSF is thus an undesirable as well as unrealistic goal, unless a test with both 100% sensitivity and 100% specificity were available. (Such a test could be based on the presence or absence of a tumor-specific antigen.) A screening test for CNS tumors might also be useful if multiple markers were used.

3.2. Determination of Presence or Absence of CNS Tumors

Limiting our test population to patients referred to neurologists or neurosurgeons with one or more of a well-defined group of symptoms or complaints that point to the possibility of a CNS tumor greatly improves our testing capability. A variety of methods including pneumoencephalography, angiography, isotope scans, computerized axial tomography, and histological examination of biopsy tissue are used for diagnosis; some of these procedures entail greater risk to the patient than lumbar puncture. A test based on the measurement of a CSF biochemical marker that has sufficient sensitivity and specificity could be used to rule out CNS tumors in many of the symptomatic patients. In addition, diagnostic tests based on radiologic visualization of the tumor are limited by a minimum detectable tumor size. A marker-based test may be able to detect tumors at an earlier stage in their growth than is now possible.

The predictive value model of Galen and Gambino[5] can be applied if there is available an estimate of the prevalence of CNS tumors in the population of patients suspected of harboring CNS tumors. No data about the prevalence of tumors in this population are available, and must be gathered. A set of symptoms that leads to a suspected diagnosis of CNS tumor must be defined. One list of the early symptoms of brain tumors has been published[9], which could serve as the starting point for compilation of a more complete set. Data must be accumulated over a number of years before a statistically valid estimate of prevalence of tumors in neurological patients can be made. As a conservative estimate, let us assume that 25% of symptomatic patients actually harbor a tumor. In this case, a test with 90% sensitivity and 90% specificity would have a predictive value of 75% for a positive result.

Such a test would be used to distinguish between patients with a particular tumor and patients who in all likelihood have some other neurologic disorder. To evaluate the test, data are required about the number of positive results obtained when the test is used in patients with neurologic disorders that share symptoms with CNS neoplasia. The specificity of a diagnostic test for CNS tumors in patients with other neurologic diseases will no doubt be somewhat lower than the specificity of the same test in a completely healthy population. If an accurate assessment of the test's clinical utility is to be made, the predictive value must be evaluated using the specificity of the test in the population of symptomatic patients.

3.3 Classifying and Grading CNS Tumors

Currently the most reliable method of classifying CNS tumors is histologic examination of biopsy specimens of surgically-removed tumor tissue. Many CNS tumors are located in regions of the brain that cannot be biopsied. A classification test for CNS tumors based on one or more biochemical markers in physiological fluids would alleviate this problem. Data relating type and grade of CNS tumor to the degree of elevation of specific markers must be obtained to construct this test. Some data of this nature are currently available; no data are available regarding mutiple marker determinations on single patients. It is possible that predictions regarding the type of CNS tumor a particular patient is suffering from can be made reliably by examining which of several CSF markers are elevated. A second possible approach would grade tumors by the magnitude of elevation of one or more of the CSF markers. If data were available, a grading test could be evaluated using the predictive value model of Galen and Gambino [5]. Each proposed predictive test would have to be evaluated independently for each type or grade of CNS tumor. It is entirely possible that different types of CNS tumors could be identified using different biochemical markers. It seems equally probable that a grading test will be based on quantitative differences in the degree of elevation of the marker(s) most reliable for a given tumor. At the present time, however, none of the markers reviewed here is a reliable replacement for, or even an adjunct to, histological examination of biopsied tumor tissue.

3.4. Long-Term Evaluation of Tumor Growth

Markers of CNS tumors may predict a decline in the clinical status of a patient, secondary to tumor regrowth, earlier and more reliably than currently available methods. Studies investigating the potential of various markers for this application depend on periodic serial determination of the marker levels in patients who have been or are currently being treated for CNS tumors. Absolute values of marker levels are not as important as changes in marker levels. Positive predictions for a marker elevated in tumor tissue include an increase in marker level accompanied by a decline in clinical status, a decrease in marker level accompanied by an improvement in clinical status, or no change in marker level accompanied by no change in clinical status. Negative, or incorrect, predictions are made when the converse of each of the above results are obtained. For markers whose levels are lower in tumor patients than in nontumor patients, this entire situation is reversed.

The sensitivity of a marker for this function can be defined as the percentage of changes in clinical status predicted correctly, i.e., the sum of the correctly predicted improvements and the correctly predicted declines divided by the total number of observed changes in clinical status. The specificity of a marker as a predictor of change in clinical status would be equal to the number of correctly predicted 'no change' results divided by the total number of no changes observed. The predictive value could be calculated as the ratio of correct predictions of change in clinical status to total number of changes predicted, while the efficiency could be calculated from the ratio of total number of correct predictions to total number of determinations.

Studies designed to evaluate the potential utility of marker determinations for such long-term predictive functions are made difficult by several factors. First, a true evaluation of change or no change in clinical status of a CNS tumor patient is, as yet, difficult to achieve infallibly. Second is the problem of obtaining fluid samples from patients who have already been discharged from the hospital. A third difficulty is posed by setting a maximum time limit within which a predicted change must occur in order for the prediction to be considered a positive one. Once sufficient data have been accumulated, however, one can determine the utility of changes in marker levels as predictors of change in clinical status by examining these changes in terms of the predictive model.

3.5. Short-Term Evaluation of the Efficacy of Therapy

When dealing with patients harboring tumors that result in short life expectancies, it is crucial to evaluate the efficacy of a particular mode of therapy within several days of administration of therapy. To evaluate the use of markers for predicting the efficacy of therapy, marker levels must be determined before therapy and then serially after therapy. Because most of the markers discussed here are produced intracellularly, and because chemotherapy or radiation therapy destroys tumor cells and causes the release of their contents into the extracellular fluid, marker levels should be transiently elevated after successful therapy; fewer tumor cells are left to produce the marker after cells have been killed by some mode of therapy. Patients who respond to therapy and show a spike in marker level and patients who do not respond to therapy and show no spike in marker levels are true predictors for the marker. The unavailability of patients for follow-up lumbar punctures, and the relatively high risk of multiple lumbar punctures, has made studies of this type almost impossible to conduct with CSF markers.

4. ENZYMATIC MARKERS OF CNS TUMORS

4.1. Lactate Dehydrogenase (E.C.1.1.1.27)

Since Warburg's initial report [1] of metabolic differences between tumor tissue and normal, nongrowing tissue from the same organ, it has been shown that the intracellular lactate dehydrogenase (LDH) activity of both human and experimental brain tumor cells is higher than that of normal brain tissue [10–14]. Assuming that the increased LDH activity is a result of an increase in the intracellular concentration of the enzyme, it would be reflected by a concommitant increase in the concentration of this enzyme in the extracellular fluid, even if the membranes of tumor cells were of no greater permeability to LDH molecules, or to proteins in general, than the membranes of normal brain cells.

LDH exists in five molecular forms [15, 16], all of which are tetramers of two different subunits in varying ratios. They can be separated by several different electrophorectic techniques (to be discussed below). As suggested by the Subcommittee on Isoenzymes of the International Union of Biochemistry, the isoenzyme that moves fastest during electrophoresis at pH 8.6—the most anodic isoenzyme—is designated as LDH-1, while the least mobile isoenzyme is designated LDH-5. All four subunits of LDH-1, referred to as the heart isoenzyme because it is the predominant subunit found in heart tissue, are identical. A number of studies have investigated the possibility that the increase in LDH activity in the CSF of patients with CNS tumors is accompanied by a shift in the CSF LDH isoenzyme distribution. Goldman et al. [11] have suggested that the shift of isoenzyme distribution from LDH-1 to LDH-5 in tumor tissue occurs because LDH-5—or muscle LDH—more actively converts pyruvate to lactate at elevated concentrations of pyruvate with the result that more nicotinamide adenine dinucleotide (NAD) is produced by LDH-5 than LDH-1. Undifferentiated tumor cells with increased glycolytic metabolism would require increased amounts of NAD for the oxidation of triosephosphate. An intracellular shift in LDH isoenzyme distribution should produce a shift of LDH isoenzymes in CSF.

Several methods have been used to determine the total LDH activity in physiological fluids such as CSF and serum. Most are based on the decrease in optical density at 340 nm of a solution of reduced nicotinamideadenine dinucleotide (NADH) that results from the oxidation of NADH in the presence of LDH and sodium pyruvate [17–20]. There are slight differences in methodology with regard to the buffers, the concentrations of the various reagents, the volume of CSF or serum, and the length of time the reaction mixture is allowed to stand before initiating the enzymatic reaction by addition of pyruvate. However, the results obtained with one method can be compared to results obtained with a second method as long as the results are reported in the same units. Unfortunately, this is not always done. Several different units have been used to report LDH activity. Currently, the most acceptable form is the International Unit (i.u.), defined as micromoles of substrate converted to product per minute per liter of serum or CSF [21]. Earlier investigations defined one unit of LDH activity as the quantity of the enzyme that would cause a decrease in optical density of 1×10^{-3} per minute per milliter of CSF or serum [17, 20]. These two units can be interconverted because one i.u. is equal to two optical density units [20].

The second major method used to measure LDH activity is based on colorimetry [22, 23]. One unit of LDH activity is defined as the amount of enzyme that would oxidize 1.0 μmole of lactate in one hour; units are usually reported per 100 ml of CSF. Multiplication of the value in colorimetric units by the conversion factor 2/3 converts them into i.u.'s [20].

LDH isoenzymes can be separated using electrophoresis in both agar gel [24, 25] and polyacrylamide gel [26]. Sano et al. [24] visualized the five LDH isoenzymes after electrophoresis on agar gel by staining the plates with nitroblue tetrazolium. Each isoenzyme was quantitated by densitometry at 520 nm, and activity of each was expressed as a fraction of the total activity.

Rabow and Kristenssen [25] used a scanning technique to estimate the ratios of LDH isoenzymes that were separated by agarose gel electrophoresis. Finally, Cunningham et al. [26], followed polyacrylamide gel electrophoresis with staining of the gel with MTT—a purple formazan dye—and quantitated the individual isoenzymes by densitometry (489 nm).

Wroblewski et al. [27] and Fleisher et al. [28] first compared CSF levels of LDH activity in patients with brain tumor to levels found in patients with other neurological diseases. An interesting aspect of the data presented in the former study and not commented on by the authors is that all three patients with primary brain tumors had CSF LDH levels below the defined cutoff point. Hain and Nutter [29] and Spolter and Thompson [30] reported a linear increase in LDH activity in the CSF of normal subjects up to age 70, which points to the necessity of using age-related normal levels for CSF LDH measurements to decide which values are elevated and which are not. One study [19] included a comparison of CSF obtained by lumbar puncture to that obtained after pneumoencephalography, which showed that samples obtained after air studies contained unpredictably elevated levels of enzyme activities.

Conflicting data on the LDH activity in the CSF of brain tumor and other neurological patients have been found. Some authors [19, 27, 31] report elevated CSF LDH levels for both brain tumor patients and patients with cerebrovascular accidents (CVA), while others [21, 32] found increases for patients with CNS tumors but not for patients who had CVA. A third group [20, 28] noted that increased CSF levels of LDH correlated with cases of CVA but not with CNS tumors. Among authors who did not examine cases of CVA, some [33–37] found increased LDH activity in the CSF correlated with brain tumors, while others [38–42] did not.

The proposed utility of measurements of LDH activity in CSF as a marker of CNS tumors can be grouped into four categories: a) useful for both primary and secondary CNS tumors [19, 31–33, 35, 37]; b) useful for primary brain tumors only [21]; c) useful for secondary intracranial metastases only [27, 34]; d) useful for neither primary nor secondary CNS tumors [20, 25, 28, 36, 38–44]. Among the non-neoplastic neurologic diseases reported to result in elevated levels of LDH activity in CSF were acute meningitis [20, 27, 31, 32], head injuries [28], degenerative CNS diseases [28, 30], convulsive disorders [28], hydrocephalus and brain abscess [37], subarachnoid hemorrhage [32], as well as CVA [19, 20, 27, 28, 31].

Although a great deal of work has been done on LDH isoenzyme distribution of brain tumor tissue [12–14], very few clinical studies of LDH isoenzyme distribution in CSF have been reported. Cunningham et al. [26] showed that fractions of LDH-2 and LDH-3 were significantly increased relative to normal controls in patients with organic structural damage to brain tissue;

they did not separate CNS tumors from other neurological diseases. Sano *et al.* [24] compared the LDH isoenzyme distribution in the CSF of 33 patients harboring brain tumor to the distributions found in CSF samples from a group of normal controls. Patients harboring glioma were characterized by a decrease in the LDH-1 fraction and marked increases of LDH-4 and LDH-5. Patients with benign intracranial tumors, on the other hand, had LDH isoenzyme distributions indistinguishable from those of the control group. Heller *et al.* [39] also reported finding differences between the LDH isoenzyme distributions of CSF samples from patients with malignant CNS tumors and patients with benign tumors. Gobiet [40], on the other hand, found no such differences in his study of 16 patients with gliomas, 26 normal controls, and 32 patients with other neurologic diseases. Finally, Rabow and Kristensson [25], reported no differences in LDH isoenzyme distribution for different types of tumor, agreeing with the findings of Gobiet [40] and not with those of Cunningham *et al.* [26] and Sano *et al.* [24].

There have been many studies of LDH activity and isoenzyme distribution in serum and/or plasma. These studies will not, however, be included in this review because elevations of serum LDH occur in many diseases other than CNS tumors. Serum LDH would not be a clinically useful marker of CNS tumors. Buckell *et al.* [45] studied the LDH activity and isoenzyme distribution of cerebral cyst fluids. They reported significant elevations of total LDH activity and of the LDH-5 isoenzyme in fluids from patients with malignant, but not benign, tumors. Patients with metastatic tumors had the highest elevations. However, because cerebral cyst fluid is most often obtained at biopsy, it is unclear what measurement of LDH in this fluid can add to histological examination of tissue samples obtained by the same procedure.

No data are available regarding changes in LDH activity in the CSF of patients with CNS tumors as a function of clinical status or of treatment. While much work has been done on the potential usefulness of LDH isoenzyme distributions of brain tumor tissue for classifying and staging CNS tumors, almost none of the investigations of total LDH activity in CSF have separated the data they presented by tumor types or grades. As a result, only the second function of Section 3, determination of presence or absence of a CNS tumor in patients that have an unknown organic CNS disease, can be evaluated for LDH.

Table 2 summarizes the data reviewed above. Data have been included only from those studies that gave CSF-LDH values for individual patients. Because we are interested in the possibility of using CSF-LDH levels to diagnose CNS tumors in patients who do show some signs of organic CNS disfunction, no data for normal populations are included in this table. For each study included, a positive result is a value for CSF-LDH activity greater than the mean plus two standard deviations for the normal population studied

Table 2. Collated data for LDH as a marker of CNS tumors.

Reference	True positives	False negatives	True negatives	False positives	Criteria for positive results and units
19	11	0	10	27	98 μm/hr/100 cm^3
20	8	5	39	37	12.4 μ (1 μ = 1/3 O.D. unit)
21	5	4	8	0	20 International Units
28	5	15	45	48	1.75 μm/hr/cm^3
29	3	5	78	21	Mean + 2 S.D. for age group
31	34	1	3	5	40 O.D. units/cm^3
32	31	5	84	22	40 O.D. units/cm^3
33	16	0	0	0	98 μm/hr/100 cm^3
34	18	18	0	0	32.9 O.D. units/cm^3
35	52	13	0	0	0.54 Bucher Units
36	11	21	0	0	40 O.D. units/cm^3
39	11	6	0	0	64 μ
42	18	22	0	0	40 O.D. units/cm^3
Totals	223	115	267	160	

Sensitivity = 223/223 + 115 = 66%
Specificity = 267/267 + 160 = 62.5%

by the same investigators. A negative result is a CSF-LDH level below this value. True positives include patients with confirmed primary or secondary CNS tumors whose CSF gave a positive result, while false negatives are those patients with confirmed tumors who gave negative results. True negatives include all patients with some CNS disease other than a tumor who had a CSF-LDH level less than the referent value, while false positives are neurologic patients that had elevated levels of LDH in their CSF. Studies excluded from this tabulation presented their data only in the form of mean values for each group of patients investigated without giving either individual values or the number of patients in each disease group above and below their referent value.

Table 3. Calculation of predictive value and efficiency of LDH as a marker of CNS tumors [1].

	No. with + test	No. with - test	Totals
Brain tumor	165	85	250
No brain tumor	291.25	468.75	750
Totals	446.25	553.75	1000

Predictive value = 165/446.25 = 37%
Efficiency = (165 + 468.75)/1000 = 63.4%

[1] Based on an assumed prevalence of 25% and the sensitivity and specificity of Table 2.

The totals in each column of Table 2 have been used to calculate the sensitivity (66%) and specificity (62.5%) of CSF levels of LDH in the diagnosis of CNS tumors, as shown at the bottom of the table. Using these values and the assumed prevalence of CNS tumors in the population discussed above, we have evaluated LDH determination in CSF as a marker of CNS tumors by the methods of Galen and Gambino[5] (Table 3). We find a predictive value for a positive result of 37% and an efficiency of 63.4%. From these calculations we conclude that LDH activity of CSF is not a very reliable marker for use in the diagnosis of CNS tumors.

4.2. Aspartate Aminotransferase (E.C.2.6.1.1.)

This enzyme, formerly called glutamic-oxaloacetic transaminase (GOT) is also called aspartate transaminase. In the overwhelming majority of studies of its activity in spinal fluid, it is referred to as GOT. We will retain this usage in this review.

Investigations of changes in the activity of CSF GOT grew out of the early work on serum levels of this enzyme in patients with myocardial infarction or liver damage. No changes in serum levels of GOT were found after cerebrovascular accidents[46]; it was hypothesized that intracellular enzymes released from damaged cells after cerebral infarction would be kept out of the serum by the blood-brain barrier, and would accumulate in the CSF. Several groups of investigators began studying variations in the level of GOT activity of CSF associated with a variety of neurologic diseases[19, 28, 33, 46–48], including CNS tumors.

The most frequently used method of measuring GOT activity in physiological fluids is that of Karmen et al. [49, 50], which is based on the GOT-catalyzed reaction of α-ketoglutarate with asparate to form glutamate and oxaloacetate. The oxaloacetate formed is then reduced by NADH in a reaction catalyzed by an excess of malic dehydrogenase. The reaction is followed spectrophotometrically at 340 nm, and actually measures the rate of disappearance of NADH. One Karmen unit is defined as a decrease in optical density of 0.001 optical density units per minute, and the results are generally reported as Karmen units per ml of CSF. Green et al. [47] have modified the original procedure of Karmen[49, 50] for measuring GOT activity of CSF samples.

In addition to the Karmen method, two colorimetric methods have been used to measure GOT activity. The first was developed by Reitman and Frankel[51], and is based on the reaction of oxaloacetate, formed from aspartate and α-ketoglutarate by GOT, with 2,4 dinitrophenylhydrazine to form a red 2,4-dinitrophenylhydrazone. The product is measured colorimetrically, with one unit of GOT activity defined as the amount of enzyme that will form 4.82×10^{-4} µmoles of glutamate per minute. GOT activity measured by the method of Reitman and Frankel can be converted into Karmen units, and some investigators who have used this colorimetric method have reported their results in this way. A second colorimetric method based on the same reactions has been described by King[52]. The units in which data obtained with King's method are generally reported are μmoles of glutamate formed per hour per 100 cm³ of serum or CSF. Data reported in King's units can be converted into Karmen units by dividing by 2.9[52].

GOT and LDH are the only two markers of CNS tumors that have been simultaneously determined on substantial patient populations. Unfortunately, neither is a very good marker of CNS tumors, as inspection of Tables 2 and 4 reveals. Green *et al.* [47] were the first to report on GOT levels in the CSF of neurological patients and found elevations associated with CVA and multiple sclerosis, but not with brain tumors. Subsequent investigations by many researchers led to conflicting results and interpretations. Four studies reported GOT activity elevations correlated with both primary and secondary CNS tumors[19, 33, 35, 36]; two papers reported that GOT measurement in CSF was a useful test only for detecting intracranial metastases[34, 53], while two others claimed it could be used to distinguish benign from malignant intracranial tumors[37, 54]. Other investigators concluded that determination of GOT activity in CSF was of no value in the diagnosis and management of CNS neoplasms[28, 38, 42, 44, 46–48].

Another finding GOT and LDH share is elevation of CSF activity in patients with a variety of neurologic diseases. As found for LDH, the disease associated with elevated CSF-GOT in the greatest number of invstigations is CVA[19, 28, 44, 46, 47, 53, 54]. The other diseases include hydrocephalus[37, 48], brain abscess[37], subarachnoid hemorrhage[46], head injury, degenerative diseases of the CNS, and convulsive disorders[28]. Both LDH and GOT have age-dependent normal CSF levels[29, 30]. It is unfortunate that a great amount of work has gone into studying a pair of markers that, in the end, have predictive values of only 37 and 30.6%, respectively. Studies of serum GOT levels are not included here because elevations of serum GOT are associated with many diseases other than CNS tumors.

Sufficient data are available to evaluate the potential use of CSF GOT determination in the CSF only with regard to the second function of Section 3. Table 4 contains data collated from twelve studies in which GOT for either individual patient levels or the numbers of patients above and below the investigators' chosen cut-off points were given. As before, studies that gave only mean GOT levels for different patient groups were not included. The sensitivity (41%) and specificity (69%) were calculated from the collated data, as shown at the bottom of Table 4. These values and an assumed 25% incidence of CNS tumors among patients with some organic neurological disease were used to calculate the predictive value (30.6%) and efficiency

Table 4. Collated data for GOT as a marker of CNS tumors.

Reference	True positives	False negatives	True negatives	False positives	Criteria for positive tests and units
19	10	14	39	71	67 μmoles/hr/100 cm^3
28	8	12	30	63	0.983 μmoles/hr/cm^3
29	1	7	95	11	Mean +2 S.D. for age group
33	9	5	0	0	67 μmoles/hr/100 cm^3
34	16	18	0	0	15.1 karmen units/cm^3
36	25	9	0	0	6 International Units
37	27	3	0	0	24.3 king units/100 cm^3
42	3	37	0	0	10 karmen units/cm^3
47	0	14	37	42	62 μmoles/hr/100 cm^3
48	3	10	37	10	32 karmen units/cm^3
53	3	10	101	33	14 karmen units/cm^3
54	10	25	197	9	27.5 sigma-frankel units/cm^3
Totals	115	164	536	239	

Sensitivity = 115/(115+164) = 41%.
Specificity = 536/(536+239) = 69%.

Table 5. Calculation of predictive value and efficiency of GOT as a marker of CNS tumors [1].

	Positive test	Negative test	Totals
Patients with CNS tumor	102.5	147.5	250
Patients without CNS tumor	232.5	517.5	750
Totals	335	665	1000

Predictive value = 102.5/335 = 30.6%
Efficiency = (102.5+517.5)/1000 = 62%

[1] Based on an assumed prevalence of 25% and the sensitivity and specificity of Table 4.

(62%) (Table 5). A test for CNS tumors based on measurement of CSF GOT apparently would not be useful. This agrees with the conclusion of Bodansky [55], who found GOT to be the least reliable marker of cancer among a variety of enzymes.

4.3. Aldolase (E.C.4.1.2.13)

Aldolase, or fructose-1,6-diphosphate aldolase, catalyzes the reversible cleavage of fructose-1,6-diphosphate (FDP) into dihydroxyacetone phosphate and D-glyceraldehyde-3-phosphate. There are three known isoenzymes of aldolase [55]: aldolase A, or muscle type; aldolase B, or liver type; and aldolase C, or brain type. Each isoenzyme is a tetramer of four identical subunits, although AC hybrids have been found in brain tissue. All three isoenzymes catalyze the cleavage of both FDP and fructose-1-phosphate (F1P), but aldolase activity measured with FDP as substrate is different from aldolase activity measured with F1P as substrate. In addition, the ratio of activity with FDP to that with F1P is different for each of the three isoenzymes: for type A, the ratio is approximately 50, for type B it is 1, and for type C it is approximately 10.

Aldolase is an enzyme in the glycolytic sequence, and the rationale for investigating aldolase activity measurments in physiological fluids is the same as for LDH. In addition, several early reports [56–59] indicated that differences in the aldolase isoenzyme distribution and in the FDP/F1P ratio exist between brain tumor tissue and normal, nongrowing brain tissue. Tsunematsu and Shiraishi [60] have shown that increases in total aldolase activity in serum associated with a wide variety of neoplasia are accompanied by an increase in the FDP/F1P ratio, while non-neoplastic diseases (e.g., acute infectious hepatitis) that also result in an increase in total aldolase activity are accompanied by a decrease in the FDP/F1P ratio. Although the overwhelming majority of investigations on aldolase and CNS tumors have been carried out on tumor tissue, some work has been done on aldolase and its isoenzymes in CSF.

Total aldolase activity in CSF has been measured [61, 62] using an adaptation of the colorimetric method of Sibley and Lehninger [63], which is based on cleavage of FDP by aldolase into triose phosphates, fixation of the triose phosphates with hydrazine, and formation of the 2,4-dinitrophenlyhydrazones of the triose hydrazides. Aldolase activity is quantitated by the intensity of the red color of the 2,4-dinitrophenylhydrazones at alkaline pH. This method can also be used to obtain the FDP/F1P ratio by repeating the measurement with F1P. Blostein and Rutter [64] reported a spectrophotometric method based on conversion of the triose phosphates formed from either FDP or F1P to α-glycerophosphate in the presence of excess triosephosphate isomerase and α-glycerophosphate dehydrogenase. The rate of this second reaction, which is determined by the activity of the aldolase reaction, measures the rate of disappearance of NADH at 340 nm.

The isoenzymes of aldolase have been separated electrophoretically on cellulose acetate membranes [65], on thin layer polyacrilamide gels [57], and on agarose gel [66]. The isoenzymes are stained with either nitroblue tetrazolium chloride [57, 65] or with amidoblack 10B [66], and quantitated by densitometry. CSF samples must be concentrated by ultrafiltration in order to detect aldolase isoenzyme patterns [66, 67], but even using concentrated CSF samples, the sensitivity of currently available techniques is insufficient for all but the most elevated samples.

Niebroj-Dobosz and Hetnarska [38] first measured total aldolase activity in the CSF of brain tumor patients, and they reported no elevation of aldolase activity in the CSF of tumor patients, compared to a control group. Tschankow and Dikow [66] reported finding no aldolase activity in the CSF of healthy subjects, while CSF obtained from patients with vascular disease and inflammation of the nervous system did have measureable levels of CSF aldolase activity. This study did not include patients with CNS tumors. Vara-Lopez and Vara-Thorbeck [35] measured aldolase activity in the CSF of 15 patients with cerebral tumors and report higher aldolase activity in the CSF of this group than found in normal controls.

Only one study has been done on aldolase isoenzyme distributions in CSF [67]. In a group of 25 patients with no CNS tumors, isoenzyme patterns were discernable in the CSF of only four patients. Of 10 patients with untreated CNS tumors, eight had demonstrable aldolase isoenzyme patterns, while two had no aldolase activity in their CSF. Seven patients from whom CSF samples were obtained shortly after surgical removal of their tumor or while on chemotherapy also had no demonstrable CSF aldolase activity.

It is evident that there are insufficient data available to allow conclusive evaluation of the potential usefulness of CSF aldolase as a marker of CNS tumors. For the rather small sample of 39 patients with tumors, total aldolase activity has a sensitivity of 53.8% as a marker of CNS tumors. While this result is not that promising, the observed specificity of 94% for 67 patients with nonneoplastic neurologic diseases indicates sufficient potential to warrant further study. Future investigations of aldolase isoenzyme distributions in CSF must, however, wait for the development of more sensitive methods for such determinations.

4.4. Other Enzymatic Markers

Glucosephosphate isomerase (E.C.5.3.1.9) or phosphohexose isomerase (PHI) catalyzes the reversible interconversion of glucose-6-phosphate and fructose-6-phosphate. Investigation of PHI as a tumor marker stems from its role in the glycolysis pathway. Based on the rate of formation of fructose-6-phosphate, it has been assayed colorimetrically as described by Bodansky [68]. Bruns et al. [18], were the first to measure PHI in CSF, but studied samples from normal individuals only. Thompson et al. [69] found elevations of PHI activity in the CSF of 21 of 33 patients with malignant CNS tumors, while six of seven patients with benign CNS tumors had normal CSF PHI levels. They also reported that only two of nine patients with CVA and four of eight patients with CNS infections had elevated PHI activity in their CSF. Buckell and Robertson [21] reported finding elevated levels of PHI in the CSF of five of eight glioma patients and two of eight patients with cerebral metastatic carcinoma. Finally, Niebroj-Dobosz and Hetnarska [38] reported elevated levels of PHI in the CSF of all ten patients with brain tumor they examined. For 67 patients with CNS tumors tested in these reports, PHI has a sensitivity of 58.2%, while for the 59 nontumor bearing neurologic patients, it had a specificity of 67.8%. Bodansky[55] noted that of all the serum enzymes whose levels have been studied in association with a variety of cancers, PHI is the one most often elevated, and elevated to the largest degree. It is evident that a great deal more work should be done on CSF levels of PHI as a function of CNS tumors, and a wider variety of non-neoplastic neurologic diseases should be tested for elevations of CSF levels of PHI.

Lysozyme (muramidase, E.C.3.2.1.17) catalyzes the hydrolysis of the β-1,4 linkage between N-acetylmuramic acid and N-acetylglucosamine. Its function is to depolymerize the mucopolysaccharide components of the cell walls of a variety of pathogenic organisms. Methods for assaying lysozyme activity in physiological fluids have been described by Wilson[70], Osserman and Lawlor[71], Parry et al. [72], Newman et al. [73], and Johansson and Malmquist[74]. All but the last of these methods use *Micrococcus lysodeikticus* as substrate, but the method of measurement is different; some rely on turbidimetry, some on densitometry, and others on measurement of the diameter of a zone of lysis surrounding a sample well on an agarose gel lysoplate[74]. The last method[74] is an immunochemical technique. These studies of CSF levels of lysozyme originated in laboratories studying markers of infectious diseases of the CNS.

A number of investigators have shown that CSF samples obtained from healthy individuals contain very low or undetectable levels of lysozyme activity[75–80]. Only one report[73] has been published claiming that CSF lysozyme determinations are useful for detection of CNS tumors. A substantial number of studies[77–82] argue against this conclusion. While some authors feel that CSF lysozyme activity can be used to diagnose and manage meningitis and other inflammatory CNS diseases, others[79, 81] argue that elevations of CSF lysozyme activity are so nonspecific that they are of no use. Among the other diseases associated with elevated CSF levels of lysozyme are neurosarcoid[81], uremia, cerebrovascular disease[78], intracranial hemorrhage, encephalitis, and cerebral atrophy[79].

Even though lysozyme may be elevated in some patients harboring CNS tumors, it is far from being a very sensitive marker of CNS neoplasms. This conclusion is borne out by the data collated from the studies. A total of 73 determinations of CSF lysozyme levels have been made in patients with CNS tumors, resulting in a sensitivity of lysozyme for brain tumors of 39.7%. The specificity of lysozyme for brain tumors is 74.2% for a sample of 314 patients with non-neoplastic neurologic diseases.

Creatine kinase (CPK, E.C.2.7.3.2.) catalyzes the transfer of a phosphate group from phosphocreatine to ADP to form ATP, and maintains the ATP levels of the peripheral tissues. Diseases accompanied by destruction of cerebral tissue or alteration of cell permeability may be reflected in elevated CPK activity in the CSF. Assay methods for CPK activity in physiological fluids have been described by Tanzer and Gilvarg [83] and Huges [84], among others. Herschkowitz and Cumings [85] reported on CPK levels in the CSF of patients with various neurological diseases, and 17 control subjects. Twenty-one of 30 patients with verified brain tumor had elevated levels of CSF CPK. Seven patients who were in the normal range harbored meningioma or craniopharyngioma. Forty-two of 71 patients with other neurological disease also had elevated CPK levels in their CSF. Niebroj-Dobosz and Hetnarska [38], on the other hand, found no elevation of CPK in the CSF of 51 patients with a variety of neurologic disorders, including 10 cases of brain tumor. While they did not report individual levels of CPK activity in the CSF of the patients included in their study, Englehardt and Avenarius [44] also observed no elevations of CPK in patients harboring CNS tumors.

For 38 patients with CNS tumors and 111 patients with other neurologic diseases [38, 85], CPK has a sensitivity of 55.3% and a specificity of 62.2%. Only one study has reported the CPK isoenzyme distributions in CSF samples [86], but no patients with primary CNS tumors were included.

Isocitrate dehydrogenase (ICD, E.C.1.1.1.42) catalyzes the conversion of isocitrate to α-ketoglutarate and is an enzyme in the tricarboxylic acid cycle. An assay method developed by Wolfson and Williams-Ashman [87] was modified for CSF by Van Rymenant and Robert [88]. They observed elevated CSF levels of ICD in 17 of 20 patients with primary or metastatic cerebral tumors. Increased ICD activity in CSF was also associated with cerebrovascular lesions, herpes zoster, and meningitis. A later study by this group found elevated ICD in the CSF of 49 of 56 brain tumor patients [89]. Elevations were also found in cases of acute encephalitis and the neurologic diseases studied in their earlier report. For 76 patients with CNS tumors and 94 patients with other neurologic diseases, ICD has a sensitivity of 86.8% and a specificity of 50% [88, 89].

Because the activity of β-glucuronidase (E.C.3.2.1.31) in tumor tissue is higher than in normal tissue from the same organ [90, 91], Anlyan and Starr [92] investigated CSF β-glucuronidase activity as a marker of CNS cancer. The method used was that of Fishman et al. [93]. Seven of 10 patients with glioblastoma multiforme had elevated β-glucuronidase activity in their CSF. Healthy subjects, 15 patients with non-neoplastic CNS disease, eight patients with benign CNS tumors, and six with metastatic CNS tumors all had normal CSF levels of this enzyme. A recent report by Fleisher et al. [94] found seven-fold elevations above the normal range for β-glucuronidase in the CSF of 20 patients with meningeal carcinomatosis, but only slight elevations for eight patients with parenchymal CNS metastases. No patients with primary CNS tumors or nontumor neurologic diseases were studied by these investigators. While the overall sensitivity of this enzyme for CNS tumors is rather low (51.9%), its sensitivity for primary malignant brain tumors is 70%; even though this result is based on a rather small sample of patients, the apparent specificity is 100% [92, 94].

Leucine aminopeptidase (LAP, E.C.3.4.1.1) has potential utility as a serum marker of pancreatic carcinoma[95]. Green and Perry modified the assay of Goldbarg[96] for LAP determinations in CSF[97]. They reported that all nine of nine patients with CNS tumors had LAP levels greater than the upper limit of their reference group, but that patients with non-neoplastic neurologic diseases also had elevated CSF levels of LAP. Because the report gives only mean values and ranges for the patient groups studied, sensitivity and specificity cannot be calculated.

Using an assay developed by Frithz et al. [98], Ronquist and coworkers[99] found no adenylate kinase (E.C.2.7.4.3) activity in the CSF of 35 healthy controls or in the CSF of both of two patients with benign brain tumors. However, all nine of nine patients with malignant tumors had measurable levels of adenylate kinase in their CSF. In a previous study[100], 11 patients suffering from transient ischemic attacks had slight but detectable levels of adenylate kinase activity in their CSF. A later report from this group found elevated CSF adenylate kinase in an additional three cases of malignant brain tumor[101]. Elevations of CSF adenylate kinase have been found in patients with multiple sclerosis, cerebral infarction, and brain hemorrhage. Getaz et al. studied CSF levels of adenylate kinase as an index of CNS involvement in hematological malignancy, but found no clear correlations and a high false positive rate[102].

Hultberg and Olsson[103] measured the activities of four lysosomal hydrolases, β-galactosidase, α-mannosidase (at both pH 4.5 and 5.5), N-acetyl-β-glucosaminidase, and acid phosphatase in the serum and CSF of 179 neurologic patients (including 20 cases of CNS tumor) and of 20 healthy controls. They report decreased activity of both serum and CSF β-galactosidase for patients with CNS tumors. Patients with multiple sclerosis had decreased activity of both β-galactosidase and N-acetyl-β-glucosaminidase, but only in CSF. Because only means and ranges for the various patient groups tested were reported, sensitivity and specificity cannot be calculated. As a result of the wide variability within all patient groups examined, the authors concluded that determinations of these enzyme activities would not be a clinically useful tool.

Cuatico and coworkers[104] used a simultaneous detection assay[105, 106] that is designed to detect RNA-directed DNA polymerase activity, supposedly of RNA tumor viruses, to examine the CSF of patients with CNS tumors; 11 of 15 patients showed positive results, while five nontumor patients showed no viral-like activity. The assay is intricate and time consuming, which limits the value of this approach as a routine diagnostic tool.

5. BIOMOLECULAR MARKERS OF CNS TUMORS

5.1. Polyamines

The polyamines spermidine and spermine and their precursor putrescine have been studied extensively. The known aspects of polyamine metabolism and function in a variety of biological systems have been well reviewed [107–117].

Increased intracellular polyamine concentrations have been linked to increased rates of cell proliferation and division [118, 119]. Higher intracellular concentrations of the polyamines have been found in neoplastic cells than in normal tissue cells. Polyamines from neoplastic cells could be released into the extracellular fluid, which may be reflected by elevated concentrations of these compounds in physiological fluids. Russell et al. [120], reported increased polyamine excretion in the urine of cancer patients. Subsequently, other investigators [121–124] confirmed these findings and extended them to polyamine levels in the serum of patients with a variety of neoplastic diseases [125–127].

Seiler [128] has recently reviewed the assay procedures now in use for measuring polyamines in urine, serum, and CSF. They include gas chromatography (GC) [129–132], gas chromatography-mass spectrometry (GC/MS) [133, 134], thin layer chromatography (TLC) [135–138], enzymatic assay [139, 140], high pressure liquid chromatography (HPLC) [141–144], ion exchange chromatography using an automated amino acid analyzer [145–147], and radioimmunoassay (RIA) [148, 149]. Good agreement between results obtained for identical samples using GC/MS, RIA, and the amino acid analyzer technique has been reported [125].

Because of limited assay techniques, early investigations [150] showing no difference in polyamine concentrations between the CSF of normal individuals and those of patients with CNS tumors are not reliable. With a more sensitive method of analysis [146], we examined the possible use of CSF polyamine measurements as markers of CNS tumors in a group of 29 non-tumor-bearing patients and 77 patients with CNS tumors [151, 152]. The data showed a statistically significant difference between the CSF polyamine levels of patients with untreated malignant CNS tumors and those of patients without neoplastic disease. Terabayashi and coworkers [153, 154] measured whole blood concentrations of polyamines for 38 CNS tumor patients and 17 controls. They reported significant elevations for the tumor patients, particularly in cases of glioma. However, they could not detect polyamines in the

CSF of the nine tumor patients investigated, undoubtedly a result of the relatively insensitive assay used. Rennert *et al.* [155] measured CSF polyamine levels in patients with acute leukemia with neuromeningeal involvement. They reported elevated levels of spermine and spermidine but not putrescine in cases of CNS relapse, while patients in relapse with no CNS involvement had elevated CSF putrescine but not spermine or spermidine. Recently it has been reported that in patients with meningeal carcinomatosis, CSF polyamine levels are elevated and may correlate with the patient's clinical status [156].

CSF polyamines are one of the few classes of markers studied for functions other than detection of CNS tumor. Preliminary studies attempted to correlate changes in CSF polyamine levels with changes in the patient's clinical status and found that significant increases in CSF polyamine levels preceded a decline in clinical status due to tumor regrowth, while in some patients improvement in clinical status was accompanied by decreased CSF polyamine concentrations [7]. Using mutliple lumbar puncture, we followed a selected group of patients during the first week of chemotherapy and observed significant rises in the CSF putrescine level of paients whose tumors responded to therapy [7]. Polyamine levels in the CSF of normal healthy volunteers were shown to be in the same range as those found in the reference group of patients with non-neoplastic neurologic disease. These results were corroborated in a larger group of patients [8]. As additional data accumulated, it became possible to evaluate the utility of CSF polyamine determinations for monitoring the clinical status of CNS tumor patients by tumor type. A total of 210 determinations were made for 32 patients with medulloblastoma [157, 158]. The polyamine assay was predictive of recurrence in 15 patients weeks to months before other tests indicated tumor regrowth. Three false negatives and no false positives were observed. In a similar study with 12 patients with glioblastoma multiforme (18 determinations) and 37 patients with anaplastic astrocytoma (76 determinations), CSF polyamines were significantly elevated in patients with recurrent tumors [159]. These elevations did not, however, appear to precede tumor recurrence, and many results were false positive or false negative. CSF polyamine levels showed no significant relationship to the degree of malignancy or to tumor size, but did correlate with proximity of the tumor to the cerebral ventricles [159].

Extensive reviews have been published evaluating the potential utility of polyamine measurement in urine and/or serum as markers of non-CNS neoplasms [4, 160–164]. Woo and his coworkers [165, 166] have formulated a mathematical model relating tumor cell number to intracellular polyamine concentrations and have shown a correlation between marker synthesis and cell cycle kinetics.

Three distinct diagnostic tests for brain tumors using measurement of polyamine concentration in CSF are possible: a test based on putrescine levels

Table 6. Sensitivity of the polyamines as markers of CNS tumors.

Patient group	Number of patients	Marker	True positives	False negatives	Sensitivity
All brain tumors	63	Putrescine	42	21	66.7%
All brain tumors	63	Spermidine	39	24	61.9%
All brain tumors	63	Combined polyamines	51	12	81%
Medulloblastoma and malignant glioma	33	Putrescine	30	3	90.9%
Medulloblastoma and malignant glioma	33	Spermidine	27	6	81.8%
Medulloblastoma and malignant glioma	33	Combined	33	0	100%

alone, on spermidine alone, and a combined polyamine test in which an elevated level of either putrescine or spermidine is considered a positive result. The data reported for a sample of 63 patients with CNS tumors[152] are summarized in Table 6. We have extracted from this sample the group of 33 patients with medulloblastoma or malignant glioma, for which the combined polyamine diagnostic test has a very encouraging 100% sensitivity. However, all patients in this study had large tumors and were in advanced stages of disease. For a group of 155 patients with neurologic diseases other than tumors, the combined polyamine test had a specificity of only 47.7%[167, 168], but a large fraction of the drop in specificity was due to patients with cerebral aneurysms and patients with a variety of back disorders. With these two groups removed a 74 patient sample was obtained in which CSF putrescine had a specificity of 75.7%, CSF spermidine had a specificity of 77%, and the combined polyamine test had a specificity of 66.2%. Because there are so many different sensitivities and specificities to be considered for polyamines, we did not calculate predictive values or efficiencies for the many possible combinations.

5.2. Desmosterol

Desmosterol (cholesta-5,24-dien-3-β-ol; Δ^{24}-cholesterol; 24-dehydrocholesterol) is the penultimate precursor in the biosynthetic pathway of cholesterol[169]. The conversion of desmosterol to cholesterol can be inhibited by triparanol (MER-29 or 1-[p-β-diethylaminoethoxyl]-phenyl-1-[p-tolyl]-2-[p-chlorophenyl]ethanol). A number of investigators have reported accumulation of desmosterol in fetal brain or CNS tumor tissue but not in normal brain tissue subsequent to triparanol treatment[170–175]. These results led to the investigation of CSF levels of desmosterol both before and after treating patients with CNS tumors and other neurological diseases with triparanol.

Colorimetric [170] and TLC [176] procedures are not sufficiently sensitive for the determination of desmosterol in CSF. Fumagalli *et al.* [177] have reported a GC method for measurement of both cholesterol and desmosterol in biological samples. Vandenheuvel *et al.* [178] have described a method for preparation of CSF samples for sterol analysis, which was modified by Fumagalli and Paoletti [179]. Weiss *et al.* [180] and Marton *et al.* [181] have described methods of CSF sample preparation that eleminate the TLC step of earlier procedures.

Patients whose CSF is to be tested for desmosterol are given a daily oral dose of triparanol (500 mg) for five days before lumbar puncture [182]. The concentrations of both cholesterol and desmosterol in the CSF are determined, and the ratio $[D]/[C] \times 100$ (desmosterol to cholesterol when cholesterol is made equal to 100) is calculated. Concentrations of desmosterol greater than 0.1 μg/ml of CSF, *or* a $[D]/[C] \times 100$ ratio of greater than 3.0 are defined as positive results. Paoletti *et al.* [183] have recently reviewed the use of the desmosterol tests as a marker of brain tumors.

A series of reports from the laboratory that developed the desmosterol test [173, 178, 179, 182] demonstrated its potential utility as a marker for CNS tumors. In the absence of triparanol treatment, no desmosterol was detected in the CSF of patients with or without CNS tumor. After triparanol administration, most patients with CNS tumors gave positive test results and most patients without CNS tumors gave negative test results. Virtually no false positives or false negatives were reported. Other groups, however, reported results that indicate a lower sensitivity for the desmosterol test than originally reported [180, 181, 184]. One study suggested replacing triparanol with 20,25-diazacholesterol because the latter was more effective as an inhibitor of the conversion of desmosterol to cholesterol [185]. The data from all the above studies have been collated and have used to calculate the sensitivity and specificity of the desmosterol test (Table 7).

Fumagalli and Paoletti also examined the relationship between the results obtained for the desmosterol test and the type of brain tumor present [179]. They concluded that CSF levels of desmosterol measured after triparanol administration correlate with the degree of malignancy of the tumor. The highest levels, however, were associated with cases of meningioma and acoustic neurinoma. The desmosterol test was also investigated as a predictor of tumor regrowth following surgical removal. Fumagalli *et al.* [186], reported that 22 of 29 patients with recurrent tumors gave positive tests, while all seven patients who did not have recurrences had negative test results. The authors do not indicate, however, the length of time between surgical removal of the original tumor and surgical verification of tumor regrowth, after which the sterol test was performed on these patients. These investigators also studied changes in CSF levels of sterols for patients being treated for brain

Table 7. Collated data for desmosterol as a marker of CNS tumors.

Reference	True positives	False negatives	True negatives	False positives
178	5	0	5	0
179	47	14	21	1
180	20	14	7	0
182	21	9	52	0
186	22	2	7	0
Totals	115	39	92	1

Sensitivity = 115/(115+39) = 74.68%
Specificity = 92/(92+1) = 98.92%

tumors with nitrosourea compounds [187, 188]. While a number of changes in CSF desmosterol levels were observed, the changes in clinical status accompanying these variations were not reported; the utility of the desmosterol test for long-term monitoring of patients with brain tumors cannot be evaluated without this information. The length of time between the end of a chemotherapy cycle and drawing the patient's CSF was not given. It is possible that the data presented in this study may be more applicable to evaluation of desmosterol as a predictor of the efficacy of chemotherapy than to long-term evaluation.

Weiss *et al.* [180] initially reported no consistent effect on the results of the desmosterol test by any of several treatments used with glioma patients. A later report, however, implied that measurement of desmosterol in the CSF may reflect the growth potential of CNS tumors [189]. There are also several reports [190, 191] on cholesterol levels in the CSF of patients with CNS tumors and other neurologic diseases, the results of which indicate little or no utility as a marker of CNS tumors.

Because necessary data have not been published, we can evaluate the desmosterol test only as a marker for the early detection of CNS tumors (Table 7). A sensitivity of 74.7% and specificity of 98.8% were calculated; assuming that 25% of patients referred for neurological diagnosis have tumors, we calculate a predictive value of 95.8% and an efficiency of 92.9% for the desmosterol test (Table 8). In contrast to the results obtained for the polyamines, the sensitivity of the desmosterol test does not change appreciably when applied solely to the more malignant types of brain tumor. Positive test results were obtained in 52 of the 71 cases of medulloblastoma or malignant glioma, for a sensitivity of 73.2%. Additionally, while a substantial number of patients without tumors have been tested (93 patients), the range

Table 8. Calculation of predictive value and efficiency of desmosterol as a marker of CNS tumors [1].

	Positive test	Negative test	Totals
Patients with CNS tumor	186.7	63.3	250
Patients without CNS tumor	8.1	741.9	750
Totals	194.8	805.2	1000

Predictive value = 186.7/194.8 = 95.84%
Efficiency = (186.7 + 741.9)/1000 = 92.86%

[1] Based on an assumed prevalence of 25% and the sensitivity and specificity from Table 7.

of diseases examined is not as extensive as those examined for LDH, GOT, or the polyamines.

5.3. Hormonal Markers

Twenty-four-hour urine levels of human chorionic gonadotropin (HCG) have been used to diagnose and manage patients with hydatiform mole and choriocarcinoma. Tashima *et al.* [192] measured CSF levels of this marker and reported that elevated CSF levels are accompanied by relatively low levels of excretion in urine, which indicates intracranial metastases from choriocarcinoma. Rushworth *et al.* [193] observed that the plasma to CSF ratio of HCG was a more accurate predictor of CNS metastases from choriocarcinoma. In their study, all patients with CNS metastases had a plasma to CSF HCG ratio below 35, while all patients without CNS metastases had ratios greater than 100. Bagshawe and Harland corroborated these results in a larger group of 78 choriocarcinoma patients with no CNS metastases and 35 patients with CNS metastases [194, 195]. Other tumors for which CNS metastases are accompanied by elevated CSF levels of HCG or low plasma to CSF ratios include malignant teratoma [196] and testicular carcinoma [197]. Allen *et al.* [198] recetly reported elevated CSF and serum levels of HCG in two cases each of intracranial embryonal carcinoma and intracranial choriocarcinoma. In all four patients, marker levels declined with therapy and rose with tumor recurrence.

For patients with pituitary tumors, Jordan *et al.* [199] have shown that elevated CSF levels of one of the pituitary hormones (corticotopin, growth hormone, thyrotropin, prolactin, luteinizing hormone, or follicle stimulating hormone) is a reliable indicator of suprasellar extension of the tumor. In four of five patients for whom CSF levels were measured before and after treatment (surgery and radiation therapy), therapy resulted in decreased CSF hormone levels. Schroeder *et al.* [200] also reported good reliability for CSF prolactin levels as an indicator of suprasellar extension of pituitary tumors. A recent report by Jordan *et al.* [201], however, reports that the CSF to plasma ratio of prolactin is a more reliable indicator of suprasellar extension than the CSF level alone.

5.4. Other Biomolecular Markers

Manno *et al.* [202] studied changes in total polysaccharide concentration in CSF of patients with a variety of neurologic diseases including 24 cases of brain tumor and 12 cases of spinal cord tumor. Eighteen patients with brain tumor and 12 patients with cord tumor had CSF polysaccharide levels above the normal range. A number of other neurologic diseases including neuropathy and inflammatory and vascular disorders were also accompanied by elevated CSF polysaccharide. The location of cerebral tumors seemed to have some relationship to the magnitude of elevation of CSF polysaccharide observed. Total CSF polysaccharide, however, appears to be insufficiently specific to serve as a marker of CNS neoplasms.

Early studies of cyclic adenosine-3',5'-monophosphate (cAMP) levels in CSF included no data on patients with CNS tumors [203–207]. Measurement of cAMP in CSF has been performed by a protein binding assay [203, 204, 207, 208] and by RIA [205, 206, 209]. Cyclic guanosine-3',5'-monophosphate (cGMP) in CSF has been measured by RIA [209, 210]. Rudman *et al.* reported elevated CSF levels of both cyclic nucleotides in patients with CNS tumors and increased intracranial pressure [209]. Patients with other neurologic diseases whose ventricular pressure was elevated also had increased CSF levels of cAMP or cGAMP. Trabucci *et al.* observed increased cGMP in the CSF of 17 of 18 patients with brain tumors, but did not report the ventricular pressure of these patients [210]. Unpublished data from this laboratory showed no clear correlations between CSF cyclic nucleotide levels and tumor type or clinical status.

Homovanillic acid, a metabolite of the catecholamines, and 5-hydroxyindoleacetic acid, a metabolite of serotonin, were measured in the CSF of brain tumor patients [211–213]. Elevated levels of both metabolites were found in patients in whom tumor caused a partial or complete block of normal CSF circulation. These measurements will probably not be of great clinical utility in early detection of CNS tumors because they reflect a secondary rather than a primary process. They may, however, be of some utility in the long-term evaluation of patients whose tumors result in impaired CSF circulation; this possibility merits further investigation.

Weisz and Mars [214] recently reported on the concentration of DNA in the CSF of 83 neurological patients. While this sample included only four patients with brain tumors, they showed the highest CSF levels of DNA. These preliminary observations should be extended to a larger sample of patients with CNS tumors and other non-neoplastic neurologic diseases.

A variety of protein fractions in CSF have been studied in patients with CNS tumors and other neurologic diseases. Cumings found elevated levels of β-globulin in both CSF and cyst fluid from patients with cerebral tumors [215]. Girke and Kovarik, on the other hand, observed elevated α_1-, α_2-, and γ-globulin fractions in the CSF of patients with malignant gliomas and cerebral metastases [216]. A recent report on a single case of cerebral glioma [217] also found elevated γ-globulin in the CSF of a patient whose levels returned to normal after cranial irradiation. Other proteins found in increased concentration in the CSF of CNS tumor patients include mucoproteins [218], β-lipoprotein and fibrinogen [219], and β-microglobulin in patients with leukemia or lymphoma with CNS involvement [220]. Primary CNS tumors do not appear to be accompanied by elevated β-microglobulin levels in CSF [221]. Lipoprotein distributions [222], IGM content [223], and plasminogen content [224] in CSF also do not appear to be clinically useful as markers.

A recent case report on a child with medulloblastoma found a 250- to 300-fold elevation of urine levels of thymine and uracil [225]. A number of other small molecules have been measured in CSF from neurological patients. These include γ-aminobutyric acid [226–230], amino acids [231–233], and polyhydric alcohols [234–236]. None of these, however, appear to be of value in diagnosis and patient management in cases of CNS tumor.

6. IMMUNOLOGICAL MARKERS

6.1. Carcinoembryonic Antigen

Carcinoembryonic antigen (CEA) was originally isolated from fetal gut and from colon carcinoma [237]. Techniques for measurement of CEA in physiologic fluids include RIA and enzyme-linked immunospecific assay; the methods have been reviewed by Egan et al. [238]. Elevated plasma levels of CEA have been found in patients with a wide variety of cancers [239]. Kido et al. [240] measured serum CEA levels in eight patients with malignant CNS tumors, 12 with CNS metastases, and 20 with benign CNS tumors. Three patients with glioblastoma had elevated serum CEA, while five patients with other malignant CNS tumors and 20 with benign tumor did not. Seven patients with CNS metastases had definite elevations and two others had slight increases. Of 49 CSF samples tested in this study, only four had demonstrable CEA and only one of these was from a patient with malignant CNS tumor. Snitzer et al. [241] reported detecting CEA in the CSF of four patients with CNS metastases; in one patient, treatment resulted in decreased CSF levels in spite of concurrent increased serum levels. Feinberg and

Hahn[242] reported that a patient with a metastatic CNS tumor had a high level of CEA in tumor cyst fluid, but did not measure serum or CSF levels of CEA in this patient. Of 62 patients with primary CNS tumors tested by Miyake *et al.* [243], only 12 had elevated serum CEA; two patients with CNS metastases had elevated levels. None of the CSF samples tested had measureable CEA content. Yap *et al.* [156, 244] reported that CSF levels of CEA are of value in detection of meningeal carcinomatosis in breast cancer patients. Fleisher *et al.* [94] also found elevated CSF CEA in patients with metastatic meningeal tumors but not in patients with metastases involving only parenchymal CNS tissue. The work to date on CEA in patients with CNS tumors indicates that this marker may be of value in detecting CNS metastases of CEA producing tumors, but is probably not useful for primary CNS tumors.

6.2. Immune Response to CNS Tumor Antigens

Haas[245] isolated a water soluble antigen from human glioblastoma tissue. However, an assay based on an antiserum was able to demonstrate the presence of this antigen in the CSF of only three of 27 patients with CNS tumors. Kornblith *et al.* [246] developed an *in vitro* microtoxicity assay to test for serum-mediated cytotoxicity to cultured astrocytoma cells, but found little antibody in patients with astrocytoma. In a subsequent study using the same assay, Phillips *et al.* [247] reported that 14 of 21 preoperative glioma patients and four of 21 normal controls had complement-dependent antibodies cytotoxic to cultured astrocytoma cells in their serum. Later reports from this group[248, 249] based on an improved version of the assay found cytotoxicity to an allogeneic glioblastoma cell line in the serum of 67 of 82 astrocytoma patients, six of 65 normal blood bank donors, one of 10 nontumor neurologic patients, and 40 of 70 patients with other CNS tumors. This cytotoxic antibody assay appears to have a sensitivity of 69.9% and specificity of 90%, with a predictive value of 70% and efficiency of 85% for detection of CNS tumors in a population of neurologic patients with an assumed prevalence of 25% for CNS tumors. Sheikh *et al.* [250] used a leukocyte adherence inhibition assay to demonstrate a cellular immune response to glioma antigens in 21 of 26 glioma patients that was absent in the 41 control subjects tested. Because demonstration of immune responses to CNS tumor antigens requires only blood samples and obviates the need for lumbar puncture, it is a most promising approach to detection of CNS tumors and merits intensive continued investigation, particularly in nontumor-bearing neurologic patients.

6.3. Glial Fibrillary Acid Protein

Glial fibrillary acid protein (GFAP) has been isolated from fibrous astrocytes[251] and has been found in human brain tumor tissue[252–254]. Eng *et al.* [255] have described an RIA for GFAP and report that 53 of 651 CSF samples contained GFAP. However, they do not list the diseases associated with GFAP in CSF. Later reports by Deck *et al.* [256] and by Eng and Rubinstein [257] demonstrated the utility of immunohistochemical localization of GFAP in biopsy specimens for classifying CNS tumors. Palfreyman *et al.* [258] have also reported an RIA for GFAP. Jacque *et al.* [259] found GFAP levels in biopsy specimens to be a reliable index of malignancy in cases of astrocytoma, with lower GFAP levels accompanying the more malignant tumors. Lowenthal *et al.* [260] found GFAP in the CSF of 67 of 649 patients, but gave no indication of the diseases accompanied by GFAP in CSF.

6.4. Astrocytin and Malignin

Astrocytin (or astroprotein) has been isolated by Bogoch [261] who developed an assay for it in serum [262, 263]. Of 74 serum samples from normal individuals and patients with non-neoplastic diseases, 71 had levels of astrocytin below a reference level, while 20 of 22 patients with malignant brain tumors had elevated levels of astrocytin in their serum. Bogoch has also isolated a second CNS tumor antigen, malignin, from cultured malignant glioma cells [264, 265]. These two antigens are immunochemically similar but have differing amino acid compositions. Measurement of antibodies to malignin in a population of 74 normal and nontumor patients and 27 CNS tumor patients reportedly resulted in a 92.6% sensitivity and 96% specificity [264]. A later report [266] of 82 patients with CNS tumor, 80 with non-CNS tumor, 51 nontumor medical and surgical patients, and 77 healthy subjects found a 95% sensitivity for CNS tumor and a 95.3 specificity in the latter two groups. The patients with non-CNS tumors, however, had mean serum levels of anti-malignin antibodies equal to the CNS tumor patients. Polypeptides similar to malignin have also been isolated from lymphoma and mammary cancer cells in culture [267], which questions the specificity of such determinations for CNS tumors. A recent report on a retrospective study of antimalignin antibody in serum of a variety of cancer patients found that patients with higher antibody levels survived longer that those with low levels [268].

Mori *et al.* [269] described an RIA for astroprotein, an antigen they report to be identical to astrocytin, and used this assay to demonstrate very high levels of astroprotein in the CSF of some, but not all, CNS tumor patients. A subsequent study [270] found elevated CSF levels of astroprotein in 10 of 17 cases of glioma, 10 of 43 cases of other brain tumors, and four of 21 cases of nontumor-bearing neurologic disease. A later report [271] found CSF astroprotein in 10 of 40 nontumor-bearing neurologic patients, 11 of 12 glioma patients and 10 of 40 nonglial brain tumor patients. Only low levels of this antigen were detected in the 85 serum samples tested.

6.5 *Miscellaneous Markers*

Several other antigens have been detected and quantitated in CSF. Myelin basic protein (MBP) can be measured by RIA [272–274], but appears to be a better marker for multiple sclerosis and other demyelinating diseases than for CNS tumors [272, 273]. Using a radial immunodiffusion technique, Galvez *et al.* [275] found elevated levels of α-1-antitrypsin in the CSF of 29 of 40 patients with intracranial tumors. No nontumor-bearing neurologic patients were investigated. Serum levels of this marker were also elevated in 15 of the 40 patients studied. CSF levels of alphafetoprotein have been measured as a potential marker of CNS metastases, but this marker does not appear to have clinical utility [196–198].

7. CONCLUSIONS

Absolute clinical utility has been demonstrated for only one marker (the polyamines), for only one function (monitoring clinical status), and for only one type of CNS tumor (medulloblastoma) [157, 158]. The remainder of the markers reviewed here have as yet not been adequately studied. With the exception of LDH and GOT, all markers have been measured on different patient populations; most of the markers discussed have not been measured in adequate numbers of tumor-free neurologic patients. For some that have, the spectrum of diseases investigated has not been sufficiently broad. Data are urgently needed about the prevalence of CNS tumors in the population of patients suspected of harboring CNS tumors, which is necessary to correctly evaluate the predictive value and efficiency of the markers for detecting the presence of CNS tumors in symptomatic patients. For some of the markers, CSF levels have been measured with assays that are not sufficiently sensitive to be reliable. Only a few of the markers have been investigated for functions other than screening or detection, and for most of the few that have, patient populations have been inadequate to yield statistically significant results. Given these limitations—and with the exception of CSF putrescine levels as a tool for monitoring patients with medulloblastoma—sufficient data are available only for some tentative statements to be made about the use of some of these markers.

As we discussed earlier, because of the very low prevalence of CNS tumors in the general population, screening for CNS tumors with a single marker is not a useful objective for continued research unless a marker with 100% specificity is found. None of the markers reviewed here meets this criterion. Thus we will not evaluate any of them for this function, in spite of the overwhelming preponderance of studies reviewed here that were designed for this purpose.

Table 9. Comparison of the sensitivities and specificities of markers of CNS tumors.

Marker	Patients with CNS tumors		Patients with other neurologic diseases		Total No. patients tested	Sensitivity (%)	Specificity (%)
	True positives	False negatives	True negatives	False positives			
Lactate dehydrogenase	223	115	267	160	756	66.0	62.5
Glutamic-oxalacetic transaminase	115	164	536	239	1054	41.0	69.0
Aldolase	21	18	63	4	106	53.8	94.0
Phosphohexose isomerase	39	28	40	19	126	58.2	67.8
Lysozyme	29	44	307	107	487	39.7	74.2
Creatine kinase	21	17	69	42	149	55.3	62.2
Isocitrate dehydrogenase	66	10	47	47	170	86.8	50
β-Glucuronidase	27	25	15	0	67	51.9	100
Adenylate kinase	23	4	27	56	110	85.2	32.5
Putrescine	42	21	56	18	137	66.7	75.7
Spermidine	39	24	57	17	137	61.9	77
Combined polyamines	51	12	49	25	137	81	66.2
Desmosterol	115	44	92	1	252	72.3	98.9
Microcytotoxicity assay (serum)	121	52	9	1	183	69.9	90.0
Anti-malignin antibody (serum)	123	6			129	95.3	?
Astroprotein (CSF)	41	71	47	14	173	36.6	77.0

The majority of the markers reviewed are at best potentially suitable for detecting the presence or absence of a CNS tumor in symptomatic patients. The calculated sensitivities and specificities of the more thoroughly investigated markers for which sufficient data could be collated are listed in Table 9. Because of these incomplete data, we will not speculate on the relative merits of the predictive values and efficiencies for markers reviewed here; this must await statistically valid evaluation of the prevalence of CNS tumors in symptomatic patients. The compilation shown in Table 9 is an updated version of earlier tables included in our two previous reviews on this subject [167, 168].

The serum antimalignin antibody test has the highest sensitivity (95.3%) for detection of CNS tumors [261–268]. There are, however, two problems with this marker. First, no data are available regarding serum levels in patients with neurologic diseases other than tumor. Second, recent reports indicate that elevated levels are also present in patients with a wide variety of non-CNS malignancies [266–268]. The two next-most-sensitive markers, isocitrate dehydrogenase (86.8%) [88, 89] and adenylate kinase (85.2%) [99–102], both have rather low specificities (50% and 32.5% respectively). Desmosterol has the highest specificity (98.9%), but this number may be unreliable because this marker has so far only been tested on patients with a limited number of non-neoplastic neurologic diseases [178–180, 182, 186]. β-Glucuronidase [92] (reported specificity = 100%) requires a much larger nontumor-bearing patient sample as well. Aldolase [35, 38, 66, 67], with a specificity of 94%, also appears promising, as does the serum microcytotoxicity assay (specificity = 90%), but many more patients must be tested for both markers. The combined polyamine test, which has been used to measure a fairly adequate population of patients with both neoplastic and other neurologic diseases, may be a reasonable compromise for a marker with high sensitivity and moderate specificity.

A number of markers may be potentially useful for detecting CNS metastases of non-CNS tumors. These include LDH [19, 27, 31–35, 37], GOT [19, 33–36, 53], β-glucuronidase [94], HCG in patients with choriocarcinoma and malignant teratoma [192–198], polyamines in cases of acute leukemia [155] or breast cancer [156], and CEA [94, 156, 240–242, 244]. Several markers have higher sensitivities for detection of specific types of CNS tumors than for all CNS tumors combined. Examples include β-glucuronidase for glioblastoma [92], the serum microcytotoxicity assay for astrocytoma [246–249], and CSF astroprotein for gliomas [269–271].

A number of studies have presented data relevant to uses for markers other than detection of tumors. Markers potentially capable of distinguishing benign from malignant CNS tumors include LDH [33] and its isoenzyme distribution [24, 39], GOT [37, 54], PHI [69], adenylate kinase [99, 101, 102], the polyamines [152], and desmosterol [179]. Prolactin appears to be of use in predicting suprasellar extension of pituitary tumors [199–201]. Markers studied to measure the efficacy of chemotherapy include LDH [32], aldolase [67], polyamines [7, 8, 152], and desmosterol [180, 184, 187], although utility for this function has not been established for any of these markers. The polyamines, as previously stated, are of proven clinical utility for monitoring patients with medulloblastoma [157, 158], but probably not for patients with glioblastoma or anaplastic astrocytoma [159]. We cannot stress too strongly the importance of evaluating each marker separately for each tumor type. Other markers studied for use in long-term monitoring include desmosterol [186, 187] and neural transmitter metabolites in instances where a CNS tumor impairs normal CSF circulation [211–213], but clinical utility for these two has not yet been demonstrated.

The research reviewed here suggests directions for future work. First, data regarding the prevalence of CNS tumors in a population of all neurological patients must be collected. Second, multiple marker determinations should be carried out simultaneously on CSF and other physiological fluid samples from patients with tumors and patients with other neurological diseases. Third, stages of tumor growth that correspond to certain marker levels should be defined, especially for patients with tumors in early growth stages, a patient group that has not been sufficiently studied. Fourth, more data are needed that define the elevation of a particular marker in patients with a particular tumor. Possibly, definition of these factors will lead to a test with which surgically inaccessible tumors can be defined and graded. Fifth, long-term serial studies on patients who have been treated for CNS tumors are needed to correlate marker levels with clinical status. Ideally, serial studies would be made on a population of patients who have a broad range of neurologic diseases, and several markers in each sample of CSF would be measured simultaneously. Sixth, short-term serial studies of patients undergoing treatment are needed to evaluate the use of markers in predicting the efficacy of therapy.

Many of these studies could be carried out conveniently in host animals large enough to supply reasonable volumes of CSF over a short period of time. Currently available rat and mouse models for CNS tumors are not satisfactory for such studies because of the small volumes of CSF that can be obtained. With animal models in larger hosts, one could study the variation of marker levels over the entire course of the disease, and the effects of radiation therapy and chemotherapy on marker levels could also be evaluated in a controlled situation, provided that trends defined in these animal models would reflect similar changes in humans. Until such a model is available, however, we must be content with the limited and often contradictory data gathered from clinical studies.

ACKNOWLEDGEMENTS

Partially supported by Public Health Service grants CA 15515 and CA 13525 from the National Cancer Institute, and by gifts from the Phi Beta Psi Sorority and the Margaret M. Anton Memorial Fund. LJM is the recipient of PHS Research Career Development Award CA 00112 from the National Cancer Institute.

We thank Ms Marilyn P. Minnaar for excellent secretarial assistance and Neil Buckley for invaluable editorial assistance.

REFERENCES

1. Warburg O: The metabolism of tumors. London: Constable, 1930.
2. Weber G: Enzymology of cancer cells. N Engl J Med 296:486–493 and 541–551, 1977.
3. Tormey DC, Waalkes TP, Ahmann D, Gehrke CW, Zumwalt RW, Snyder J, Hansen H: Biological markers in breast carcinoma. Cancer 35:1095–1100, 1975.
4. Bachrach U: Polyamines as chemical markers of malignancy. Ital J Biochem 25:77–93, 1976.
5. Galen RS, Gambino SR: Beyond normality: the predictive value and efficiency of medical diagnosis. New York: John Wiley, 1975.
6. Galen RS: The normal range: a concept in transition. Arch Pathol Lab Med 101:561–565, 1977.
7. Marton LJ: Polyamines and brain tumors. J Natl Cancer Inst (Monog) 46:127–131, 1977.
8. Marton LJ: The potential of cerebrospinal fluid polyamine determinations in the diagnosis and therapeutic monitoring of brain tumors. In: Advances in polyamine research, vol 2, Campbell RA, Morris DR, Bartos D, Daves GD, Bartos F (eds). New York: Raven Press, 1978, pp 257–263.
9. Herrschaft H: Zur Fruherkennung der Gehirntumoren. Fortschr Neurol Psychiat 45:383–404, 1977.
10. Wollemann M: Biochemistry of brain tumors. Baltimore: University Park Press, 1974.
11. Goldman RD, Kaplan NO, Hall TC: Lactic dehydrogenase in human neoplasmatic tissues. Cancer Res 24:389–399, 1964.
12. Viale GL: Biochemical patterns in brain tumors. I. Enzymes of the glycolysis pathway. Acta Neurochir 20:263–272, 1969.
13. Haglid K, Carlsson CA, Thulin CA: Lactate dehydrogenase isoenzymes and proteins in human gliomas. Neurochirurgica (Stuttgart) 13:19–28, 1970.
14. Timperley WR: Lactate dehydrogenase isoenzymes in tumors of the nervous system. Acta Neuropathol (Berlin) 19:20–24, 1971.
15. Kaplan NO: Symposium on multiple forms of enzymes and control mechanisms. I. Multiple forms of enzymes. Bacteriol Rev 27:155–169, 1963.
16. Markert CL: Developmental genetics. Harvey Lect 59:187–218, 1965.
17. Wroblewski F, LaDue JS: Lactic dehydrogenase activity in blood. Proc Soc Exp Bio Med 90:210–213, 1955.
18. Bruns FH, Jacob W, Weverinck F: Phosphohexoisomerase, Phosphoriboisomerase und Milchsauredehydrogenase in Liquor cerebrospinalis. Clin Chim Acta 1:63–66, 1956.

19. Green JB, Oldewurtel HA, O'Doherty DS, Forster FM: Cerebrospinal fluid transaminase and lactate dehydrogenase activities in neurologic disease. Arch Neurol Psychiatr 80:148–156, 1958.

20. Jakoby RK, Jakoby WB: Lactic dehydrogenase of cerebrospinal fluid in the differential diagnosis of cerebrovascular disease and brain tumor. J Neurosurg 15:45–51, 1958.

21. Buckell M, Robertson MC: Enzyme studies in cerebral tumors: lactate dehydrogenase, glucose phosphate isomerase, acid and alkaline phosphatase in plasma, ventricular CSF, and tumor cyst fluid from cases of glioma and cerebral secondary carcinoma. Br J Cancer 19:83–91, 1965.

22. King J: A routine method for the estimation of lactic dehydrogenase activity. J Med Lab Tech 16:265–272, 1959.

23. King J: Practical clinical enzymology. London: Van Nostrand, 1965.

24. Sano K, Chigasaki H, Takakura K: Diagnostic value of LDH isozyme studies in intracranial tumors. In: Proc 3rd Int Congr of Neurological Surgery, DeVet AC, (ed.). Copenhagen Denmark, August 1965. Amsterdam: Excerpta Medica Foundation, 1966, pp 575–579.

25. Rabow L, Kristensson K: Changes in lactate dehydrogenase isoenzyme patterns in patients with tumors of the central nervous system. Acta Neurochir 36:71–81, 1977.

26. Cunningham VR, Phillips J, Field EJ: Lactic dehydrogenase isoenzymes in normal and pathological spinal fluid. J Clin Pathol 18:765–770, 1965.

27. Wroblewski F, Decker B, Wroblewski R: Activity of lactic dehydrogenase in spinal fluid. Am J Clin Pathol 28:269–271, 1957.

28. Fleisher GA, Wakim KG, Goldstein NP: Glutamic oxalacetic transaminase and lactic dehydrogenase in serum and cerebrospinal fluid of patients with neurologic disorders. Mayo Clin Proc 32:188–197, 1957.

29. Hain RF, Nutter J: Cerebrospinal fluid enzymes as a function of age. Arch Neurol 2:331–337, 1960.

30. Spolter H, Thompson HG: Factors affecting lactic dehydrogenase and glutamic oxalacetic transaminase in cerebrospinal fluid. Neurology (Minneap) 12:53–59, 1962.

31. Wroblewski F: The significance of alterations in lactic dehydrogenase activity of body fluids in the diagnosis of malignant tumors. Cancer 12:27–39, 1959.

32. Wroblewski F, Decker B, Wroblewski R: The clinical implications of spinal fluid lactate dehydrogenase activity. N Engl J Med 258:635–639, 1958.

33. Green JB, Oldewurtel HA, Forster FM: Glutamic oxalacetic transaminase and lactic dehydrogenase activities. Neurology (Minneap) 9:540–544, 1959.

34. Davies-Jones GAB: Lactate dehydrogenase and glutamic oxalacetic transaminase of the cerebrospinal fluid in tumors of the central nervous system. J Neurol Neurosurg Psychiatr 32:324–327, 1969.

35. Vara-Lopez R, Vara-Thorbeck R: Modifications in the activity of some enzymes of the cerebrospinal fluid in patients with intracranial tumors. J Neurosurg 34:749–752, 1971.

36. Konshod F: Enzyme activity of cerebrospinal fluid in brain tumors. Med Arch 29:577–584, 1975.

37. Dharker SR, Dharker RS, Chaurasia BD: Lactate dehydrogenase and aspartate transaminase of the cerebrospinal fluid in patients with brain tumors, congenital hydrocephalus, and brain abscess. J Neurol Neurosurg Psychiatr 39:1081–1085, 1976.

38. Niebroj-Dobosz, I, Hetnarska L: The activity of enzymes in the cerebrospinal fluid in diseases of the nervous system. Pol Med J 8:451–455, 1969.

39. Heller W, Oldenkott P, Driesen W, Elies W, Blankenhorn H: Clinical chemical examinations for the early diagnosis of malignant brain tumors. Arztliche Forsch 25:44–47, 1971.

40. Gobiet W: Der diagnostische Wert der LDH-Bestimmung und ihrer Isoenzyme bei intrakrraniellen Prozessen. Z Neurol 202:247–250, 1972.

41. Stiffel M, Dittman J, Faulhauer K, Loew F: Liquorenzyme in normalen Proben, bei Hirntumoren und anderen neurologischen Erkrankungen. Wien Z Nervenheilkunde 31:325–333, 1973.
42. Hildebrand J: Early diagnosis of brain metastases in an unselected population of cancerous patients. Eur J Cancer 9:621–626, 1973.
43. Hildebrand J, Levin S: Enzymatic activities in cerebrospinal fluid in patients with neurological diseases. Acta Neurol Belg 73:229–240, 1973.
44. Engelhardt P, Avenarius HJ: Der diagnostische Wert von Enzymebestimmungen im Liquor cerebrospinalis. Med Klin 71:699–702, 1976.
45. Buckell M, Crompton MR, Robertson MC, Barnes GK: Lactate dehydrogenase in cerebral cyst fluids: total activity and isoenzyme distributions as an index of malignancy. J Neurosurg 32:545–552, 1970.
46. Katzman R, Fishman RA, Goldensohn ES: Glutamic oxalacetic transaminase activity in spinal fluid. Neurology (Minneap) 7:853–855, 1957.
47. Green JB, Oldewurtel HA, O'Doherty DS, Forster FM, Sanchez-Longo LP: Cerebrospinal fluid glutamic oxalacetic transaminase activity in neurologic disease. Neurology (Minneap) 7:313–322, 1957.
48. Miyazaki M: Glutamic oxalacetic transaminase in cerebrospinal fluid. J Nerv Ment Dis 126:167–175, 1958.
49. Karmen A, Wroblewski F, LaDue JS: Transaminase activity in human blood. J Clin Invest 34:126–131, 1955.
50. Karmen A: A Note on the spectrophotometric assay of GOT in human blood serum. J Clin Invest 34:131–133, 1955.
51. Reitman S, Frankel S: A colorimetric method for the determination of serum glutamic oxalacetic and glutamic pyruvic transaminases. Am J Clin Pathol 28:56–63, 1957.
52. King J: A study of human serum transaminases. J Med Lab Tech 17:1–21, 1960.
53. Mann SH, DePasquale N, Patterson R: Cerebrospinal fluid glutamic oxalacetic acid transaminase in patients receiving electroconvulsive therapy and in neurologic disease. Neurology (Minneap) 10:381–390, 1960.
54. Mellick RS, Basset RL: The cerebrospinal fluid glutamic oxalacetic transaminase activity in neurological diseases. Lancet 1:904–906, 1964.
55. Bodansky O: Biochemistry of human cancer. New York: Academic Press, 1975.
56. Sugimura T, Sato S, Kawabe S, Suzuki N, Chien TC, Takakura K: Aldolase C in brain tumor. Nature 222:1070, 1969.
57. Kumanishi T, Ikuta F, Yamamoto T: Aldolase isozyme patterns of representative tumors in the human nervous system. Acta Neuropathol 16:220–225, 1970.
58. Sato S, Sugimura T, Chien TC, Takakura K: Aldolase isozymes patterns of human brain tumors. Cancer 27:223–227, 1971.
59. Chein TC: Aldolase isozymes of human brain tumors. Brain and Nerve (Tokyo) 23:625–635, 1971.
60. Tsunematsu K, Shiraishi T: Aldolase isozymes in human tissue and serum. Cancer 24:637–642, 1969.
61. Schapira F: The normal aldolase activity of the CSF. Clin Chim Acta 7:566–571, 1962.
62. Wolintz AH, Jacobs LD, Christoff N, Solomon M, Chernick N: Serum and cerebrospinal fluid enzymes in cerebrovascular disease. Arch Neurol 20:54–61, 1969.
63. Sibley JA, Lehninger AL: Determination of aldolase in animal tissues. J Biol Chem 177:859–872, 1949.
64. Blostein R, Rutter WJ: Comparative studies of liver and muscle aldolase. II. Immunochemical and chromatographic differentiation. J Biol Chem 238:3280–3285, 1963.
65. Matsushima T, Kawabe S, Shibuya M, Sugimura T: Aldolase isozymes in rat tumor cells. Biochem Biophys Res Comm 30:565–570, 1968.

66. Tschankow IA, Dikow Al: Isoenzymes der Fructose-phosphate aldolase im Liquor cerebro-spinalis bei organischen Erkrankungen des Nervensystems. Z Klin Chem Klin Biochem 8:33–34, 1970.
67. Man EY: Development of an electrophoretic method for the determination of aldolase isoenzyme patterns in cerebrospinal fluid. Master's thesis, University of California, San Francisco, 1976.
68. Bodansky O: Serum Phosphohexose isomerase in cancer. I. Method of determination and establishment of range of normal values. Cancer 7:1191–1199, 1954.
69. Thompson HG, Hirschberg E, Ornos M, Gellhorn A: Evaluation of phosphohexose isom-erase activity in cerebrospinal fluid in neoplastic disease of the central nervous system. Neurology (Minneap) 9:545–552, 1959.
70. Wilson AT: Urinary lysozyme. I. Identification and measurement. J Pediatr 36:39–44, 1950.
71. Osserman EF, Lawlor DP: Serum and urinary lysozyme in monocytic and monomyelocytic leukemia. J Exp Med 124:921–951, 1966.
72. Parry RM, Chandan RC, Shahani KM: A rapid and sensitive assay of muramidase. Proc Soc Exp Biol Med 119:384–386, 1965.
73. Newman J, Josephson AS, Cacatian A, Tsang A: Spinal fluid lysozyme in the diagnosis of central nervous system tumors. Lancet II: 756–757, 1974.
74. Johansson BG, Malmquist J: Quantitative immunochemical determination of lysozyme in serum and urine. Scand J Clin Lab Invest 27:255–261, 1971.
75. Rabe EF, Curnen EC: The occurence of lysozyme in the cerebrospinal fluid and serum of infants and children. J Pediatr 38:147–153, 1951.
76. Hankeiwicz J, Swierczek E: Lysosyme in human body fluids. Clin Chim Acta 57:205–209, 1974.
77. DiLorenzo N, Palma L: Spinal fluid lysozyme in diagnosis of central nervous system tumors. Lancet 1:1077, 1976.
78. Reitamo S, Klockars M: Lysozyme activity in cerebrospinal fluid. Acta Med Scand 199:321–325, 1976.
79. Constantopoulos A., Antonakakis K, Matsaniotis N, Kapsalakis Z: Spinal fluid lysozyme in the diagnosis of central nervous system tumors. Neurochirurgie 19:174–178, 1976.
80. DiLorenzo N, Palma L, Ferrante L: Cerebrospinal fluid lysozyme activity in patients with central nervous system tumors. Neurochirurgie 20:19–22, 1977.
81. Mason DY, Roberts-Thompson P: Spinal fluid lysozyme in diagnosis of central nervous system tumors. Lancet II:952–953, 1974.
82. Hansen NE, Karle H, Jensen A, Bock E: Lysozyme activity in cerebrospinal fluid. Acta Neurol Scand 55:418–424, 1977.
83. Tanzer ML, Gilvarg C: Creatine and creatine kinase measurement. J Biol Chem 234:3201–3204, 1959.
84. Hughes BP: A method for the estimation of serum creatine kinase and its use in comparing creatine kinase and aldolase activities in normal and pathological serum. Clin Chim Acta 7:597–603, 1962.
85. Herschkowitz N, Cumings JN: Creatine kinase in cerebrospinal fluid. J Neurol Neurosurg Psychiatr 27:247–250, 1964.
86. Bell RD, Rosenberg RN, Ting R, Mukherjee A, Stone MJ, Willerson JT: Creatine kinase BB isoenzyme levels by radioimmunoassay in patients with neurologic disease. Anal Neurol 3:52–59, 1978.
87. Wolfson SK, Williams-Ashman HG: Isocitric and 6-phosphogluconic dehydrogenase in human blood serum. Proc Soc Exp Biol Med 96:231–234, 1957.

88. Van Rymenant M, Robert J: Enzymes in cancer. II. The isocitrate dehydrogenase of the cerebrospinal fluid in various cancerous and noncancerous conditions. Cancer 13:878–881, 1960.

89. Van Rymenant M, Robert J, Otten J: Isocitrate dehydrogenase in the cerebrospinal fluid—clinical usefulness of its determination. Neurology (Minneap) 16:351–354, 1966.

90. Anylan AJ, Gamble J, Hoster HA: β-Glucuronidase activity of the white blood cells in human leukemias and Hodgkin's disease. Cancer 3:116–123, 1950.

91. Fishman WH, Anlyan AJ: β-Glucuronidase activity in human tissues. Cancer Res 7:808–817, 1947.

92. Anlyan AJ, Starr A: β-Glucuronidase activity of spinal and ventricular fluids in humans. Cancer 5:578–580, 1952.

93. Fishman WH, Springer B, Brunetti R: Application of an improved glucuronidase assay method to the study of human blood β-glucuronidase. J Biol Chem 173:449–456, 1948.

94. Fleisher M, Schold C, Schwartz MK, Posner J: Tumor markers in cerebrospinal fluid for the differential diagnosis of central nervous system metastasis. Clin Chem 24:1002, 1978.

95. Rutenberg AM: LAP activity-observations in patients with cancer of the pancreas and other disease. N Engl J Med 259:469–472, 1958.

96. Goldbarg JA: The colorimetric determination of LAP in urine and serum of normal subjects and patients with cancer and other diseases. Cancer 11:283–291, 1958.

97. Green JB, Perry M: Leucine aminopeptidase activity in cerebrospinal fluid. Neurology (Minneap) 13:924–926, 1963.

98. Frithz G, Ericsson P, Ronquist G: Serum adenylate kinase activity in the early phase of acute myocardial infarction. Upsala J Med Sci 81:155–158, 1976.

99. Ronquist G, Ericsson P, Frithz G, Hugosson R: Malignant brain tumors associated with adenylate kinase in cerebrospinal fluid. Lancet I:1284–1286, 1977.

100. Frithz G, Ericsson P, Ronquist G: Adenylate kinase activity in cerebrospinal fluid in connection with transitory ischemic attacks. Upsala J Med Sci 82:11–14, 1977.

101. Ronquist G, Frithz G: Adenylate kinase activity and glutathione concentration of cerebrospinal fluid in different neurological disorders. Eur Neurol 18:106–110, 1979.

102. Getaz EP, Bhargava A, Fitzpatrick J: Adenylate kinase in central nervous system malignancy. Lancet II: 146, 1979.

103. Hultberg B, Olsson JE: Diagnostic value of determinations of lysosomal hydrolases in CSF of patients with neurological diseases. Acta Neurol Scand 57:201–215, 1978.

104. Cuatico W, Woldron R, Tyschenko W: Biochemical evidence for viral-like characteristics in CSF of brain tumor patients. Cancer 39:2240–2246, 1977.

105. Cuatico W, Cho JR, Spiegelman S: Particles with RNA of high molecular weight and RNA-directed DNA polymerase in human brain tumors. Proc Natl Acad Sci USA 70:2789–2793.

106. Cuatico W, Cho JR: Preliminary evidence for the existence of RNA-directed DNA polymerase and high molecular weight RNA in human brain tumor tissue culture supernatants. Biochem Exp Biol 12:161–165, 1976.

107. Bachrach U: Function of naturally occurring polyamines. New York: Academic Press, 1973.

108. Caldarera CM: A tribute to G. Moruzzi. Ital J Biochem 25:5–114, 1976.

109. Cohen SS: Introduction to the polyamines. Englewood Cliffs, N.J.: Prentice Hall, 1971.

110. Janne J, Poso H, Raina A: Polyamines in rapid growth and cancer. Biochim Biophys Acta 473:241–293, 1978.

111. Morris DR, Fillingame RH: Regulation of amino acid decarboxylation. Ann Rev Biochem 43:303–325, 1974.

112. Raina A, Janne J: Physiology of the natural polyamines putrescine, spermidine, and spermine. Med Biol 53:121–147, 1975.

113. Russell DH: Polyamines in normal and neoplastic growth. New York: Raven Press. 1973.

114. Stevens I: The biochemical role of naturally occurring polyamines in nucleic acid synthesis. Biol Rev 45:1–27, 1970.

115. Tabor H, Tabor CW: Spermine, spermidine and related amines. Pharmacol Rev 16:245–300, 1964.

116. Tabor H, Tabor CW: Biosynthesis and metabolism of 1,4-diaminobutane, spermidine, spermine, and related amines. Adv Enzymol 36:203–268, 1972.

117. Tabor CW, Tabor H: 1,4-diaminobutane (putrescine), spermidine, and spermine. Ann Rev Biochem 45:285–306, 1976.

118. Heby O, Marton LJ, Wilson CB, Martinez HM: Polyamine metabolism in a rat brain tumor cell line: its relationship to the growth rate. J Cell Physiol 86:511–522, 1975.

119. Heby O, Marton LJ, Zardi L, Russell DH, Baserga R: Accumulaton of Polyamines after stimulation of cellular proliferation in human diploid fibroblasts. In: The cell cycle in malignancy and immunity, Hampton JD (ed.). Springfield, Va: National Technical Information Service, 1975, pp 50–66.

120. Russell DH, Levy CC, Schimpf SC, Hawk IA: Urinary polyamines in cancer patients. Cancer Res 31:1555–1558, 1971.

121. Dreyfuss F, Chayen R, Dreyfuss G: Polyamine excretion in the urine of cancer patients. Isr J Med Sci 11:785–795, 1975.

122. Sanford EJ, Drago JR, Rohner TJ: Preliminary evaluation of urinary polyamines in the diagnosis of genitourinary tract malignancy. J Urol 113:218–221, 1975.

123. Townsend RM, Banda PW, Marton LJ: Polyamines in malignant melanoma; urinary excretion and disease progress. Cancer 38:2088–2092, 1976.

124. Waalkes TP, Gehrke CW, Tormey DC, Zumwalt RW, Hueser JN, Kuo KC, Lakings DB, Ahmann DL, Moertel CG: Urinary excretion of polyamines by patients with advanced malignancy. Cancer Chemother Rep 59:1103–1116, 1975.

125. Bartos F, Bartos D, Grettie DP, Campbell RA, Marton LJ, Smith RG, Daves GD: Polyamine levels in normal human serum: comparison of analytical methods. Biochem Biophys Res Comm 75:915–919, 1977.

126. Marton LJ, Vaughn JG, Hawk IA, Levy CC, Russell DH: Elevated polyamine levels in serum and urine of cancer patients: detection by a rapid automated technique utilizing an amino acid analyzer. In: Polyamines in normal and neoplastic growth, Russell DH (ed.). New York: Raven Press, 1973, pp 367–372.

127. Nishioka K, Romsdahl MM: Elevation of putrescine and spermidine in sera of patients with solid tumors. Clin Chim Acta 57:155–161, 1974.

128. Seiler N: Assay procedures for polyamines in urine, serum, and cerebrospinal fluid. Clin Chem 23:1519–1526, 1977.

129. Denton MD, Glazer HS, Zellner DC, Smith FG: Gas chromatographic measurement of urinary polyamines in cancer patients. Clin Chem 19:904–907, 1973.

130. Gehrke CW, Kuo KC, Zumwalt RW, Waalkes TP: The determination of polyamines in urine by gas liquid chromatography. In: Polyamines in normal and neoplastic growth, Russell DH (ed.). New York: Raven Press, 1973, pp 343–354.

131. Makita M, Yamamoto S, Kono M: Rapid determination of di- and polyamines human urine by electron capture gas chromatography. Clin Chim Acta 61:403–405, 1975.

132. Seiler N, Weichmann M: Die Mikrobestimmung von Spermin und Spermidin als 1-Dimethylamino-naphthalin-5-sulfonsaure-derivate. Hoppe Seyler's Z Physiol Chem 348:1285–1290, 1967.

133. Smith RG, Daves GD: Gas chromatography-mass spectrometry analysis of polyamines using deuterated analogs as internal standards. Biomed Mass Spectrom 4:146–151, 1977.

134. Walle T: Gas chromatography-mass spectrometry of di- and polyamines in human urine. In: Polyamines in normal and neoplastic growth, Russell DH (ed.). New York: Raven Press, 1973, pp 355–366.

135. Abe F, Samejima K: A new fluorometric method for the determination of spermidine and spermine in tissues by thin layer chromatography. Anal Biochem 67:298–308, 1975.

136. Dreyfuss G, Dvir R, Harell A, Chayen R: Determination of polyamines in urine. Clin Chim Acta 49:65–72, 1973.

137. Heby O, Andersson G: Simplified micro method for the quantitative analysis of putrescine, spermidine, and spermine in urine. J Chromatog 145:73–80, 1978.

138. Seiler N, Wiechmann M: TLC analysis of amines as their DANS-derivatives. In: Progress in thin-layer chromatography and related methods, Niederwieser A, Pataki G (eds.) Ann Arbor, Mich.: Humphrey Science, 1970, pp 94–144.

139. Bachrach U, Reches B: Enzymatic assay for spermine and spermidine. Anal Biochem 17:38–48, 1966.

140. Harik SI, Pasternak GW, Snyder SH: An enzymatic isotopic microassay for putrescine. Biochem Biophys Acta 304:753–764, 1973.

141. Abdel-Monem MM, Ohno K: Separation of the DNS derivatives of polyamines and related compounds by thin layer and high pressure liquid chromatography. J Chromatog 107:416–419, 1975.

142. Hayashi T, Sugiura T, Kawai S, Ohno T: High speed liquid chromatographic determination of putrescine, spermidine, and spermine in human urine. J Chromatog 145:141–146, 1978.

143. Newton NE, Ohno K, Abdel-Monem MM: Determination of diamines and polyamines in tissues by high pressure liquid chromatography. J Chromatog 124:277–285, 1976.

144. Seiler N, Knodgen B: Determination of di- and polyamines by high-performance liquid chromatography separation of their 5-dimethylaminonaphthalene-1-sulfonyl derivatives. J Chromatog 145:29–39, 1978.

145. Gehrke CW, Kuo KC, Ellis RL: Polyamines: an improved automated ion exchange method. J Chromatog 143:345–361, 1977.

146. Marton LJ, Heby O, Wilson CB: A method for the determination of polyamines in cerebrospinal fluid. FEBS Lett 46:305–307, 1974.

147. Marton LJ, Lee PLY: More sensitive automated detection of polyamines in physiological fluids and tissue extracts with o-phthaldehyde. Clin Chem 21:1721–1724, 1975.

148. Bartos D, Campbell RA, Bartos F, Grettie DP: Direct determination of polyamines in human serum by radioimmunoassay. Cancer Res 35:2056–2060, 1975.

149. Bartos F, Bartos D: Antipolyamine antibodies. In: Advances in polyamine research, vol 2, Campbell RA, Morris DR, Bartos D, Davies GD, Bartos F (eds). New York: Raven Press, 1978, pp 65–70.

150. Kremzner LT:Polyamine metabolism in normal and neoplastic neural tissue. In: Polyamines in normal and neoplastic growth, Russell DH (ed.). New York: Raven Press, 1973, pp 27–40.

151. Marton LJ, Heby O, Wilson CB: Increased polyamine concentrations in the CSF of patients with brain tumors. Int J Cancer 14:731–735, 1974.

152. Marton LJ, Heby O, Levin VA, Lubich WP, Crafts DC, Wilson CB: The relationship of polyamines in cerebrospinal fluid to the presence of central nervous system tumors. Cancer Res 36:973–977, 1976.

153. Terabayashi T: Blood levels of polyamines in patients with brain tumor. Neurol Med Chir (Tokyo) 16:43–50, 1976.

154. Terabayashi T, Tanimura K: Determination of blood polyamines in patients with brain tumor. Neurol Surg (Tokyo) 4:1051–1056, 1976.

155. Rennert OM, Lawson DL, Shukla JB, Miale TD: Cerebrospinal fluid polyamine monitoring in CNS leukemia. Clin Chim Acta 75:365–369, 1977.
156. Yap BS, Yap HY, Nishioka K, Bodey GP: Cerebrospinal fluid polyamines and carcinoembryonic antigen in meningeal carcinomatosis. Proc Am Assoc Cancer Res 20:187, 1979.
157. Marton LJ, Edwards MS, Levin VA, Lubich WP, Wilson CB: Predictive value of cerebrospinal fluid polyamines in medulloblastoma. Cancer Res 39:993–997, 1979.
158. Marton LJ, Edwards MS, Levin VA, Lubich WP, Wilson CB: CSF polyamines: a new and important means of monitoring medulloblastoma. Cancer (in press).
159. Fulton DS, Levin VA, Lubich WP, Wilson CB, Marton LJ: Cerebrospinal fluid polyamines in patients with glioblastoma multiforme and anaplastic astrocytoma. Cancer (in press).
160. Cohen SS: Conference on polyamines in cancer. Cancer Res 37:939–942, 1977.
161. Durie BGM, Salmon SE, Russell DH: Polyamines as markers of response and disease activity in cancer chemotherapy. Cancer Res 37:214–221, 1977.
162. Russell DH, Durie BGM, Salmon SE: Polyamines as predictors of success and failure in cancer chemotherapy. Lancet II: 797–799, 1975.
163. Russell DH: Clinical relevance of polyamines as biochemical markers of tumor kinetics. Clin Chem 23:22–27, 1977.
164. Schimpff SC, Levy CC, Hawk IA, Russell DH: Polyamines: potential role in the diagnosis, prognosis, and therapy of patients with cancer. In: Polyamines in normal and neoplastic growth, Russell DH (ed.). New York: Raven Press, 1973, pp 395–403.
165. Woo KB, Simon RM: A quantitative model for relating tumor cell number to polyamine concentrations. In: Polyamines in normal and neoplastic growth, Russel DH (ed.). New York: Raven Press, 1973, pp 381–393.
166. Woo KB, Enagonio RD: A quantitative analysis of biological marker synthesis in tumor cell cycle. Clin Chem 23:1409–1415, 1977.
167. Seidenfeld J, Marton LJ: Biochemical markers of central nervous system tumors in cerebrospinal fluid. Ann Clin Lab Sci 8:459–466, 1978.
168. Seidenfeld J, Marton LJ: Biochemical markers of central nervous system tumors measured in cerebrospinal fluid and their potential use in diagnosis and patient management: a review. J Natl Cancer Inst 63:919–931, 1979.
169. Steinberg D, Avigan J: Studies of cholesterol biosynthesis. II. The role of desmosterol in the biosynthesis of cholesterol. J Biol Chem 235:3127–3129, 1960.
170. Avigan J, Steinberg D, Vroman H, Thompson MJ, Mosettig E: Studies of cholesterol biosynthesis. I. The identification of desmosterol in serum and tissue of animals and man treated with MER-29. J Biol Chem 235:3123–3126, 1960.
171. Fumagalli R, Grossi E, Paoletti P, Paoletti R: Studies on lipids in brain tumors. I. Occurrence and significance of sterol precursors of cholesterol in human brain tumors. J Neurochem 11:561–565, 1974.
172. Weiss JF: Sterols and other lipids in tumors of the nervous system. Prog Biochem Pharmacol 10:227–268, 1975.
173. Paoletti P, Fumagalli R, Grossi-Paoletti E: Drugs acting on brain tumor sterols. In: The experimental biology of brain tumors, Kirsch WM, Grossi-Paoletti E, Paoletti P (eds). Springfield, Ill.: Charles C. Thomas, 1972, pp 457–479.
174. Fumagalli R, Grossi-Paoletti E, Paoletti P, Paoletti R: Lipids in brain tumors. II. Effect of triparanol and 20,25-diazacholesterol on sterol composition in experimental and human brain tumors. J Neurochem 13:1005–1010, 1966.
175. Fumagalli R, Grossi-Paoletti E, Paoletti R, Paoletti P: Sterol metabolism in brain tumors and cerebrospinal fluid. Ann N Y Acad Sci 159: 472–479, 1969.
176. Wolfman L, Sachs BA: Separation of cholesterol and desmosterol by thin layer chromatography. J Lipid Res 5:127–128, 1964.

177. Fumagalli R, Capella P, Vandenheuvel WJA: Gas chromatographic determination of cholesterol-desmosterol ratios. Anal Biochem 10:377–386, 1965.
178. Vandenheuvel FA, Fumagalli R, Paoletti R, Paoletti P: A possible biochemical procedure for the diagnosis of human brain tumor. Life Sci 6:439–444, 1967.
179. Fumagalli R, Paoletti P: Sterol test for human brain tumors: relationship with different oncotypes. Neurology (Minneap) 21:1149–1156, 1971.
180. Weiss JF, Ransohoff J, Kayden HJ: Cerebrospinal fluid sterols in patients undergoing treatment for gliomas. Neurology (Minneap) 22:187–193, 1972.
181. Marton LJ, Gordan GS, Barker M, Wilson CB, Lubich W: Failure to demonstrate desmosterol in spinal fluid of brain tumor patients. Arch Neurol 28:137–138, 1973.
182. Paoletti P, Vandenheuvel FA, Fumagalli R, Paoletti R: The sterol test for the diagnosis of human brain tumors. Neurology (Minneap) 19:190–197, 1969.
183. Paoletti P. Fumagalli R, Weiss JF, Pezzotta S: Desmosterol: a biochemical marker of glioma growth. Surg Neurol 8:399–405, 1977.
184. Weiss J, Ransohoff J, Kayden H: Evaluation of patients undergoing therapy for gliomas by examination of CSF sterols after triparanol treatment. Trans Am Neurol Assoc 96:324–326, 1971.
185. Weiss JF, Cravioto H, Bennet K, Weiss E, Ransohoff J: Desmosterol in human and experimental brain tumors in tissue culture. Arch Neurol 33:180–182, 1976.
186. Fumagalli R, Paoletti P, Pezzotta S: The desmosterol test in the diagnosis of recurrent cerebral tumors. Acta Neurol (Naples) 28:268–274, 1973.
187. Fumagalli R, Pezzotta S, Racca AR, Paoletti P: Sterols in cerebrospinal fluid during nitrosourea chemotherapy of human brain tumors. Pharmacol Res Comm 8:127–141, 1976.
188. Paoletti P, Pezzotta S, Racca AR, Fumagalli R: Chemotherapy of human nervous system tumors: influence on cerebrospinal fluid sterols. Natl Cancer Inst Monogr 46:125–126, 1977.
189. Ransohoff J, Weiss J: Cerebrospinal fluid sterols in the evaluation of patients with gliomas. Natl Cancer Inst Monogr 46:119–124, 1977.
190. Tichy J: Cholesterol in the cerebrospinal fluid: an analysis of 447 neurological patients. Rev Czech Med 12:265–271, 1966.
191. Fleisher JH, Marton LJ, Bachur NR, Mann-Kaplan RS: Cholesterol in cerebrospinal fluid of brain tumor patients. Life Sci 13:1517–1526, 1973.
192. Tashima CK, Timberger R, Burdick R, Leavy M, Rawson RW: Cerebrospinal fluid titer of chorionic gonadotrophin in patients with intracranial metastatic choriocarcinoma. J Clin Endocrinol Metab 25:1493–1495, 1965.
193. Rushworth AGJ, Orr AH, Bagshawe KD: The concentration of HCG in the plasma and spinal fluid of patients with trophoblastic tumors in the central nervous system. Br J Cancer 22:253–257, 1968.
194. Bagshawe, KD, Harland S: Detection of intracranial tumors with special reference to immunodiagnosis. Proc Roy Soc Med 69:51–53, 1976.
195. Bagshawe KD, Harland S: Immunodiagnosis and Monitoring of gonadotropin producing metastases in the central nervous system. Cancer 38:112–118, 1976.
196. Kaye SB, Bagshawe KD, McElwain TJ, Peckham MJ: Brain metastases in malignant teratoma: a review of four years' experience and an assessment of the role of tumor markers. Br J Cancer 39:217–223, 1979.
197. Vugrin D, Nisselbaum J, Schold C, Posner J, Cvitkovic E, Schwartz M, Golbey R: Blood and cerebrospinal fluid tumor markers in the diagnosis of brain metastases from testicular carcinoma. Proc Am Assoc Cancer Res 20:115, 1979.
198. Allen JC, Nisselbaum J, Epstein F, Rosen G, Schwartz MK: Alphafetoprotein and human chorionic gonadotropin determination in cerebrospinal fluid: an aid to the diagnosis and management of intracranial germ-cell tumors. J Neurosurg 51:368–374, 1979.

199. Jordan RM, Kendall JW, Seaich JL, Allen JP, Paulsen CA, Kerber CW, Vanderlaan WP: Cerebrospinal fluid hormone concentration in the evaluation of pituitary tumors. Ann Intern Med 85:49–55, 1976.

200. Schroeder LL, Johnson JC, Malarkey WB: Cerebrospinal fluid prolactin: a reflection of abnormal prolactin secretion in patients with pituitary tumors. J Clin Endocrinol Metab 43:1255–1260, 1968.

201. Jordan RM, McDonald SD, Stevens EA, Kendall JW: Cerebrospinal fluid prolactin: a reevaluation. Arch Intern Med 139:208–211, 1979.

202. Manno NJ, McGuckin WF, Goldstein NP: Cerebrospinal fluid total polysaccharide in diseases of the nervous system. Neurology (Minneap) 15:45–55, 1965.

203. Cramer H, Goodwin FK, Post RM, Bunney WE Jr: Effects of probenecid and exercise on cerebrospinal fluid cyclic AMP in affective illness. Lancet I:1346-1347, 1972.

204. Cramer H, Ng LKY, Chase TN: Adenosine-3',5'-monophosphate in cerebrospinal fluid: effect of drugs and neurologic disease. Arch Neurol 29:197–199, 1973.

205. Heikkinen ER, Myllyla VV, Vapaatalo H, Hokkanen E: Urinary excretion and cerebrospinal fluid concentration of cyclic adenosine-3',5'-monophosphate in various neurological diseases. Eur Neurol 11:270–280, 1974.

206. Myllyla VV, Heikkinen ER, Vapaatalo H, Hokkanen E: Cyclic AMP concentration and enzyme activities of cerebrospinal fluid in patients with epilepsy or central nervous system damage. Eur Neurol 13:123–130, 1975.

207. Heikkinen ER, Myllyla VV, Hokkanen E, Vappaatalo H: Cerebrospinal fluid concentration of cyclic AMP in cerebrovascular diseases. Eur Neurol 14:129–137, 1976.

208. Furman MA, Shulman K: Cyclic AMP and adenyl cyclase in brain tumors. J Neurosurg 46:477–483, 1977.

209. Rudman S, O'Brien MS, McKinney AS, Hoffman JC Jr, Patterson JH: Observations on the cyclic nucleotide concentrations in human cerebrospinal fluid. J Clin Endrocinol Metab 42:1088–1097, 1976.

210. Trabucci M, Cerri C, Spano PF, Kumakura K: Guanosine-3',5'-monophosphate in the CSF of neurological patients. Arch Neurol 34:12–13, 1977.

211. Porta M, Bareggi SR, Collice M, Ferrara M, Calderini G, Morselli PL: Determination of HVA and 5-HIAA in ventricular CSF of patients with brain tumors. J Neurosurg Sci 18:157–163, 1974.

212. Collice M, Porta M, Ferra M, Castelli A: Mediatori cerebralli, e neoplasie endocraniche. Acta Neurol (Naples) 30:71–77, 1975.

213. Bareggi SR, Porta M, Collice M, Calderini G, Ferrara M, Morselli PL: Monoamine acid metabolites in ventricular CSF of patients with brain tumors. Acta Neurochir 35:161–170, 1976.

214. Weisz R, Mars H: Deoxyribonucleic acid determination in human cerebrospinal fluid. Ann Neurol 2:357, 1977.

215. Cumings JN: The examination of the cerebrospinal fluid and cerebral cyst fluid by paper strip electrophoresis. J Neurol Neurosurg Psychiatr 16:152–157, 1953.

216. Girke W, Kovarik J: Electrophoretic investigations on protein components in the cerebrospinal fluid of brain tumor patients. Arch Psychiatr Nervenkr 214:72–79, 1971.

217. Neuwelt EA, Garcia JH, Kolar O, Rao K, Ducker T: Elevated CSF gamma globulins with cerebral glioma. Surg Neurol 8:107–110, 1977.

218. Zlotnick A, Weisenberg E, Chowers I: Mucroproteins of cerebrospinal fluid and blood in neurologic disorders. J Lab Clin Med 54:207–212, 1959.

219. Dencker SJ, Bronnestam R, Swahn B: Demonstration of large blood proteins in cerebrospinal fluid. Neurology (Minneap) 11:441–444, 1961.

220. Alsabti E, Keating M, Cabanillas F, Mavligit G: Early diagnosis of central nervous system leukemia and lymphoma by radioimmunoassay of β-microglobulin in the cerebrospinal fluid. Proc Am Assoc Cancer Res 20:190, 1979.
221. Starmans JJP, Vos J, Vanderhelm HJ:The β_2-microglobulin content of the cerebrospinal fluid in neurological disease. J Neurol Sci 33:45–49, 1977.
222. Swahn B, Bronnestam R, Dencker SJ: On the origin of the lipoproteins in the cerebrospinal fluid. Neurology (Minneap) 11:437–440, 1961.
223. Schuller E, Delasnerie N, Helary M, Lefevre M: Serum and cerebrospinal fluid IGM in 203 neurological patients. Eur Neurol 17:77–82, 1977.
224. Wu KK, Jacobsen CD, Hoak JC: Plasminogen in normal and abnormal human cerebrospinal fluid. Arch Neurol 28:64–66, 1973.
225. Berglund G, Greter J, Lindstedt S, Steen G, Waldenstrom J, Wass U: Urinary excretion of thymine and uracil in a two year old child with a malignant tumor of the brain. Clin Chem 25:1325–1328, 1979.
226. Enna SJ, Stern LZ, Wastek GJ, Yamamura HI: Cerebrospinal fluid γ-aminobutyric acid variations in neurologic disorders. Arch Neurol 34:683–685, 1977.
227. Bohlen P, Schechter PJ, Van Damme W, Coquillat G, Dosch J-C, Koch-Weser J: Automated assay of γ-aminobutyric acid in human cerebrospinal fluid. Clin Chem 24:256–260, 1978.
228. Wood JH, Gleaser BS, Enna ST, Hare TA: Verification and quantification of GABA in human cerebrospinal fluid. J Neurochem 30:291–293, 1978.
229. Faull KF, DoAmaral JR, Berger PA, Barchas JD: Mass spectrometric identification and selected ion monitoring quantification of γ-aminobutyric acid in human lumbar cerebrospinal fluid. J Neurochem 31:1119–1122, 1978.
230. Bala Manyam NV, Hare TA, Katz L, Glaeser BS: Huntington's disease: cerebrospinal fluid GABA levels in at-risk individuals. Arch Neurol 35:728–730, 1978.
231. Pye IF, Stonier C, McGale EHF: Double enzymatic assay for determination of glutamine and glutamic acid in cerebrospinal fluid and plasma. Anal Chem 50:951–953, 1978.
232. Iigima K, Tabase S, Tsumuraya K, Endo M, Itahara K: Changes in free amino acids of cerebrospinal fluid and plasma in various neurological diseases. Tohoku J Exp Med 126:133–150, 1978.
233. Heiblim DI, Evans HE, Glass L, Agbayani MM: Amino acid concentrations in cerebrospinal fluid. Arch Neurol 35:765–768, 1978.
234. Servo C, Palo J, Pitkanen E: Gas chromatographic separation and mass spectrometric identification of polyols in human cerebrospinal fluid and plasma. Acta Neurol Scand 56:104–110, 1977.
235. Servo C, Palo J, Pitkanen E: Polyols in the cerebrospinal fluid and plasma of neurological, diabetic, and uraemic patients. Acta Neurol Scand 56:111–116, 1977.
236. Smith SL, Novotny M, Weber EL: Gas-chromatographic determination of polyol profiles in cerebrospinal fluid. Clin Chem 24:545–548, 1978.
237. Gold P, Freedman S: Specific carcinoembryonic antigens of the human digestive system. J Exp Med 122:467–481, 1965.
238. Egan ML, Engvall E, Ruoslahti EI, Todd CW: Detection of circulating tumor antigens. Cancer 40:458–466, 1977.
239. Reynoso G, Chu TM, Holyoke D, Cohen E, Nemoto T, Wang JJ, Chuang J, Guinan P, Murphy GP: Carcinoembryonic antigen in patients with different cancers. JAMA 220:361–365, 1972.
240. Kido DK, Dyce BJ, Haverback BJ, Rumbaugh CL: Carcinoembryonic antigen in patients with untreated central nervous system tumors. Bull Los Angeles Neurol Soc 41:47–54, 1976.

241. Snitzer LS, McKinney EC, Tejada F, Sigel MM, Rosomoff HL, Zubrod CG: Cerebral metastases and carcinoembryonic antigen in CSF. N Engl J Med 293:1101, 1975.

242. Feinberg SB, Hahn JF: Carcinoembryonic antigen in a metastatic brain tumor. Neurosurgery 2:266–268, 1978.

243. Miyake E, Yamashita M, Kitamura K, Ishigami F: Carcinoembryonic antigen levels in patients with brain tumors. Acta Neurochir 46:53–57, 1979.

244. Yap BS, Yap HY, Benjamin RS, Bodey GP, Freireich EJ: Cerebrospinal fluid carcinoembryonic antigen in breast cancer patients with meningeal carcinomatosis. Proc Am Assoc Cancer Res 19:98, 1978.

245. Hass WK: Soluble tissue antigens in human brain tumors and cerebrospinal fluid. Arch Neurol 14:443–447, 1966.

246. Kornblith PL, Dohan FC Jr, Wood WC, Whitman BO: Human astrocytoma: Serum mediated immunologic response. Cancer 33:1512–1519, 1974.

247. Phillips JP, Sujatanond M, Martuza RL, Quindlen EA, Wood WC, Kornblith PL, Dohan FC Jr: Cytotoxic antibodies in preoperative glioma patients: a diagnostic assay. Acta Neurochir 35:43–52, 1976.

248. Wood WC, Kornblith PL, Quindlen EA, Pollock LA: Detection of humoral immune response to human brain tumors: specificity and reliability of microcytotoxicity assay. Cancer 43:86–90, 1979.

249. Kornblith PL, Pollock LA, Coakham HB, Quindlen EA, Wood WC: Cytotoxic antibody responses in astrocytoma patients. J Neurosurg 51:47–52, 1979.

250. Sheikh KMA, Apuzzo MLJ, Weiss MH: Specific cellular immune responses in patients with malignant gliomas. Cancer Res 39:1733–1738, 1979.

251. Eng LF, Vanderhaeghen JJ, Bignami A, Gerstl B: An acidic protein isolated from fibrous astrocytes. Brain Res 28:351–354, 1971.

252. Delpech B, Delpech A, Vidard MN, Girard N, Tayot J, Clement JC, Creissard P: Glial fibrillary acid protein in tumors of the nervous system. Br J Cancer 37:33–40, 1978.

253. Jacque CM, Vinner C, Kujas M, Racadot J, Baumann NA: Determination of glial fibrillary acid protein in human brain tumors. J Neurol Sci 35:147–155, 1978.

254. Maunoury R, Delpech A, Delpech B, Bidard MN, Vedrenne C, Constans JP, Hillereau J: Localization de la protein gliofibrillaire (GFAP) pare immunocytochimie dans les tumeurs cerebrales humaines. Neuro-Chirurgie 23:173–185, 1977.

255. Eng LF, Lee YL, Miles LEM: Measurement of glial fibrillary acid protein by a two-site immunoradiometric assay. Anal Biochem 71:243–259, 1976.

256. Deck JHN, Eng LF, Bigbee J, Woodcock SM: The role of glial fibrillary acidic protein in the diagnosis of central nervous system tumors. Acta Neuropathol (Berlin) 42:183–190, 1978.

257. Eng LF, Rubinstein LJ: Contribution of immunohistochemistry to diagnostic problems of human cerebral tumors. J Histochem Cytochem 26:513–522, 1978.

258. Palfreyman JW, Thomas DGT, Ratcliffe JG, Graham DI: Glial fibrillary acid protein: purification from human fibrillary astrocytoma, development and validation of a radioimmunoassay for GFAP-like immunoactivity. J Neurol Sci 41:101–113, 1979.

259. Jacque CM, Kujas M, Poreau A, Raoul M, Collier P, Racadot J, Baumann N: GFA and S100 protein levels as an index for malignancy in human gliomas and neurinomas. J Natl Cancer Inst 62:479–483, 1979.

260. Lowenthal A, Noppe M, Gheuens J, Karcher D: α-Albumin (glial fibrillary acid protein) in normal and pathological human brain and cerebrospinal fluid. J Neurol 219:87–91, 1978.

261. Bogoch S: Brain glycoprotein 10B: further evidence of the 'sign-post' role of brain glycoproteins in cell recognition, its change in brain tumor, and the presence of a 'distance factor' Adv Exp Med Biol 32:39–52, 1972.

262. Bogoch S: Brain glycoproteins and recognition functions: recognins and cancer. Adv Exp Med Biol 68:555–566, 1976.

263. Bogoch S: The detection of malignant gliomas in brain by the quantitative production *in vitro* of TAG (target attaching globulins) from human serum. In: Biological diagnosis of brain disorders, Bogoch S (ed.). New York: Spectrum-Wiley 1973, pp 358–361.

264. Bogoch S: Astrocytin and malignin: two polypeptide fragments (recognins) related to brain tumor. Natl Cancer Inst Monogr 46:133–137, 1977.

265. Harris JH, Gohara A, Bogoch S: New immunodiagnostic techniques for CNS tumors. J Neuropath Exp Neurol 37:623, 1978.

266. Bogoch S, Bogoch ES, Fager CA, Goldensohn ES, Harris JH, Hickok DF, Lowden JA, Lux WE, Ransohoff J, Walker MD: Elevated serum anti-malignin antibody in glioma and other cancer patients: a seven-hospital blind study. Neurology (Minneap) 29:584–585, 1979.

267. Bogoch S, Bogoch ES: Production of two recognins related to malignin: recognin M from mammary MCF-7 carcinoma cells and recognin L from lymphoma P_3G cells. Neurochem Res 4:465–472, 1979.

268. Bogoch S, Bogoch ES: Disarmed anti-malignin antibody in human cancer. Lancet I:987, 1979.

269. Mori T, Morimoto K, Ushio Y, Hayakawa T, Mogami H: Radioimmunoassay of astroprotein (an astrocyte-specific cerebroprotein) in cerebrospinal fluid from patients with glioma: a preliminary study. Neurol Med Chir 15:23-25, 1975.

270. Mori T, Morimoto K, Hayakawa T, Ushio Y, Mogami H, Sebiguchi K: Radioimmunoassay of astroprotein (an astrocyte-specific cerebroprotein) in cerebrospinal fluid and its clinical significance. Neurol Med Chir 18:25–31, 1978.

271. Morimoto K, Hayakawa T, Ushio Y, Mogami H, Mori T: Radioimmunoassay of astroprotin (an astrocyte-specific cerebroprotein) in cerebrospinal fluid and its clinical significance. Adv Neurol Sci 22:75–81, 1978.

272. Cohen SR, Herndon RM, McKhann GM: Radioimmunoassay of myelin basic protein in spinal fluid: an index of active demyelination. N Engl J Med 295:1455–1457, 1976.

273. McPherson TA, Gilpin A, Seland TP: Radioimmunoassay of CSF for encephalitogenic basic protein: a diagnostic test for MS. Can Med Assoc J 107:856–859, 1972.

274. Schmid G, Thomas G, Hempel K, Gruninger W: Radioimmunological determination of myelin basic protein (MBP) and MBP-antibodies. Eur Neurol 12:173–185, 1974.

275. Galvez S, Farcas A, Monari M: The concentration of alpha-1-antitrypsin in cerebrospinal fluid and serum in a series of 40 intracranial tumors. Clin Chim Acta 91:191–196, 1979.

6. Non-Chemotherapeutic Approaches to Uncontrolled CNS Tumors

W.L. BANKS JR., H.F. YOUNG, S.S. JENNINGS and A.M. KAPLAN

1. INTRODUCTION

The American Cancer Society predicted that there would be 11,900 new cases of primary central nervous system cancers and 9800 deaths in the U.S. during 1980 [1]. Tumors of the central nervous system are the second most common cancer in children of both sexes under the age of 15 years, surpassed only by the incidence of leukemias. The etiology of intracranial tumors is unknown, although trauma has often been discussed as a possible cause [2–4], even though there is, as yet, no clear demonstration that trauma is involved in the generation of primary brain cancers. A few relatively rare forms of central nervous system tumors such as acoustic neuromas and neurofibromas appear to follow hereditary patterns. Different forms of primary brain cancers have different biological, kinetic and metabolic characteristics, making it difficult to discuss the oncology of this organ site as a single entity.

In the adult, the most common form of primary brain cancer is glioblastoma multiforme, which has a predominant age distribution between 40 and 60 years, and is rare in children [5]. This tumor is the most important of the glioma or astrocytoma series which comprises 50% of all primary intracranial cancers. Astrocytomas of lower grades, often cystic in the cerebellum, constitute about 50% of intracranial cancers in children. The other potentially lethal tumor of childhood is the medulloblastoma for which patient survival patterns of approximately 50% in three years, 40% in five years, and 30% at ten years after the original diagnosis have been documented [6]. This tumor may recur many years after therapy and survivors continue to be at risk of relapse indefinitely. Recurrence or metastasis of medulloblastoma is nearly always fatal and further therapy under those circumstances is usually palliative in nature. After radiation therapy, the recurrence rate for medulloblastoma, in most studies, appears to peak in the first two years with diminished recurrence rates noted thereafter [7]. An intriguing recent report is strongly sugges-

tive of a viral etiology for medulloblastoma [8]. Craniophryngiomas are the
commonest non-glial tumor in children, accounting for approximately 99% of
all intracranial tumors [9].

Anaplastic astrocytoma grades III and IV (glioblastoma multiforme) remain
at this time resistant to the combinations of surgery, radiation and chemotherapy that have been employed in their treatment. Radical cancer operations
cannot be performed on patients with primary brain tumors without the
penalty of increasing or producing severe neurological deficits. Nearly all
surgical procedures for astrocytoma leave viable tumor tissue in the operated
site. The Brain Tumor Study Group (BTSG) has clearly shown that patients
with anaplastic astrocytomas who receive 5500 to 6000 rads of radiation to
the head live significantly longer than those receiving 5000 rads or less [10].
These data show that radiation therapy following conventional surgical resection increases median survival time from 17 weeks to 38 weeks following
surgical resection of the tumor. Thus, radiation therapy appears to be a
partially effective treatment for primary brain tumors, but it certainly is not
curative. Furthermore, there is both clinical [11, 12] and experimental [13] evidence of host cellular damage when 6000 rads are administered to the normal
brain. The most commonly used chemotherapeutic agents, currently the
nitrosoureas, add only slightly increased median survival times when used
with radiation therapy following conventional surgery, i.e., 38–43
weeks [10, 14]. However, for those 25% of patients that tolerate the initial
courses of chemotherapy, survival is often extended beyond 18 months
although no claims of cure have been reported using these agents. In fact,
reports are now appearing in the literature of pulmonary toxicity of nitrosoureas when given in long-term administration [15, 16]. If patients with anaplastic
astrocytoma are to have increased survivals and eventually cures, it is imperative to seek new forms of therapy which may be used alone or possibly in
combination with our present forms of therapy. For instance, it is imperative
to seek new forms of therapy which may be used alone or possibly in
combination with our present forms of therapy. For instance, it is most
probable that in the future, lower doses of irradiation to the brain will be
given and chemotherapy will be reduced or alternated with other forms of
therapy in order to optimize their combined effects. It is with this viewpoint
that we explored two novel approaches to therapy of primary brain cancers: 1)
the use of differential nutritional therapy involving dietary restriction of an
essential amino acid, and 2) the direct infusion of lymphocytes into the brain.
Our protocols and preliminary results of these two independent approaches
with adult patients are described below.

2. DIET THERAPY STUDIES

2.1. Background

From a nutritional point of view, the growing tumor presents a complex and intricate set of interrelationships with respect to the host and the diet. One must keep in mind that in many cases the host may become catabolic at the same time as the tumor is growing or anabolic. In one view, the host may serve as a proximal supplier of essential nutrients when the dietary source is insufficient to meet the needs for tumor growth. Thus, there is a potential competition for nutrient supply between the host and the cancer for maintenance and growth, respectively. The long-range goal for the study described below is to establish whether dietary restriction of a single essential amino acid is a safe and effective new treatment modality for cancers and specifically, for primary brain cancers in adults. The patient with an anaplastic astrocytoma is a very useful clinical model in which to test the feasibility of this approach, because the prognosis is for relatively short expected life time with current therapies and therefore, the outcome can be ascertained within a reasonably short period. Secondly, the tumor is always small in size relative to the host, so that the host's competition for nutrient supply should be optimized. Finally, we believe current therapies are generally associated with significant toxicities, whereas dietary restriction of an essential amino acid offers a new approach that should, when correctly monitored, be associated with minimal untoward side effects. By and large the rationale for this approach was developed as a result of animal model studies.

Munro[17] has recently reviewed the status of our understanding of cancer and host relationships with respect to their competition for nutrient supply. He concluded, as is generally accepted, that with regard to amino acids and proteins, the tumor can serve as a 'nitrogen trap' which, under certain circumstances, draws amino acid nitrogen from the host to maintain the continued growth of the cancer. The cachexic state, whether due solely to anorexia or partly to underlying metabolic alterations, might be viewed as a condition of semi-starvation, since many of the same metabolic changes are seen in cancer-related cachexia and in starvation of a non tumor-bearing host. Numerous studies with respect to the effects of dietary protein deprivation on tumor and host behavior have been published. Among them, White and Belkin[18] reported that a transplantable mammary adenocarcinoma grew almost as fast in mice on a low nitrogen diet as compared to those receiving adequate dietary protein (18% casein). They found a 26% decrease in tumor size owing to protein restriction, but the body weights of the animals were also reduced by 25%. In another study, White[19] reported that the low nitrogen fed animals bearing the mammary adenocarcinoma were in negative nitrogen balance, thus suggesting that the host served as a nutrient supply for the tumor. White further suggested that once the tumor is established in the body, it was not greatly affected by dietary protein restriction. Based on tissue nitrogen and protein contents, the data obtained by Sherman et al. [20], using a rat Walker 256 carcinoma model, and Babson [21], using a rat sarcoma R-1 model, suggested that carcass, presumably skeletal muscle protein, provided a major reservoir of essential amino acids to maintain tumor growth when dietary protein intakes were reduced or absent. Babson found that Flexner-Jobling carcinoma growth was more affected by dietary protein level than was R-1 sarcoma growth. This, and other findings, led Munro [17] to conclude that various experimental tumors responded differently to alterations in diminished dietary protein levels. In general, although a diet free of protein will limit tumor growth, it would be of no great benefit since the host tissues will be detrimentally affected.

We are therefore led to the following question: 'What effect does a diet deficient in a single essential amino acid have on tumor and host behavior?' Skipper and Thompson [22] showed that diets devoid of either VAL, LEU, ILE, PHE, HIS, or MET inhibited growth of sarcoma 180 in mice. Sugimura et al. [23] tube-fed diets lacking one essential amino acid to rats carrying Walker 256 carcinoma and found diets devoid of either MET, ILE or VAL slowed tumor growth, those devoid of either PHE, HIS or TYR only slightly retarded tumor growth, and a diet devoid of LYS had no effect on tumor growth. However, in each case the host suffered severe weight loss when an essential amino acid was missing completely. Thus, it appears that diets either devoid of protein or an essential amino acid may reduce tumor growth, but this benefit must be balanced by the generally unfavorable effects on the host. In this condition, host skeletal muscle protein presumably becomes catabolic and provides a source of the essential amino acids missing from the diet.

The next logical question that emerges is: 'Is there a level of restriction of the dietary intake of an essential amino acid at which tumor growth is inhibited, but at which the host tissues are not compromised?' As a result of the development of commercial dietary formulations low in PHE for use in the treatment of phenylketonuria, there are reports of the effects of diets restricted, but not devoid in PHE on cancer and host behavior in animal models and humans. Lorincz et al. [24] reviewed their own findings as well as those from Demopoulos' laboratory using these commercial formulations low in PHE and/or TYR. Using the Mead-Johnson product 'Lofenolac', which is nutritionally adequate in all respects except that it has lowered levels of PHE, Lorincz found significant tumor growth inhibition with small host weight loss for BW7756 transplanted mouse hepatoma and C3HBA mouse mammary adenocarcinoma models. They also found that the growth of sarcoma 180 in mice was not affected by the low PHE dietary regimen. Although the food intake of the mice was reduced in the models where tumor growth inhibition was noted, the tumor inhibition could not be explained solely on the basis of reduced caloric intakes. Further, they reported (anecdotally) some benefit in patients with advanced cancers in which they utilized PHE restriction. In this review, they described the case history of one patient with differentiated bilateral papillary serous cystadenocarcinoma who was treated beneficially with a low PHE regimen. Demopoulos found that diets low in PHE and TYR would inhibit S91 melanoma growth, but not S37 sarcoma growth in mice[25]. In addition, Demopoulos[26], reported that he obtained regression of metastatic disease in three of five patients with advanced malignant melanoma by feeding a diet low in PHE and TYR.

In an extensive animal model study, Theurer[27] examined the effects on tumor weight and tumor-free weight (host weight) of feeding diets containing various levels of each of the essential amino acids to C57BL female mice bearing BW10232 implanted adenocarcinomas. In this study, he used synthetic diets in which the concentrations of each of the essential amino acids were varied from zero to optimal levels. He then determined the effect on the tumor weights and the tumor-free weights for each group of animals compared to these weights in animals fed a control synthetic diet of all of the essential amino acids at their optimal levels. He reported that low levels of PHE, VAL, or ILE decreased tumor weight with no significant detrimental effect on host weight loss; low leves of TYR, THR, LEU, or MET also produced decreased tumor weights but host weights were decreased as well; and low LYS diets did not affect either weight change. He did not evaluate dietary HIS levels in this study. Thus, his results revealed that a favorable balance between reduced tumor weight combined with no greater reduction in host weight when compared to host weights of the control groups was achieved only with diets low in PHE, VAL, and ILE. These findings suggest that regulation of dietary levels of some, but not all of the essential amino acids might be useful in reducing the tumor growth without compromising the host's weight.

Recently, Pine[28] reported the effects of low dietary levels of PHE on survival of mice bearing L1210 leukemia. Using 'Lofenolac' and other similar Mead-Johnson formulations low in PHE and TYR, he reported a near doubling of the survival time for the mice when the low PHE diet was provided between 16 days before to 1 day after tumor implantation in DBA/2HaDD mice. Survival was still somewhat increased when the diet was started 4 days after implantation; whereas, no benefit was observed when the diet was started at 5 days after the tumor challenge. Furthermore, dietary restriction of PHE did not prolong survival in strains of mice that have diminished host defenses against L1210. Low dietary PHE levels increased survival of P388 leukemia only if the diet was begun prior to tumor implantation. TA/3 mammary tumors and EL4 leukemia survivals were not increased by dietary restriction of PHE in this study. Thus, beneficial effects of dietary modulation were not the same for all the model systems studied. The major thrust of this paper, however, dealt with the mechanism by which PHE restriction exerted its beneficial effects. Pine's results, along with those of Jose and Good [29], suggested that the beneficial effect of dietary restriction of PHE on tumor growth and/or survival in those systems where it was effective, might be mediated by host response of the immune system rather than by a direct effect on tumor growth *per se*.

In contrast to several of the above findings, Worthington *et al.* [30] recently reported that synthetic diets containing a 25% reduction in ILE, LEU or PHE-TYR were of no benefit in reducing tumor incidence or long term survival (54–57 weeks) in female Balb/C AN mice when methylcholanthrene (MCA) was implanted when compared to a control group of MCA implanted mice fed a complete synthetic amino acid mixture. They concluded that reduction in the diet of these essential amino acids was ineffective in altering the carcinogenic progression in this MCA 1409/3 myosarcoma model system. However, they only fed their groups of animals at a single level of restriction of the essential amino acids and thus, extrapolation of these findings over the broad range of possible dietary reduction of these essential amino acids must be viewed with some caution. However, they indicated that the body weights of the restricted animals were generally somewhat lower than the control group's weights throughout, although only the ILE deficient group appeared to show deficiency signs. In a second experiment, they assessed the impact of the various dietary restrictions on the growth of a second transplantable tumor challenge to animals fed the optimal diet after surgical removal of the primary tumor. They reported no differences in survival between the control and experimental groups in terms of tumor incidence from this experiment. Moreover, they found that the blood levels of the restricted essential amino acids were reduced in the ILE and PHE-TYR restricted groups, but not in the LEU restricted group. They also noted that the tumor free essential amino acid pools of the diet-restricted amino acids were not altered as a result of the dietary restriction when expressed on a mg/mmole basis. These latter findings are difficult to evaluate, but the authors indicate that it is suggestive evidence that the dietary restriction of at least this set of essential amino acids in their model system resulted in a lowering of the blood levels without a concomitant decrease in their tumor pool concentrations. However, they did not report the amino acid composition of the tumor protein compartment.

Finally, recent work by Lowrey *et al.* [31], indicates that the survival rate of MCA tumor-bearing mice was reduced when the host's nutritional status was compromised. Thus, it is important for survival, that the dietary regimen does not place the host tissue in a catabolic state. An appropriate summation from all of the above animal studies would be that favorable reductions in tumor growth without unfavorable effects on the host may be obtained by diets low in an essential amino acid, but is dependent upon the specific essential amino acid being restricted, the level of its restriction in the diet, and the model system employed.

In terms of identifying the best 'target' essential amino acid for dietary modulation, Rogers and Woodhall [32] have developed an assay procedure using human cancer tissues that attempts to identify the essential amino acid which is taken up disproportionately greater by tumor (in this case, human astrocytomas) than any of the other essential amino acids. This assay procedure, described in detail in the following section, actually assesses the net change in essential amino acid composition of a tissue culture media after a three hour period of incubation with minced tumor tissue. Thus, when there is a net uptake from the media of an essential amino acid it is believed to be required by the tumor. However, the results of the assay are probably due to a composite of factors including 1) the transport of the amino acid into the cell, 2) the rate of its conversion into protein, 3) the rate of its metabolism to other intermediates and 4) its uptake into the interstitial spaces. Rogers and Robertson [33] have suggested that the group of astrocytomas grades III and IV that they have studied could be subdivided according to the specific essential amino acids lost from the media to the greatest extent by the method described above. They found groups that preferred either HIS and MET, PHE and TYR, MET (with little HIS), or ILE, VAL and LEU. We also have employed this technique in our laboratory and the results we have obtained (which will be discussed in a later section) are not very different from those reported by Rogers and Robertson. In any event, it is clear that there are distinct differences in the degrees of uptake of the individual essential amino acids by human brain tumors using this assay procedure.

On the basis of the above literature, as well as a preliminary clinical experience with three patients, the Diet, Nutrition and Cancer Program of the National Cancer Institute contracted with our group and the Neurosurgery group at the University of Tennessee Medical Units in Memphis for an exploratory study to define the feasibility of limiting one essential amino acid in the diet on the host and tumor of a limited number of glioblastoma patients as a potential new form of therapy either singally or in combination with chemotherapy. The experimental protocol which was followed is outlined in the next section.

2.2. Diet Therapy Protocol

2.2.1. Patient Selection and Interventions

Surgical operation. Surgical decompression of the tumor mass was performed with as much tumor removed as possible. Frozen sections were prepared for initial pathological evaluation and additional tissue was fixed for permanent sections for subsequent confirmation. The adjacent remaining tumor specimen was examined in our laboratory by the Rogers and Woodall procedure [32] described in the next section.

2.2.2. Determination of the 'Tumor Dependent' Amino Acid. The tumor specimen that was obtained by the laboratory was minced into fine particleš, and weighed into 50 mg portions, which were each placed into 25 ml Erlenmeyer flasks. Then, 3.0 ml Difco Media TC-199 was added and the flasks covered with a 10 ml beaker. The minced tumor tissue and media were incubated at 37 °C for 3 hours in a Dubnoff metabolic shaker. The essential amino acid concentrations of the media were determined by elution chromotagraphy using an automated amino acid analyzer [34, 35]. In addition, samples of the pre-incubation media were chromatographed in order to determine the change in media essential amino acid concentrations over the incubation period. Thus, the 'tumor dependent' amino acids were identified as those essential amino acids whose concentrations were decreased in the media during this incubation period. The one that was decreased to the greatest extent was the one which was modulated in the diet of patients that randomized to a diet therapy arm of the study as described below.

2.2.3. Criteria Evaluation. The following criteria were used to determine whether a patient was suitable to be entered into the study:
   i) anaplastic astrocytoma Grades III or IV as determined pathologically from the permanent tissue section,
  ii) ages between 21 and 66 years, either sex,
 iii) no atypical dietary habits or restrictions as determined from a nutritional history conducted by a registered dietitian,
  iv) no significant food allergies as determined from the nutritional history,
   v) clearly identifiable 'tumor dependent' amino acid as determined by the procedure described above.

2.2.4. Randomization. Each patient that qualified for entry into the study was then randomized into one of four groups:
   i) No Additional Therapy (Control),
  ii) BCNU Only,
 iii) Diet Therapy Only,
  iv) Diet Therapy and BCNU.

2.2.5. Radiation Therapy. After approximately a one week recovery period following surgery, all patients started the radiation therapy phase of the protocol which began when the patients were in the hospital and was completed on an out-patient basis for those patients that completed the full course of therapy. The specific radiation therapy protocol involved a total dose of 6000 rads administered 5 days per week for 6–7 weeks.

2.2.6. BCNU Therapy.

1, 3 bis-(2-chloroethyl)-1-nitrosourea (BCNU) treatment was performed according to the BTSG protocol for those patients that randomized into either the BCNU Only or Diet Therapy and BCNU groups. In this protocol, BCNU was administered intravenously, over three successive days at a total dose of 80 mg per m^2 body surface area every 8 weeks unless signs of toxicity developed. When toxicity symptoms were noted, the dose was decreased incrementally or discontinued completely depending on the severity of alterations in the platelet, WBC and hematocrit values. In some cases, BCNU therapy was discontinued at points further into the study due to sclerosis and/or collapse of the veins.

2.2.7. Diet Therapy

Diet planning. During the radiation therapy phase of the study, the planning for the diet therapy was accomplished for those patients that randomized to a group requiring this intervention. The diet plan was based on restriction of the 'tumor dependent' essential amino acid identified by the procedure described above. The dietary regimen included a synthetic formulation devoid of the essential amino acid that was restricted plus normal foods to be patterned to meet the following criteria:

1) The restricted essential amino acid concentration was specified in milligrams.
2) All other essential amino acids met the minimum requirements as ascertained by Rose for men [36] and Leverton for women [37].
3) The protein, energy (Calorie), vitamins and mineral content of the diet were established and specified according to the 1974 National Research Council Recommended Daily Allowances [38].

2.2.8. Composition of the Diet.

The diet contained:
i) a synthetic amino acid formula which was devoid in the restricted essential amino acid,
ii) a variety of natural foods, in prescribed quantities to meet the requirements for the restricted essential amino acid, taking into consideration the patient's food preferences as much as possible,
iii) vitamin and mineral supplements as needed,
iv) sufficient fluids,
v) free foods, including oils, fats and sugar, as desired and needed to provide adequate calories,
vi) proprietary products to provide additional calories as needed.

The formula was prepared using Mead-Johnson product 80056 as the vitamin, mineral, and non-protein caloric portion of the formula to which was added all the essential amino acids except the one which was restricted. Occasionally, when the patient was not consuming adequate additional protein or calories from foods, the formula for that patient was supplemented with skim milk powder and/or 'Polycose' to supply the restricted amino acid and/or sufficient calories to meet the specified requirements. Thus, each dietary formulation was prepared specifically for a given patient so that adequate nutriture could be achieved principally via the formula when a patient had difficulty complying with the overall diet.

The diet was also composed of a variety of natural foods organized into exchange lists which are similiar in concept to exchange lists used for diabetic meal planning. Foods on each list were grouped according to the average amount of the restricted amino acid per serving.

2.2.9. Instruction of the Diet. The patient, or the appropriate individual responsible for the patient's food preparation, was provided with the diet plan, and the components of the formula and a complete explanation of the use of these by the dietitian. Each patient (and/or the individual responsible for their food preparation) was instructed to keep daily food records when on an out-patient basis as a reminder to the patient of the importance of compliance with the regimen. During the follow-up phase, food records for the three days prior to the periodic visits were recorded by the patient (and/or the individual preparing the food for the patient) and given to the dietitian who assessed their nutritional adequacy. Nutritional deficiencies were brought to the patient's attention and ways to correct these would be discussed by the dietitian.

The initial phase of the diet therapy program was begun at approximately two weeks following the completion of the radiation therapy treatments in the MCV Clinical Research Center (CRC) where the patient was admitted for a 1 to 2 week period to adjust to the regimen and for intensive dietary instruction. Food intakes during this period were recorded, and computerized nutrient analysis of these were obtained using the information provided in the USDA Handbook No. 8 [39]. During this particular phase of the study, the nature of the protein containing foods that the diet therapy patients could consume was regulated using those foods for which amino acids compositional analysis is available. However, during the subsequent out-patient phases some difficulty was encountered in obtaining data on the essential amino acid compositional analysis of some foods that are not currently available in food composition tables. Currently, the USDA is updating Handbook No. 8 to expand it considerably to include the essential amino acid composition of a variety of foods. To date, four volumes (8-1 through 8-4) which cover 'Spices and Herbs,' 'Dairy and Eggs' and 'Baby Foods' and 'Fats and Oils' are available.

After the 1 to 2 week period in our CRC, the diet therapy patients were discharged. Upon discharge from the hospital, the dietary therapy instruction was provided on a periodic basis to all patients regardless of the specific arm of the study in which they were enrolled when they returned for follow-up evaluation.

2.3. Follow-Up Evaluation

2.3.1. The Plan. All groups of patients were generally seen on a monthly basis as out-patients and the following assessments were made:

Blood and urine assessments:
 i) routine blood and urine chemistry,
 ii) complete blood count (CBC),
 iii) plasma amino acid analyses,
 iv) immunological evaluation.

Neurological evaluations:
 i) Karnofsky ratings,
 ii) computerized axial tomography scans (CT scans).

Anthropometric measurements:
 i) height,
 ii) body weight,
 iii) mid-triceps skinfold thickness,
 iv) mid-upper arm circumference.

With the exception of the immunology and CT Scans, which were determined every 2 months, all other evaluations were planned to be made on a monthly basis.

2.3.2. The Procedures. The following procedures were utilized to obtain what appeared *a priori* to be useful follow-up data.

Blood and urine assessments:
From the blood samples, routine blood (SMAC systems analyses) and urinary creatinines were assayed by the MCV Hospital Laboratories using standard methods. In addition a CBC was determined by the MCV Hospital Laboratories as a clinical assessment parameter over the long term as well as to identify toxicities related to BCNU therapy each time prior to subsequent administration of the drug.

In addition, a sample of fasting plasma was withdrawn from all the patients, a protein free filtrate prepared and the plasma amino acid profile determined using the amino acid analyzer [34, 35].

Every 2 months, blood was withdrawn for immunological evaluation in which the number of peripheral T-lymphocytes were assayed by the sheep erythrocyte rosette formation procedure [40]. T-cell blastogenesis to PHA and Con A mitogens was estimated both in the presence of normal pooled human plasma and with the patient's plasma as we have previously described elsewhere [41, 42]. Lymphocytes from normal individuals were always run as controls, both in the presence of normal pooled plasma as well as with the patient's own plasma. To minimize daily variations within the test samples and the problems of different lymphocyte populations having different reactivity to the mitogens, the data were calculated as the ratio's of the maximum point on the dose-response curve for:

$$\frac{\text{Patient's lymphocytes in normal pooled plasma}}{\text{Normal lymphocytes in normal pooled plasma}} \times 100$$

and

$$\frac{\text{Normal lymphocytes in patient's plasma}}{\text{Normal lymphocytes in normal pooled plasma}} \times 100.$$

Monocyte chemotaxis to a lymphocyte-derived chemotactic factor was assayed in blind-well chambers as previously described by Snyderman et al. [43, 44]. Mononuclear cells migrating to the lower filter surface were counted under oil with an eyepiece grid and the results expressed as a ratio of:

$$\frac{\text{Mean cells per grid area (patient)}}{\text{Mean cells per grid area (control)}} \times 100.$$

Neurological evaluations:

Routine evaluations of each patient's clinical performance status were performed monthly and quantitated by the Karnofsky scale in order to identify changes in the level of the patient's capabilities. The status of the tumor remaining after the surgical procedure was assessed every 2 months by CT Scans.

Anthropometric measurements:

Anthropometric measurements were performed by the dietitian using standard procedures [45] in both the in-patient and out-patient phases of the study. In each case, multiple measurements were made and averaged. These included:

i) *Height* — the patient's height without shoes was recorded in centimeters.

ii) *Body weight* — the patient was weighed before breakfast and after the bladder had been emptied and the body weight was recorded accurately in kilograms. It was compared to the ideal body weight according to the 1974 Recommended Allowance suggested weights for heights and a percentage of ideal body weight calculated.

iii) *Mid-triceps skinfold* — triplicate measurements on the non-dominant arm using the Lange caliper were performed by standard methods and read to the nearest 0.5 mm.

iv) *Mid-upper arm circumference* — was measured on the non-dominant arm, using flexible steel tape by the standard methods and the measurement recorded to the nearest millimeter.

v) *Derived mid-arm parameters* — the following quantities were derived from the mid-arm circumference and the mid-triceps skinfold measurements above using the equations of Gurney and Jelliffe [46].

Cross-sectional fat area (cm^2) =

$$\frac{\text{(Mid-triceps skinfold)} \quad \text{(Mid-upper arm circumference)}}{2} - \pi \frac{\text{(Mid-triceps skinfold)}^2}{4}$$

Cross-sectional muscle area (cm^2) =

$$\frac{\text{(Mid-upper arm circumference} - \pi \text{ mid-triceps skinfold)}^2}{4\pi}.$$

F/M = ratio of cross sectional fat area to cross sectional muscle area.

2.3.3. The Results. Even though this study was only an exploratory excursion to determine the feasibility and potential usefullness of dietary restriction therapy as an adjunct to current treatment modalities for gliomas, results that we have assembled to date will be described.

Since the design of the specific diet therapy was dependent upon the identification procedures [32] for the 'tumor dependent' essential amino acid, we assayed tissues from a total of 32 patients with anaplastic astrocytomas. This group included 11 patients that did not qualify for further study in addition to 21 patients involved in the clinical protocol study outlined above. We hoped to determine whether any pattern or trend emerged from this group in terms of amino acids that were preferentially extracted from the media as a result of incubation with the cancer tissues. The assay procedure involved estimation of the relative change in the concentrations of various essential amino acids in the tissue culture media following incubation with pieces of minced tumor tissue. The 'tumor dependent' amino acids were identified as those for which there was a decrease in the media concentration of that amino acid over the period of incubation. Thus, the term 'tumor dependent' in this context does not imply a specific mechanism for the effects noted, but rather, refers simply to a decreased media concentration of a specific amino acid that is depleted in the presence of the minced tumor tissue.

The results we obtained for this group of patients are listed in Table 1. The table indicates the number of patients for each of the amino acids as 'First,' 'Second,' or 'Third' with respect to the relative percentage loss from the media according to the assay procedure. For example, the first row of the table indicates that for 10 of the 32 patients studied, HIS concentration showed the greatest loss from the media in comparison to the other essential amino acids, in three patients HIS concentrations were decreased by the second greatest percentage, and in one patient of 30 HIS was lowered in the media by the third greatest amount when incubated with the tumor tissue. The fact that there are only 30 cases in the 'Third' column illustrates that not all tissues examined had more than two amino acids that showed a loss from the media by this procedure. The relative differences between the 'First,' 'Second,' and 'Third' amino acids, as far as the mean ($\pm$ standard error in the mean) change in media concentrations were $29\pm4\%$, $19\pm3\%$ and $17\pm3\%$, respectively. These figures imply that there was a clearer distinction between 'First' and 'Second' than between 'Second' and 'Third' which was most often the case for individual determinations. However, we must quickly add that the rank-order for each specimen assayed is probably more useful than the mean percentage change due to the homogeneity of the sampling techniques. We were able to assay small amounts of 'normal' brain tissue in

Table 1. Frequency and rank order of amino acids for anaplastic astrocytoma patients by the assay procedure of Rogers and Woodall [32].

Amino acid	Rank order		
	First *	Second *	Third *
HIS	10	3	1
MET	8	6	3
LYS	5	4	4
THR	4	2	4
ILE	2	5	6
LEU	2	4	8
PHE	1	3	3
VAL	0	3	1
ARG	0	2	0
n	32	32	30

* These terms refer to the ranking of the amino that was lost from the media, the most, next most, etc., by the assay procedure (see text).

two patients when it was removed as part of the surgical procedure. In both of these cases, there was a difference in the rank-order obtained between the tumor and 'normal' tissues in the same patients.

There was quite a considerable variability in the behavior of the specific tumor tissues in terms of whether one, two, three or more of the amino acids were decreased in concentration in the media by this procedure. Some patient's assays did not show a loss of any of the essential amino acids from the media following incubation whereas, in others, there were decreases in the concentrations of all of the essential amino acids. Furthermore, in almost every case there was at least one amino acid, different for individual patients that gave an increased concentration in the media following incubation with the minced tumor tissue by this method. The assay, however, was remarkably consistent between the three replicates we ran each time in terms of the order of which essential amino acids ranked 'First,' 'Second,' 'Third' and thereafter. In one patient, sufficient tumor was removed and dissected into four zones from the central core to the periphery and the rank-order of the first three essential amino acids was quite similar among the four zones.

In Table 1, some diversity is noted between patients in terms of the amino acids that ranked 'First,' 'Second' and 'Third.' With the exception of VAL and ARG, all of the other amino acids in the list ranked 'First' for at least one patient. VAL and ARG were considered 'Second' in five of 32 patients in this series. Thus, there seems to be some degree of heterogeneity between the results from different patients although HIS and MET ranked 'First' in more than 50% of the patients of our series. Rogers and Robertson[33] noted similar, but not identical, results in their series. However, we did not see the PHE-TYR and VAL-ILE-LEU categories that these investigators have described. Yet, there was agreement about the prominance of HIS and MET, a finding that should be kept in mind in any future studies. In particular, the consistent identification of HIS by this assay in disproportionate number of patients from two separate laboratories is interesting. It is all the more provocative, since HIS has long been considered a non-essential amino acid for adults but recent evidence suggests that it now should be considered as essential for adult humans[47–49]. This point of whether HIS is essential is crucial for the design of the diet for those patients for whom HIS was identified as 'First' by this assay method. We opted to consider HIS as essential for adults as well as children and found subsequently that we were indeed able to lower the plasma HIS levels in patients whose diets were low in HIS, at least for varying periods of time.

In theory, however, it should be possible to achieve similar clinical results by modulating the 'Second,' 'Third' or any selected essential amino acid in the diet, as there is no evidence to suggest that biosynthesis of the tumor proteins would not require all of the essential amino acids. Thus, although this assay is not obligatory to design the specific diet therapy, it might serve as useful guidance in the design of this therapy, particularly, if subsequent studies prove that HIS and/or MET are unique essential amino acids for at least a subset of glioma patients. No data is currently available to us with regard to gliomas (or other primary brain cancers) of childhood. This area most certainly should be explored as the diet–host–tumor interrelationships would be even more complex in children, since the host has requirements for essential amino acids for growth over and above those needed for maintenance in the adults.

It is difficult at this point to evaluate the efficacy of the diet therapy intervention from our experience because the outcome for several patients is currently in doubt. Furthermore, the number of evaluable patients from our study is too small to draw clear statistical conclusions as to the relative value of the four treatment arms of the study. It is clear, however, that the diet therapy interventions were not curative. We would prefer to evaluate the results to date from the perspective of whether the diet therapy intervention, either alone or in combination with BCNU, was at least as safe as currently acceptable therapies. In doing this, we will describe our preliminary survival results, the performance status, the immunologic changes and the anthropometric changes we observed for these patients. It is our opinion that these results demonstrate that this type of dietary intervention did not increase the risk to our patients.

The mean age, mean initial Karnofsky status, and mean survival times for 15 evaluable patients at this time are listed in Table 2. It appears that mean ages of the four groups were comparable; the initial Karnofsky status was lower for the patients that randomized to the 'no additional therapy' (Control) group than the other three groups and that the Control group mean survivals were somewhat shorter than the BCNU group, with the two diet therapy groups intermediate between these. Statistical evaluation of each of the three

Table 2. Age, Karnofsky status and survival of MCV diet therapy study patients.

Group	n	Mean age (yr)	Mean initial Karnofsky status (%)	Mean survival time (days)
No additional therapy	3	42 ± 2 *	58 ± 14 *	331 ± 152 *
BCNU only	4	40 ± 8	70 ± 4	603 ± 129
Diet therapy only	4	44 ± 9	70 ± 9	477 ± 180
Diet therapy and BCNU	4	46 ± 4	80 ± 4	471 ± 56

* Mean ± standard error of the mean

columns reveals that there are no significant differences between the four groups. The apparent increased survivals of the BCNU group is partially due to one patient, age 24, who was a long term survivor, which is not unexpected. Nevertheless, the survival results to date with this limited number of patients do not indicate a meaningful increased risk due to diet therapy, either alone or in combination with chemotherapy, over the Control group. When these results are compared to the BTSG major trial of BCNU [10, 14] the length of survival of our patients who received diet therapy are in about the same survival range as the BCNU group from that study (e.g., median survival = about 300 days for the BCNU arm). Furthermore, five of our eight patients that received diet therapy (two 'Diet Therapy' and three 'Diet Therapy and BCNU') have survived beyond 400 days to date. On the other hand, four out of seven of the non-diet therapy groups (three 'BCNU' and one 'Control') have survived beyond 400 days to date. The early deaths in most cases were older patients that were at lower performance levels when they entered the study. Perhaps, when our results are combined with those from the University of Tennessee and each patient normalized for pre-treatment characteristics more definite treads may emerge.

In terms of follow-up evaluations, certain trends emerged when various assessment parameters were examined for each patient over the period of time for which measurements were taken. For the purpose of the following discussion, we have separated two distinct periods in time for comparing several of the assessment parameters, the pre-dietary treatment phase in which the patients were either receiving chemotherapy or not and the post-dietary treatment phase in which the patients were then finally sub-divided by therapy into the four arms of the study. During the pre-treatment phase, those patients receiving BCNU showed a mean Karnofsky status of 73% for all of individual observations combined for that period, whereas in the post-treatment phase the 'BCNU' group dropped to 62% and the 'BCNU and Diet Therapy' group returned to 74%. This is somewhat surprising since the BCNU group showed the longest mean survival (Table 2) and had many survivors beyond 400 days. For the non-BCNU patients the changes in Karnofsky status from 59% in the pre-treatment period to 62% for the Control group and 72% for the Diet Therapy group.

In terms of the anthropometric measurements, the percent of ideal body weights were increased in the Diet Therapy and the BCNU groups and somewhat decreased for the Control and the Diet Therapy and BCNU groups when the post-diet therapy period was compared to the pre-diet therapy period. Although the ideal body weight is a useful clinical assessment, it does not provide any information about the *quality* of weight changes in terms of fat or lean body mass (muscle), which are the major determinants of body weight changes in the absence of massive edema. When the fat to muscle ratio of the mid-upper arm circumferences were determined by the equations noted previously, the post diet therapy period showed decreases in these ratios for all groups as compared to the pre-diet therapy period. The greatest decreases were noted in the Control group and the Diet Therapy and BCNU group which was due to the fat circumference since the muscle circumferences were essentially unchanged for all four groups. Thus, the body weight changes described above appear to be primarily attributed to changes in the fat composition. No clear explanation emerges as to the relative contributions of the diet therapy and/or BCNU therapy to these changes. Nevertheless, the important consideration is that, at least by this indirect procedure, diet therapy appeared not to stimulate a loss in muscle even though one essential amino acid was lowered (but not devoid) in the regimen.

The immunologic parameters that were assessed from the pre-operative period (where we obtained data for these factors) through the treatment and follow-up periods were % T rosettes, monocyte chemotaxis and Con A and PHA induced blastogenesis. Prior to surgery, T rosettes were 78% of normal and fluctuated independent of diet and/or chemotherapy between 58% and 80% of normal throughout the study. Chemotaxis values were normal prior to surgery, depressed during X-ray treatment and generally fluctuated between 80% and 140% of normal, again independent of treatment group. The T-cell response to Con A and PHA was initially 70% of normal and remained relatively constant in the Control patients. In contrast, the blastogenic response in both the BCNU group and Diet and BCNU group decreased until the Con A response was less than 40% and the PHA response was less than 50% of normal control lymphocytes. Concomitant with the decrease in blastogenesis in the BCNU and Diet Therapy group and the BCNU group was a gradual rise in the blastogenic response of the Diet Therapy group which reached 125% of normal in the follow-up period. Plasma inhibitory activity for blastogenesis was present prior to surgery, decreased in the Diet Therapy and BCNU group and the BCNU group in the cumulative post-surgery X-ray therapy period and then remained near normal throughout the remainder of the follow-up period. Evaluation of longitudinal studies on each patient did not indicate any obvious trends other than the marked suppression of blastogenesis in those administered chemotherapy whether they also received diet therapy or not. These latter results would suggest that BCNU therapy, with or without diet therapy, reduced the blastogenic response to these mitogens. However, the diet therapy alone did not appear to compromise these immunological parameters. If the diet therapy produced a nutritional deficit, in the patients, then one would expect to note some adverse effects on their immunological status. The results obtained, therefore, add further support for the contention that the diet restriction therapy did not produce a notable compromise of host protein status.

Other parameters such as blood and urine chemistries and CT scans provided additional clinical assessments of the patient status. These were not altered by diet and/or chemotherapy specifically but generally were predictive of the failure of the therapy. There were no specific changes in these parameters that could be ascribed to the diet theapy *per se*.

The results from these selected assessment parameters, taken together, would support the contention that the diet therapy appeared to be associated with no increased risk to the group of patients we studied. We are of the opinion that this point is certainly meaningful in the process of evaluation of the potential of this novel adjunct to current therapies.

As is the case for many self-administered therapies, compliance is a major concern with this form of diet-restriction therapy. We attempted to monitor this by two means, the diet records and the plasma amino acid levels. Neither of these methods proved to be satisfactory. The patient and/or individual responsible for the patient's food preparation, provided records for the periods between out-patient visits, but, in general these type of records are notoriously inaccurate. The situation is further complicated in some patients by neurological deficits due to the disease and/or surgical procedure. The quality of the records varied considerably as a function of the patients or their family educational level and motivation. Some records were complete and meticulous, whereas, other patients failed to keep records during some periods of the diet therapy. Evaluation of the records was slowed by the current lack of information concerning the essential amino acid composition of a wide variety of foods. As stated earlier, this latter problem should be corrected in the near future when the USDA completes its *Handbook 8* revisions.

The plasma amino acid results should provide some estimate of compliance at least for the immediate period prior to the out-patient visit. These values did fluctuate, even in patients that we knew were complying with the dietary regimen over periods when they were re-admitted to the CRC. Nevertheless, we were able to lower the plasma amino acid concentration of the restricted amino acid in most diet therapy patients over reasonably long periods during the out-patient phase. In comparison to their pre-treatment levels, we established an average 60% reduction in these levels during the follow-up period for the two groups of patients receiving the diet therapy. The non diet therapy groups showed no lowering in the plasma amino acid levels of their 'tumor dependent' amino acids. Furthermore, we studied two patients on the CRC for lenghty periods who were fed constant diets at periods when their plasma amino acid levels began to rise sharply and we suspected they might be cachexic. However, nitrogen balance studies revealed that these patients were in nitrogen equilibrium even though the plasma level of a given amino acid is a function of the diet, the rates of extraction and addition by the tumor and the host and the rate its excretion from the body. The host serves as a large reservoir for essential amino acids and the success of this form of diet restriction therapy rests with balancing the host's need to maintain this reservoir intact when the tumor's needs are compromised. Therefore, it is difficult to simply explain an elevation in the plasma amino acid level in a diet restricted patient on a constant diet that is in nitrogen equilibrium. A great deal concerning the diet–host–tumor interactions must be clarified in the future.

Regarding the plasma amino acids, another point should be addressed and that is the HIS diets. At the start of the study, it was not clear whether HIS was an essential amino acid in the diet of adults, which still continues to be a somewhat of a controversial issue. However, we fed HIS restricted diets to four patients and their plasma amino acid levels averaged 73% of their initial values during the follow-up period. This finding supports the notion that HIS is an essential amino acid, since we should not have been as successful in lowering these levels were it a non-essential amino acid. We, as well as Rogers and Robertson [33], have found a substantial number of tumors that appear to be HIS 'dependent,' whether 'First,' 'Second' or 'Third' by the minced tissue assay. Thus, the disproportionate number of apparently HIS 'dependent,' tumors may be an important clue to exploit in the future.

2.3.4. Conclusions and The Future. This particular study was exploratory in nature; nevertheless, certain interesting and encouraging trends can be noted that could be explored in the future. Among these is the consistency of observing a sub-set of patients for which HIS and/or MET appear to be identified as 'tumor dependent' for anaplastic astrocytoma tissues by the procedure developed by Rogers and Woodhall [32]. This observation has been made in two cooperating, but independent, laboratories. By the measures of survival, Karnofsky status, anthropometric measurements and immunological profiles, our diet restriction therapeutic intervention appeared to be without additional risk to the limited number of our patients studied. The type of dietary restriction therapy that we employed, either alone, or in combination with chemotherapy, was not a curative modality for the group of patients we studied who have a very poor prognosis by current therapies as well.

For the future, it remains to be determined whether this adjunct to the currently available surgery, radiation therapy and chemotherapy will be useful in prolonging survival and/or the quality of life of this group of patients. The quality of life question can be debated at great length, since this form of diet restriction therapy severely limits an important facet of life, e.g., the food one can consume. On the other hand, our experience demonstrated that acceptance of this rigorous regimen can be achieved by most patients after a limited trial period in which the diet change is graduated from normal eating habits to the restricted dietary regimen. Much help was offered to the patient's in this transition by the type of dedicated, supportive and competent team members that we had.

Many questions have been developed as a result of this experience. How long should the patient receive the diet therapy? Should it be started earlier, perhaps following the surgical procedures? Can the same results be achieved by limiting the same essential amino acid for all patients? What better methods of nutritional status assessment can be developed? Can this adjunct form of therapy be useful for other types of cancers? Would it be useful in management of primary brain cancers in children?

3. LYMPHOCYTE STUDIES

3.1. Background
3.1.1. *General.* Lymphocytic infiltration around gliomas has been noted by Bertrand and Mannen in 1960 but without consideration of its relevance [50]. In a post mortem study, Ridley and Cavanaugh studied 93 cases of glioma and found that 30% of gliomas showed significant lymphocytic infiltration; 28%, slight infiltration and 42% showed no lymphocytic reaction [51]. They discussed evidence which supports the idea that the response may represent an attempt by the host to reject the tumor. More recently, in a review of lymphocytic infiltrates in 228 cases of primary glioblastomas, Palma [52] found that the group that exhibited a definite lymphocytic infiltration had significantly longer preoperative histories and post operative survivals ($p < 0.01$) than the other two groups that presented slight or no infiltration. Palma further noted that severe lymphocytic infiltration is a rare immunological reaction which significantly improves the prognosis of a patient with a brain cancer and seems not be influenced by time, local X-ray therapy, or sterioid therapy. Furthermore, Brooks *et al.* [53] have reviewed the hospital records of 149 patients harboring primary brain tumors and found that lymphocytic infiltration confined to the perivascular spaces was the only histological finding that correlated significantly with prognosis in gliomas. They concluded that perivascular lymphocytes at the advancing edge of an infiltrating glioma may be immunological in nature and could account for prolonged survival through retardation of tumor growth. A further possibility suggested that that cellular response represented an autoimmune reaction similar to experimental allergic encephalitis.

We have been studying the host-immune response in glioma patients and we have been able to demonstrate inhibition of cell-mediated immunity in patients with high-grade gliomas [42]. An *in vitro* technique of lymphocyte blast transformation to the mitogens conconavalin A (Con A) and phytohemagglutinen (PHA) was used. Much of the impetus for this work derives from the observation that the gross morphological and biochemical characteristics of mitogen-induced lymphocyte responses *in vitro* are very similar to antigen induced immune reactions *in vivo*. It is, therefore, generally considered that the lymphocyte activation phenomenon *in vitro* offers not only a means of analyzing the biochemical events involved in cellular de-repression [42, 54] but is also of considerable value as a clinical tool for monitoring the immunologic competence of lymphocytes from patients with various immunological disorders and those undergoing immunosuppressive therapy [54]. The degree of inhibition of blastic response *in vitro* correlates well with the condition of the patient.

In patients with low-grade astrocytomas (Grade I and II) and doing well clinically, we have found no evidence of inhibition of lymphocyte blast transformation. This suggests that immunosuppressive (inhibitory) factors are not present in patients with astrocytomas. Patients with glioblastomas (22 total patients) responded to the mitogens in one of three patterns, 1) normal response at all concentrations of mitogens; 2) markedly impaired response to low mitogen concentrations, but normal response at high concentrations; 3) markedly impaired response at all mitogen concentrations. These patterns correlated well with the clinical status of the patients. Those patients who were both physiologically and neurologically well demonstrated normal response at all concentrations of mitogens as in 1) above. Patients who had neurologic deficits or were bedridden tended to show the second pattern. Terminal patients had impaired responses throughout or high titers of immunosuppressive plasma factors. Our data indicates the inhibitory (immunosuppressive) factor impairing cell-mediated immunity is in the serum [54]. This adds weight to Cobb's [55] work, wherein he used a glioma explant and found the tumor was markedly stimulated to grow in autologous serum. Brooks [56] likewise demonstrated this same impairment of cell-mediated immunity in glioma patients with the *in vitro* mitogen technique. He stated a heat-stable factor in the patient's sera blocked cell-mediated tumor immunity.

In 1978, Levy reported finding that serum from 80% of patients with gliomas had significant blocking activity against lymphocyte-mediated cytotoxicity to tumor target cells. He suggested the blocking factor seems to be an immunoglobulin G and that *in vivo* these blocking factors may abrogate lymphocyte-mediated cytotoxicity against tumor cells [57].

In another study, Levy studied lymphocyte-mediated cytotoxicity in 41 patients with CNS gliomas and in 25 patients with primary CNS tumors not of glial origin [58]. He found specific tumor-directed lymphocyte-mediated cytotoxicity in 85% of patients with gliomas and in 96% of patients with nonglial tumors (meningiomas and acoustic neuromas). These studies demonstrate that consistent and specific lymphocyte-mediated cytotoxicity exists in the vast majority of patients with gliomas. Our laboratory, as well, is currently attempting to identify the plasma inhibitory factor. Therefore, our laboratory research agrees with that of others in that glioblastoma patients have a factor in their serum which inhibits the normal lymphocyte response to the glioblastoma, and thereby may 'enhance' the tumor. The lymphocyte, as long as it remains in the serum, may be inhibited from destroying the tumor.

3.1.2. Immunotherapy of Brain Tumors. Previous and on-going trials of immunotherapy in brain tumors are few and the results not encouraging. The pioneering work of Mahaley *et al.* [59], was instrumental in establishing a firm basis for the immunotherapy of primary CNS tumors. Bloom *et al.* [60] reported a randomized prospective clinical trial carried out to assess the value of specific active immunotherapy using irradiated autologous tumor cells in patients with glioblastoma multiforme treated by radical surgery and postoperative irradiation. The results in 62 patients showed no statistically significant difference in survival between the group receiving adjuvant autologous tumor cells and those treated with surgery and radiotherapy alone. The results were considered sufficiently discouraging to abandon the trial on the grounds that administration of irradiated autologous cells were of no benefit to patients with high-grade astrocytomas.

Combined chemotherapy and immunotherapy for malignant gliomas has been reported by A.K. Ommaya and Leland A. Albright [61]. This protocol consists of BCG immunization to enhance systemic nonspecific cellular immune response mechanisms, PPD injections into the tumor cyst to excite a local nonspecific cellular immune response and glioma cell inoculations to induce active immunization of the patient against his own glioma. It was anticipated that within three years a more definitive answer to glioma management was to be expected. Twelve patients treated in this way were initially reported at the Neurosurgical Research Society of America Meeting at the Medical College of Virginia in Richmond in March of 1974, without statistical significance in terms of survival. Takakura *et al.* [62] have demonstrated enhanced survival in a small series of glioma patients when autogenous white blood cells were placed into the tumor cavity. In 1978 Neuwelt *et al.* [63] reported on four patients with malignant gliomas who had repeated intrathecal lymphoid cell infusions. No toxicity was observed and in one patient examined at autopsy, the lymphoid cells appeared to have gained access to the tumor bed as well as the rest of the subarachnoid space. No conclusions could be made from this latter study, either in support of or against the efficacy of intrathecal autologous lymphocyte infusions in patients with primary CNS tumors.

In an immunotherapeutic trial using a glial tumor model in rats, Lim *et al.* [64] presented data that immunotherapy did result in slower tumor growth although complete rejection was not observed. In this tumor immunotherapy model, rats were challenged with astrocytoma cells and treated with neuraminidase treated tumor cells mixed with BCG. In 1975, Albright *et al.* [65] reported on immunotherapy in an intracerebral murine glioma model to evaluate various combinations of preimmunization, immunotherapy and chemotherapy. For preimmunization and immunotherapy experiments, tissue cultured tumor cells were used from the culture which produced the intracerebral tumors. Cells were mechanically harvested, counted and treated with mitomycin C and with *Vibrio cholera* neuraminidase to remove cell surface sialic acid. Animals receiving preimmunization were injected subcutaneously with cells emulsified in complete Freund's adjuvant. Animals receiving immunotherapy were injected subcutaneously with cells and reconstituted Pasteur BCG continuing for 45 days or until the animal's death. Animals receiving chemotherapy were injected once, intra-peritoneally with CCNU. In this tumor system, immunotherapy alone was not an effective treatment.

3.1.3. Clinical Immunotherapy. The relative safety of intratumoral puncture and the opportunity afforded by the confined nature of brain tumors and their independent spinal fluid (CSF) circulation may permit white cell diffusion largely independent of the circulation and the presence of serum blocking factors. We, as well as others, have demonstrated *in vitro* an inhibitory (blocking) factor in serum of patients with gliomas. The tissue culture studies of Levy [57] strongly suggest that some patients have lymphocytes which are cytotoxic to autologous glioblastoma cells. Thus, we reasoned, a plan of therapy where lymphocytes were removed from the serum and placed directly into the tumor may offer the best opportunity for success. Such a method may diminish the effectiveness of the serum blocking factor and allow direct contact between the lymphocyte and tumor cell as in tissue culture.

3.2. Methods
3.2.1. Selection of Patients. All patients had confirmation of diagnosis by resection or biopsy information and were classified as having grade III and IV astrocytoma (glioblastoma multiforme). Table 3 outlines the character of response and quantity of leukocytes administered to each patient and summarizes the experience in both nonresponder and responders.

Fifteen of 17 patients selected for this study showed progressive clinical signs of disease following surgical resection, radiotherapy and/or chemotherapy with BCNU, carmustine, 1-(2-chloroethyl)-3-cyclohexyl-1-nitrosourea (CCNU), or lomustine. Patients had also failed to respond significantly to dexamethasone or were showing disease progression despite an adequate trial of this steroid (at least 6 mg dexamethasone every 4 hours for 4 days). Only one patient had received radiotherapy or chemotherapy within 6 weeks of this

Table 3. Glioblastoma: treatment and survival.

Patient	Age	Sex	Rx *	Recurrence (months from Rx)	Clinical status	Autologous leukocytes (cell No.)	Results	Post-lymph survival (months)	Total survival (months from diagnosis)
R.N.	52	M	6000R	11	Hemiparesis, confusion, memory loss	5×10^7	Unchanged	1 week	11
W.D.	60	M	6000R	2	Comatose, dilated pupil	2×10^7	Unchanged	1 week	2
J.S.	58	M	Biopsy Steroids +	—	Confused, aphasic	1.4×10^7	Unchanged	3	3
S.W.	57	M	Steroids +	1	Hemiparesis	1.8×10^7	Unchanged	3	3
J.H., II	58	M	6000R †	12	Hemiparesis	4.2×10^8	Unchanged	4	16
M.C.	48	F	—	—	Comatose	3×10^6	Unchanged	5	5
J.R.	63	M	6000R	8	Hemiparesis, aphasic	1.5×10^9 7×10^8	Unchanged	5	13
R.M.	67	F	Radiation	5	Ataxia, memory loss, incontinent	2×10^7	Hydrocephalus (shunt, mild improvement)	5	10
J.L.	64	M	6000R Steroids +	2	Blind, confused, aphasic	2.6×10^7	Unchanged	12	14
					Clinical improvement (responders)				
Case 1 W.R.	49	M	6500R CCNU Steroids +	6	Semicomatose, incontinent	5.0×10^7	Fully, functional, 16 months	17	23

* All patients had original subtotal resection of tumor, except biopsy only where indicated.
+ Five patients had maintenance Decadron (4 mg i.m. or p.o. q6hr) until death. No increased dosage during Rx.
† Repeat subtotal tumor resection 2 months and 1 month prior to lymphocyte treatment.

Table 3. (continued)

Patient	Age	Sex	Rx *	Recurrence (months from Rx)	Clinical status	Autologous leukocytes (cell No.)	Results	Post-lymph survival (months)	Total survival (months from diagnosis)
Case 2 M.P.	20	M	6000R	4	Memory loss, headache	5.8×10^8 1.8×9	Improved, functionally independent working	25	29
Case 3 A.T.F.	59	M	5040R § BCNU	10	Aphasic, hemiparetic	1.2×10^9 1.8×10^9 1.2×10^9	Improved 1 month	10	20
Case 4 J.A.	57	M	6500R	3	Aphasic, hemiparetic, confusion	4.5×10^8	Alert, speech improvement (shunted), walks	20 6 (post-shunt)	23
Case 5 R.S.	49	F	6000R	36	Seizure, confusion, mild hemiparetic	1.8×10^8 1.8×10^9 1.7×10^9	Functionally independent	26	62
Case 6 J.H.	25	M	5000R CCNU Steroids +	36	Aphasic, incontinent, drowsy, hemiparetic	3×10^7 3×10^7 4.2×10^8	Alert, functional, self-feeding	12	72
Case 7 R.S.	56	M	6000R +	12	Drowsy, aphasic	2×10^9	More alert	6	19
Case 8 A.M.	63	M	6000R	4	Aphasic, hemiparetic	1.9×10^8 1.8×10^9 1.7×10^9	Returned to work 1 month	4	8

* All patients had original subtotal resection of tumor, except biopsy only where indicated.

+ Five patients had maintenance Decadron (4 mg i.m. or p.o. q6hr) until death. No increased dosage during Rx.

† Repeat subtotal tumor resection 2 months and 1 month prior to lymphocyte treatment.

program. Baseline brain scans were obtained on all patients and where possible, arteriographic and CT data were also obtained.

Objective responses were defined as marked and durable (at least 4 weeks) with improvement of at least one neurologic symptom without deterioration of any other neurologic sign or appearance of a new neurologic deficit. Decrease in intracranial pressure, as suggested by relief of headache or resolution of papilledema, and decrease in tumor mass as defined by brain scan, were additional criteria. All improvements had to be maintained for a period greater than 1 month and, to qualify as improvement, had to be seen in the absence of objective progression or new neurologic symptoms or deficits.

Patients receiving steroid medication at the time of treatment were either maintained on Decadron 4 mg q.i.d., or steroids were reduced or discontinued. No patient had steroid dosage increased after treatment. Most patients had original surgical subtotal tumor removal and two patients had a second subtotal tumor removal within 1 to 2 months prior to lymphocyte treatment. One patient had a second surgical subtotal tumor removal between the first and second lymphocyte treatment.

3.2.2. Procedure. Patients treated in this program were admitted to the Neurosurgical Service at MCV, and a brain scan or CT scan was done, the neurological examination was carefully recorded, and the patient was examined and followed at regular intervals.

The patient, resting in his bed or transported to the clinical pathology blood processing unit, was attached to the Latham leukophoresis (Haemonetic) cell separator, and a lymphocyte concentrate was removed and the plasma and erythrocytes were infused back into the patient. The cell separation technique for this differential centrifuge has been well established, and the autologous fraction removal from the cell separator had a ratio of lymphocytes to granulocytes of 60:40 or 50:50. In some cases, the white blood cell concentrate obtained from the Haemonetics separator was washed three times in sterile RPMI 1640 tissue culture media to remove any residual serum factors. The cells were concentrated by centrifugation at 1000 rpm with removal of the buffy coat into a syringe under steriles technique, to bring the final volume of cell suspension to less than 10 ml. The cells finally obtained had a ratio of lymphocytes to granulocytes of 1:1. These cells were then injected through previous craniotomy sites into the tumor bed using a 22 spinal needle with localization established by brain scan and CT scan data. Alternatively, injection was made into a Rickham reservoir attached to indwelling catheters going directly into the tumor. The lymphocytes were injected slowly at a rate of 1 cm^3/minute while the patient's condition was carefully monitored. To determine absolute lymphocyte counts, a sample from the leukocyte bag was taken for differential and total count. The one major complication of this program has been *Klebsiella* meningitis which contributed to the death of our first patient. Increased efforts to maintain strict sterility of the autologous cells has resulted in no subsequent infections in the remaining 16 patients.

An occasional side effect of injection of leukocytes has been transient increase of intracranial pressure due to increase of the intracranial volume too rapidly. This has been avoided in the majority of our patients by concentrating the cells into a small volume (less than $10\,cm^3$) and by slow injection ($1\,cm^3$ per minute). The largest volume of cells given has been $12\,cm^3$ with an average volume of $10\,cm^3$ administered to each patient. Two patients had aspirations of $10\,cm^3$ of tumor cyst fluid at the time of injection of an equal volume of lymphocytes.

3.3. Results and Discussion

This was a non-controlled, non-randomized trial of intratumoral lymphocyte injections. However, it should be noted that of the 17 patients in this study, the first five listed were considered preterminal and one of them improved dramatically and returned to a functional state for 16 months. There was no cyst fluid obtained at the lymphocyte injection site and clinical improvement with decrease of tumor size could not be attributed to remote effects of radiation therapy. In reviewing the results from patients considered non-responders, it was noted that there was only a 4.5 month mean survival time from the time of treatment (surgery, radiotherapy and chemotherapy) suggesting that they had biological aggressive tumors resistant to the usual modalities of therapy. The eight responders had a mean survival to recurrence of 13.9 months after treatment, which might imply that these patients may have had less biologically aggressive tumors. Nonetheless, where there was relapse or tumor recurrence following treatment, deterioration is usually rapid despire further chemotherapy [67]. Though we cannot argue strongly for definite statistical benefit from intra-tumoral lymphocyte injection, repeated biopsies in two patients and, autopsy studies in four patients at various time intervals from injection failed to reveal evidence of toxicity related to the lymphocyte injection. Sepcifically, there was no evidence of acute allergic encephalitis. The lack of toxicity of these limited injections is in complete agreement with Neuwelt's laboratory and clinical studies [63, 66]. He found no toxicity when syngeneic lymphocytes were injected intrathecally in rabbits, but did observe choroid plexitis when xenogenic (human) lymphocytes were injected into rabbits. In two of four patients receiving multiple intrathecal lymphocytes injections, he observed that CSF glucose decreased in two patients. He suggested that this decrease of glucose (hypoglycorrhachia) might be a reflection of lymphocytes undergoing blastogenesis and subsequently exerting a tumoricidal effect.

Furthermore, our study is extremely preliminary. The optimum number of lymphocytes necessary for a tumoricidal effect is unknown. In one *in vitro* study, Levy [68] demonstrated that 10^5 lymphocytes appear necessary to show optimum evidence of cytotoxicity against 100 tumor target cells. In 14 of our 17 patients there was clearly more than 1 cm² of tumor tissue or at least 10^8 cells. We therefore did not achieve the optimal ratio of lymphocyte/tumor ratio in most of our patients. It appears, though, that clinical results were seen with only 10^7 and 10^9 cells given, and thus far only a maximum of three infusions have been given per patient. Many of the patients in this study had lymphopenia secondary to chemotherapy, but it was possible to increase the volume of packed autochthonous lymphocytes to 10^{10} lymphocytes or more by extending the period of infusion with a slow pump (i.e., Harvard pump), while closely monitoring CNS pressure. Furthermore, cells can be given daily, or weekly, though access to a leukaphoresis machine is necessary.

The impetus for the above study is derived from the pioneering work of the Hellstroms [69] who indicated that cancer patients have lymphocytes cytotoxic for their autochthonous tumor or allogenic tumor of the same histologic type. Similarly, patients with gliomas have been shown now by a number of investigators to have varying numbers of circulating tumor specific killer lymphoid cells [63]. There is both *in vitro* and *in vivo* evidence for this. As mentioned previously Levy [57, 58] reported specific lymphocyte toxicity *in vitro* in 5% of 41 glioma patients in a well controlled study. *In vivo*, lymphocytes appear to be relevant in patients with gliomas according to the previously mentioned studies of Brooks and Palma [52, 53, 57]. This is the rationale for exposing the tumor in patients with gliomas to autologous lymphoid cells, as was done in our study.

3.4. The Future of Immunotherapy of Brain Tumors

The possible use of immunology in the treatment of patients must be vigorously explored. At this time we know neither the initiator nor the promoter of cerebral cancers. It often appears that even after radical (grossly complete) removal of a glioma via lobectomy, there is an initiating factor or promoting factor which is operative in causing recurrence of the tumor. This may be because of a defect in the immunesurveilance system. As immune mechanisms become increasingly better explored and known, we may be able to better control this currently fatal disorder.

Immunotherapy will almost certainly play a role in the armamentaria of the treatment of patients with brain cancers. Radical cancer operations cannot be performed in the brain. Irradiaton and chemotherapy are toxic to cerebral tissue in dose currently necessary to control the cancer. Potentially, immunotherapy will not have these limiting effects.

4. OVERALL CONCLUSIONS

We have attempted to investigate two novel lines of therapy, one using diet restriction therapy and the other lymphocyte infusion to alter the course of growth of anaplastic astrocytomas in two independent exploratory studies. Although results of both studies are clinically inconclusive, there were some encouraging signs from the information developed in them. This group of gliomas are tumors that cannot be removed completely by surgery, can be treated with some life extension by radiation therapy and somewhat longer when chemotherapy is added, but are invariably fatal. New ideas and approaches are needed and we feel that each of these avenues of approach that we have tried offers some promise for development in the future either alone or in combination with other modalities. Clearly, we have provided no answers, but these investigators may have uncovered clues to formulating the right questions.

ACKNOWLEDGEMENTS

The diet therapy studies described above were supported in part by a contract from the Diet, Nutrition and Cancer Program (NCI), NO 1 CP 75881, and a grant from the NIH, MO 1 RR 000-65, for the CRC.

The diet-therapy studies involve a team effort to execute and we wish to thank Dr. Winnie M.Y. Chan, Joan Dobek, R.D. Patty Clarke and Majorie Imberg for their important contributions to this work.

REFERENCES

1. American Cancer Society, Cancer facts and figures 1980. New York: American Cancer Society, p 9.
2. Annegers JF, Laws ER, Kurland LT, Grabow JD: Head trauma and subsequent brain tumors. Neurosurgery 4:203–206, 1979.
3. Cushing H, Eisankardt L: Meningiomas: their classification, regional behavior, life history and surgical end results. Springfield, Ill.: Charles C. Thomas, 1938.
4. Parker HL, Kernohan JW: The relation of injury and glioma of the brain. J Am Med Assoc 97:535–540, 1931.
5. Wilson CB, Boldery EB, Enot KJ: Bis (2-chloroethyl)-1-nitrosourea (NSC-409962) in the treatment of brain tumors. Cancer Chemother Rep 54:273–281, 1970
6. Venes JL, McIntosh S, O'Brien RT, Schwartz AD: Chemotherapy as an adjunct in the initial management of cerebellar medulloblastoma. J Neurosurg 50:721-724, 1979.
7. Crafts DC, Levin VA, Edwards MS, Pisher TL, Wilson CB: Chemotherapy of recurrent medulloblastoma with combined procarbazine. CCNU and vincristine. J Neurosurg 49:589–592, 1978.

8. Farwell JR, Dohrmann GJ, Marrett LD, Mergs JW: Effect of SV40 virus-contaminated folio vaccine on the incidence and type of CNS neoplasms in children. Ann Neurol 6: 166–167, 1979.

9. Russell DS, Rubinstein LJ: Pathology of tumors of the nervous system, 3rd edn. London: Edward Arnold, 1970.

10. Walker MD, Hunt WE, Mahaley MS, Norrell HA, Ransohoff J, Gehan EA: Evaluation of BCNU and/or radiotherapy in the treatment of anaplastic gliomas. J Neurosurg 49:333–343, 1978.

11. Kusske JA, Williams JP, Garcia JH, Pribram HW: Radiation necrosis of the brain following radiotherapy of extracerebral neoplasms. Surg Neurol 6:15–20, 1976.

12. Sogg RL, Donaldson SS, Yorke CH: Malignant astrocytoma following radiotherapy of a craniopharyngioma. J Neurosurg 48:622–627, 1978.

13. Caveness WF: Pathology of radiation damage to the normal brain of the monkey. Natl Cancer Inst Monogr 46:57–76, 1976.

14. Shapiro WR: Management of primary malignant brain tumors. Neurol Neurosurg Update. Princeton, N.J.: Biomedia, 1978.

15. Hologe PY, Jenkins EE, Greenberg SD: Pulmonary toxicity in long term administration of BCNU. Cancer Treatment Rep 60:1691–1694, 1976.

16. Jones MPH, Marsden HB, Bailey CC: Fatal pulmonary fibrosis following 1,3-bis (2-chloroethyl)-nitrosourea (BCNU) therapy. Cancer 42:74–76, 1978.

17. Munro HM: Tumor-host competition for nutrients in the cancer patient. J Am Dietetic Assoc 71:380–384, 1977.

18. White FR, Belkin M: Source of tumor protein. I: Effect of a low-nitrogen diet on the establishment and growth of a transplanted tumor. J Natl Cancer Inst 5:261–263, 1945.

19. White ER: Source of tumor proteins. II: Nitrogen-balance studies of tumor bearing mice fed a low nitrogen diet. J Natl Cancer Inst 5:265–270, 1945.

20. Sherman CD Jr, Morton JJ, Midler GB: Potential sources of tumor nitrogen. Cancer Res 10:374–378, 1950.

21. Babson AL: Some host–tumor relationships with respect to nitrogen. Cancer Res 14:89–93, 1954.

22. Skipper HE, Thomson JR: Amino acids and peptides with antimetabolic activity. Boston: Little Brown, 1958, pp 38–53.

23. Sugimura T, Birnbaum SM, Winitz M, Greenstein JP: Quantitative nutritional studies with water-soluble, chemically defined diets. VII. The forced feeding of diets lacking one essential amino Acid. Arch Biochem Biophys 81:448–455, 1959.

24. Lorincz AB, Kuttner RE, Brandt MB: Tumor response to PHE-TYR limited diets. J Am Dietetic Assoc 54:198–205, 1969.

25. Demopoulos HB: Effects of low phenylalanine-tryrosine diets on S 91 mouse melanomas. J Natl Cancer Inst 37:185–190, 1966.

26. Demopoulos HB: Effects of reducing the phenylalanine-tyrosine intake of patients with advanced malignant melanoma. Cancer 19:657–664, 1966.

27. Theuer RC: Effect of essential amino acid restriction on the growth of female C57BL mice and their implanted BW 10232 adenocarcinomas. J Nutr 101:223–232, 1971.

28. Pine MJ: Effect of low phenylalanine diet on murine leukemia L1210. J Natl Cancer Inst 60:633–641, 1978.

29. Jose DJ, Good RA: Quantitative effects of nutritional essential amino acid deficiency upon immune responses to tumors in mice. J Exp Med 137:1–9, 1972.

30. Worthington BS, Syrotock JA, Ahmed SI: Effects of essential amino acid deficiencies on syngeneic tumor immunity and carcinogenesis in mice. J Nutr 108:1402–1411, 1978.

31. Lowery SF, Goodgame T, Norton JA, Jones DC, Brennan MF: Effect of chronic protein malnutrition on host–tumor composition and growth. Surg Res 26:79–86, 1979.

32. Rogers S, Woodhall B: Rapid method of metabolically characterizing individual tumors. Proc Soc Exp Biol Med 98:874–877, 1958.

33. Rogers S, Robertson JT: Biochemical subclassification of astrocytoma grade IV, and its utilization in therapy. Proc Am Assoc Cancer Res 19:98, 1978.

34. Spackman DH, Stein WH, Moore S: automatic recording apparatus for use in chromatography of amino acids. Anal Chem 30:1190–1198, 1958.

35. Hamilton PB: Ion exchange chromatography of amino acids—micro determination of free amino acids in serum. Ann N Y Acad Sci 120: 55–67, 1962.

36. Rose WC: Amino acid requirement of man. Fed Proc 8:546–552, 1949.

37. Leverton RM, Gram MR, Chaloupka M, Brodousky E, Mitchel A: The quantitative amino acid requirements of young women, I. Threonine. J Nutr 58:59–81, 1955.

38. National Academy of Sciences: Recommended dietary allowances, 8th ed. Washington, DC, 1974, 128 pp.

39. USDA: Handbook No, 8 revised—composition of foods. Washington, DC.: U S Govt Printing Office, 1963, 190 pp.

40. Jondal M: In Lymphocytes: isolation, fractionation and characterization, Natvig JB, Perlman P, Wizzel H (eds). Oslo: Universititsforlaget, 1977, pp 69–76.

41. Young HF, Sakalas R, Kaplan AM: Inoculation of cell-mediated immunity in patients with brain tumors. Surg Neurol 5:19–23, 1976.

42. Young HF, Sakalas R, Kaplan AM: Immunologic depression in cerebral gliomas. Adv Neurol 15:327–335, 1976.

43. Snyderman R, Pike MC, Altman LC: Abnormalities of leukocyte chemotaxis in human disease. Ann NY Acad Sci 256:386–392, 1974.

44. Snyderman R, Pike MC: An inhibitor of macrophage chemotaxis produced by neoplasms. Science 192:370–373, 1976.

45. Blackburn GL, Bistrian BR, Maini BS, Schlamm HT, Smith MF: Nutritional and metabolic assessment of the hospitalized patient. J Parenteral Enteral Nutr 1:11–22, 1977.

46. Gurney JM, Jelliffe DB: Arm anthropometry in nutritional assessment: nomogram for rapid calculation of muscle circumference and cross-sectional muscle and fat areas. Am J Clin Nutr 26:912–915, 1973.

47. Bergstrom J, Furst P, Josephson B, Norée LO: Factors affecting the nitrogen balance in chronic uremic patients receiving essential amino acids intravenously or by mouth. Nutr Metabol 14 (Suppl): 162–170, 1972.

48. Kopple JD, Swendseid ME: Evidence that histidine is an essential amino acid in normal and chronically uremic man. J Clin Invest 55:881–891, 1975.

49. Anonymous: Histidine: an essential amino acid for normal adults. Nutr Rev 33:200–202, 1975.

50. Bertrand I, Mannen H: Etude des reactions vasculaires dans les astrocytomas. Rev Neurol 102:3–19, 1960.

51. Ridley A, Cavanaugh JB: Lymphocytic infiltration in gliomas. Evidence of possible host resistance. Brain 94:117–124, 1971.

52. Palma L, DiLorenzo N, Grudetti B: Lymphocyte infiltrates in primary glioblastomas and recidivous gliomas. Incidence. fate and relevance to prognosis in 228 operated cases. J Neurosurg 49:854–861, 1978.

53. Brooks WH, Markesbery WR, Gupta GD, Roszman TL: Relationship of lymphocyte invasion and survival of brain tumor patients. Ann Neurol 4:219–224, 1978.

54. Young HF, Kaplan AM: Immunotherapy of human gliomas. In: The handbook of cancer immunology, Waters H. (ed.), New York: Garland Press, 1978, pp 357–382.

55. Cobb JP, Walker DG: Effect of heterologous, homologous and autogenous serums on human normal and malignant cells in vitro. J Natl Cancer Inst 27:1–9, 1961.

56. Brooks WH, Netsky MG, Normansell DE, Horwitz DA: Depressed cell-mediated immunity in patients with primary intracranial tumors. J Exp Med 136:1631–1647, 1972.
57. Levy NL: Specificity of lymphocyte-mediated cytotoxicity in patients with primary intracranial tumors. J Immunol 121: 903–915, 1978.
58. Levy NL: Cell-mediated cytotoxicity and serum mediated blocking: evidence that their associated determinants on human tumor cells are different. J Immunol 121:916–922, 1978.
59. Mahaley MS Jr: Immunological considerations and the malignant glioma problem. Clin Neurosurg 15:175–189, 1968.
60. Bloom HJ, Peckham MJ, Richardson AE, Alexander PA, Payne PM: Glioblastoma Multiforme: A controlled trial to assess the value of specific active immunotherapy in patients treated by radical surgery and radiotherapy. Br J Cancer 27:253–267, 1973.
61. Ommaya Ak, Albright L: Immunochemotherapy of gliomas. Excerpta Medica Int Congr 293:314, 1973.
62. Takakura K, Miki Y, Kubo O, Ogawa N, Matsutani M, Sano K: Adjuvant immunotherapy for malignant brain tumors. Jap J Clin Oncol 12:109–120, 1972.
63. Neuwelt EA, Clark K, Kirkpatrick JB, Toben H: Clinical studies of intrathecal autologous lymphocyte infusions in patients with malignant gliomas. A toxicity study. Ann Neurol 4:307–314, 1978.
64. Lim R, Kluskens L: Immunological specificity of astrocytoma antigens. Cancer Res 32:1667–1670, 1972.
65. Albright L, Madigan JC, Gaston MR, Houchens DP: Therapy in an intracerebral murine glioma model, using Bacillus Calmette Guerin, neuraminidase-treated tumor cells and 1-2-chloroethyl)-3-cyclohexyl-1-nitrososurea. Cancer Res 35:658–665, 1975.
66. Neuwelt EA, Doherty D: Toxicity kinetics and clinical potential of subarachnoid lymphocyte infusions. J Neurosurg 47:205–217, 1977.
67. Rosenblum MI, Reynolds AF, Smith KA, Rumack BH, Walker MD: Chloroethyl-cyclohexyl-nitrosourea (CCNU) in the treatment of malignant brain tumors. J Neurosurg 39:306–314, 1973.
68. Levy NL, Mahaley MS, Day ED: *In vitro* demonstration of cell-mediated immunity to human brain tumors. Cancer Res 32:477–482, 1972.
69. Hellstrom I, Sjogren Ho, Warner G: Blocking of cell-mediated immunity by sera from patients with growing neoplasma. Int J Cancer 7:226–237, 1971.

7. Advantages and Disadvantages of Adjuvant Chemotherapy in the Treatment of Primary CNS Tumors

WILLIAM M. WARA

1. INTRODUCTION

Primary brain tumors are the most common solid tumors seen in children[1]. They vary from the curable suprasellar germinoma to the lethal malignant glioblastoma multiforme. In addition to the histologic variations, the clinical effects and management of CNS tumors differ according to location, extent of tumor, biologic characteristics and a knowledge of the value and limitations of surgery, irradiation and chemotherapy used singly or in combination for therapy. Because of the complex management decisions required we have evolved an experienced neuro-oncology team which includes the pediatrician, the pediatric neurologist, the neurosurgeon, the pediatric neuro-oncologist, the radiation oncologist and the pediatric endocrinologist.

For most primary brain tumors surgery is the first modality of treatment, both for diagnosis and for tumor debulking with preservation of neurological function. After surgery, irradiation is recommended for all incompletely removed lesions. Modern radiation therapy is largely limited to megavoltage irradiation, i.e., energy greater than one million electron volts. As compared with kilovoltage, megavoltage irradiation has the advantages of greater penetration, less bone absorption, decreased side scatter and reduced dose to skin and subcutaneous tissues. Particularly important in the treatment of children, collimators, blocks, wedge filters and individually designed tissue-compensating filters may be utilized to shape the high dose volume and to protect sensitive normal tissues. After selecting the best physical distribution of dose, the maximum absorbed dose consistent with an acceptable risk for critical normal structures is given. The risk of radiation injury must be balanced against expected benefit and the risk of uncontrolled tumor. In general, normal tissue sensitivity limits radiation therapy, especially for tumors of the central nervous system which only rarely metastasize outside its confines.

Toxicity and risk from irradiation has not been established. Available liter-

G. B. Humphrey et al. (eds.), Pediatric oncology 1, 199–211. All rights reserved.

ature is anecdotal and usually fails to provide pertinent factors such as total dose at the exact site of necrosis, size and number of individual treatment fractions, overall treatment time, arrangement of fields and volume irradiated. Few investigators have supplied the number of patients which have been evaluated for an adequate amount of time to achieve the described morbidity with and without chemotherapy in order to determine the exact incidence of injury. Caveness [2], who treated monkeys with irradiation alone in a clinical regimen (200 rad per day, 5 fractions per week to a total whole brain dose of 4000, 6000 and 8000 rad), has supplied information which is helpful in extrapolating to human data. His data provide insight into the limitations of total dose and fractionation which has proved useful in designing clinical protocols.

Historically the changes seen have been divided into acute reactions, early delayed reactions and late reactions with or without concurrent leukoencephalopathy. Although there may be overlap the clinical endpoints differ and may be influenced by chemotherapy; therefore, they should be distinguished and may play a role in determining a rational treatment program.

Associated with high dose cranial irradiation is a syndrome of somnolence thought to be secondary to transient irradiation myelopathy [3]. Boldrey and Sheline [4] have described this syndrome which consists of symptoms mimicking the original tumor and usually resolves within 3 months post irradiation. The symptoms have been interpreted by some investigators as tumor recurrence but in fact resolve spontaneously or with steroid therapy.

Late delayed reactions constitute the major hazard of CNS exposure to therapeutic irradiation. Onset may be from several months to years after exposure. It is generally irreversible, progressive and often fatal. Signs and symptoms depend upon the area and volume of brain irradiated and frequently are those of an intracranial mass. The injury tends to be more severe in white matter and may present as an area of gliosis or frank necrosis. Recently, Gangji et al. [5] found elevated CSF myelin levels within months after cranial irradiation of children with ALL and overt leukoencephalopathy. It is probable that multiple mechanisms are involved and that their relative importance differs with radiation dose and latent interval. The weight of evidence suggests that demyelination is important in the early delayed reaction and that vascular changes become progressively more important with time.

Other late delayed effects after cranial irradiation include pituitary–hypothalamic dysfunction and decreased intellectual ability. Serum hormone levels may be depressed by irradiation of the pituitary-hypothalamic axis, especially in children [6–9]. The incidence of radiation induced hypopituitarism as a function of radiation dose is unknown, but most studies of patients who have received incidental sellar irradiation have shown a latent period of several years, a dose–effect relationship, and that growth hormone production is most sensitive [7, 9]. Often the effect is subclinical and found only by detailed biochemical studies [10]. More difficult to quantitate is the effect of cranial irradiation on intellectual function. After prophylactic irradiation with doses of 1200–2400 rad in children with ALL, psychometric tests have failed to demonstrate loss of function [11]. Investigators of patients with brain tumors, who may have had pre-irradiation neurological damage from tumor and/or increased intracranial pressure, have shown minimal to major impairment of intellectual function, especially in children, after cranial irradiation (4000–6000 rad) [12–15]. Eisner described 28 children with acute lymphocytic leukemia studies retrospectively [16]. Nine children had received no irradiation, 10 received irradiation within 2 months of diagnosis and nine received prophylactic cranial irradiation ≥6 months after diagnosis. Those irradiated (2400 rad/12 fractions) within 2 months showed significant impairment with poor performance of quantitative mathematical tests and of tasks involving abstract material; this group was irradiated during the injection period which utilizes a different set of chemotherapeutic agents than is used during the later maintenance period. The author concluded the differences were not due to lack of school attendance or family stresses but failed to discuss the possible interaction and timing of irradiation and chemotherapy. This study points out the need for prospective, carefully controlled intelligence testing to define the incidence and interaction of various therapeutic modalities.

Patients with brain tumors are often treated with cranial irradiation and/or various combinations of chemotherapeutic drugs, many of which can cross the blood–brain barrier. Numerous case reports have described clinical and pathologic changes that mimic radiation damage but which have occurred in patients receiving chemotherapy alone [17–23]. It is probable, as has been described for other normal tissues [24–28], that some of these agents will also sensitize or enhance radiation damage in the CNS.

Under the auspices of the Brain Tumor Study Group (BTSG), several hundred patients had whole brain irradiation with doses of 5000–6000 rad. 170–200 rad per fraction. Burger et al. [29] reported five instances of necrosis among 24 brains from BTSG patients examined at postmortem. Three of the five also had had multicourse chemotherapy. Unfortunately, the low autopsy rate and absence of information regarding selection of patients undergoing autopsy prevents an estimate of necrosis incidence or determination of possible synergistic effects from the chemotherapeutic agents. Burger et al. found a predilection for necrosis in the white matter adjacent to neoplasms suggesting a role mediated by the tumor itself. Perhaps local sensitivity was enhanced by cerebral edema or the concentration of chemotherapeutic agent was increased in the area surrounding the tumor. Based upon anecdotal reports, it is likely that chemotherapeutic agents, such as BCNU, Procarbazine, Methotrexate and Vincristine will enhance the radiation effects on the CNS.

2. ASTROCYTOMAS

In order to determine which histological type of tumor might be suitable for adjuvant chemotherapy it is necessary to examine the results with conventional surgery and irradiation alone; only in those tumor types in which the results are poor should additional chemotherapy be considered. Therapy should result in the minimal neurological disability possible in order to achieve the best control rate.

Although astrocytomas are a common pediatric tumor, the necessity of radiation therapy is controversial [30–33]. Most reports in the literature are inconclusive because they lack unirradiated control groups, study patients have undergone inadequate radiotherapy, mixed tumor types have been pooled in the data reports, and descriptions of the irradiation treament are incomplete. Presently, there is no randomized controlled study to evaluate the effectiveness of irradiation in the control of differentiated astrocytomas.

In order to determine a rational treatment basis we reviewed our experience with all cases of astrocytomas treated between 1942 and 1967 [34] (Table 1). Each patient underwent craniotomy with biopsy and surgical removal of as much tumor as possible. One hundred and twenty-two patients were evaluable and were separated into groups by type of treatment.

Fourteen patients underwent total surgical resection and none of these were recurrent at 10 years after surgery. Nine of the tumors which were totally resected were cystic cerebellar astrocytomas of childhood. The only death in this group occurred in an elderly patient who died of congestive heart failure 12 years post resection without recurrence of the tumor. Therefore, because of these and other results we do not recommend postoperative irradiation when total surgical removal has been accomplished.

Seventy-one patients with incompletely removed astrocytomas were treated without irradiation and the 5-year recurrence-free survival rate was 19%. This result may be compared with a 46% relapse-free survival rate after partial

Table 1. Relapse-free survival for astrocytomas.

Complete surgical resection			Incomplete surgical resection			
Survival (year)	No. patients	% survival	Without irradiation		With irradiation	
			No. patients	% Survival	No. patients	% Survival
1	14	100	37	51	71	80
5	14	100	37	19	71	46
10	12	100	37	11	54	35

resection plus irradiation. When only well-differentiated astrocytomas were considered the 5-year survival rate with irradiation was 58% but was 25% without irradiation. For astrocytoma, grade 2 the 5-year survival rate was 25% with irradiation and 0% without irradiation. The difference in favor of postoperative radiation persisted throughout the period of observation. Fazekas[35] had similar survival results following irradiation, i.e., 54% at 5 years and 10-20% at 10 years. These data indicate that radiation therapy increases the disease free interval when given postoperatively and delays recurrence for at least 20 years in patients with incompletely resected astrocytomas. With the microsurgical techniques which are now available, it is probable that more extensive resections can be performed without an increase in morbidity; these techniques, combined with aggressive radiation therapy, may yield further improvement in survival rates.

It is our policy to irradiate any incompletely excised astrocytoma. Treatment is initiated when the patient has recovered from surgery and the wound is well-healed. Daily fractions of 180-200 rad are given to a total tumor dose of 5000-5500 rad. Because of these encouraging results adjunctive chemotherapy is not recommended for these patients at the present time.

3. GLIOMAS

Malignant gliomas constitute a more difficult therapeutic problem and must be differentiated histologically into groups of tumors consisting of malignant astrocytomas; undifferentiated astrocytomas, or astrocytoma grade 3, referred to as malignant gliomas; and astrocytomas grade 4 or glioblastoma multiforme, which should be grouped and reported as glioblastoma multiforme. There is no question from the literature that postoperative radiation therapy increases the survival of these patients. As shown in Table 2, pooled data

Table 2. Surgery and irradiation for malignant gliomas.

	No. patients	% survival	
		1 yr	5 yr
Malignant astrocytoma			
Surgery alone	63	12	2
Surgery + irradiation	128	40	16
Glioblastoma Multiforme			
Surgery alone	145	8	0
Surgery + irradiation	90	24	0

from the Mayo Clinic [36], the University of California, Los Angeles [37], Thomas Jefferson University [38] and the University of California, San Francisco [39] show an improvement in 1–5 year survival rates after irradiation. At 5 years the average survival for the four series of patients was one of 63 with resection only and 16% when irradiation was added. The patients who survived had a diagnosis of malignant astrocytoma. No patients survived with the diagnosis of glioblastoma multiforme at 5 years.

During the past decade several prospective randomized studies of radiation therapy and/or various combinations of chemotherapeutic agents have been undertaken in order to improve this poor therapeutic result. The BTSG compared radiation therapy, BCNU (carmustine), and radiotherapy plus BCNU. Other studies with BCNU, procarbazine, vincristine, CCNU (lomustine), high dose corticosteroids, hydroxyurea, hypoxic cell radiosensitizers and various combinations thereof are ongoing. The BTSG found that total doses of postoperative radiotheapy of 5000–6000 rad increased immediate survival from 14 weeks with surgery alone to 36 weeks [40]. The addition of BCNU chemotherapy apparently improved survival time but the increase in median survival was small. Median survival was directly related to age and to initial functional status. The improvement in survival appeared dose related with median survival of 28, 36 and 42 weeks for radiation doses of approximately 5000, 5500 and 6000 rad, respectively [41].

Other groups have investigated 'hyperfractionated' (more than one treatment per 24 hours) radiotherapy, irradiation in combination with immunotherapy [42], or hypoxic cell radiosensitizers [43]. Using historical controls, Douglas [44] reported a 1-year survival of 44% for treatment with three fractions per day compared with 27% for conventional single daily fracionated radiotherapy. Urtasun et al. [43] found that with relatively low doses of radiation (3000 rad in fractions) the hypoxic cell radiosensitizer metronidazole increased the 50% probability of survival from 110 to 210 days. Perhaps higher doses will further improve survival.

We recommend doses of 6000 rad with daily fractionation to generous fields, usually with concurrent chemotherapy for gliomas. The fields often, but not always, include the entire intracranial contents. Kramer [38] has used either 6000 rad to the whole brain or 5000 rad to the whole brain plus a 1500 rad boost to the tumor volume.

While most tumor sites inside the calvarium can be surgically approached to obtain histological diagnosis and for the initial step in treatment, tumors of the brain stem are usually not resectable because of the risk to the patient's life or neurologic functional loss. The exact incidence of brain stem tumors is not known. An estimate of the number of new cases annually can be obtained from the number of patients treated at radiotherapy centers. A reasonable estimate would be 100 to 150 new cases per year, based upon data that high-grade gliomas elsewhere in the brain occur with equal frequency as do brain stem tumors [45–47]. Because of the tightly packed tracts and nuclear groups in the brain stem, symptoms occur early [48]; frequently the progress of the clinical neurologic deficit is rapid and lethal [49, 50]. Thus the natural course of brain stem gliomas should show changes with intensive therapy.

Surgical resection plays little or no role in the therapy of brain stem tumors. The condition of patients who receive no radiation therapy deteriorates rapidly and they expire more than 95% of the time, although steroids and irradiation may modify the neurologic deficit briefly. Radiotherapy centers report a 10–20% 5-year survival when high doses of irradiation are employed [46, 51, 52]. It is believed that a few of these patients have high-grade gliomas, but the majority of these patients probably have other neoplastic and non-neoplastic lesions.

Little data specific to the management of brain stem lesions with chemotherapy is reported. However, since the vast majority of these lesions are ultimately diagnosed as high-grade gliomas, the data reported for therapy of high-grade gliomas of other sites in the central nervous system seem appropriate [53–55].

Various chemotherapy agents and several different dose schedules have been tried in patients with brain tumors. Much of the early work was accomplished in patients with recurrences after conventional therapy methods (surgery and/or radiotherapy) had been employed. Hydroxyurea, intrathecal methotrexate, Vincristine (VCR), the nitrosoureas, procarbazine and halogenated pyrimidines have been used, and preliminary results have been published. Most reports show that tumor response does occur with some frequency (from 20% up to 40% objective response); however, long-term survival has changed very little.

Because of the poor results from previous therapeutic regimens for brain stem gliomas, we are initiating aggressive treatment which consists of chemotherapy prior to and during radiation therapy. Fluorouracil (FU) prior to CCNU experimentally has enhanced CCNU activity [56]. The results attained with hydroxyurea, radiation therapy and BCNU were better than those for BCNU and radiation therapy for glioblastoma [57]. Misonidazole, a radiosensitizer, should improve the radiation therapy response in brain stem tumors, which quite likely have low blood flow and considerable hypoxia based on the normal vessel patterns in the brain stem and the clinical course of these tumors. Therefore, all of these chemotherapeutic agents have been combined in a pilot protocol to determine their toxicity and efficacy.

4. EPENDYMOMAS

Ependymomas are relatively sensitive to irradiation. Thus, the usual treatment course is subtotal resection and postoperative irradiation. Table 3 illustrates the increase in survival when irradiation is given. Bouchard and Peirce [58] and Phillips et al. [59] had 50% and 62% 10-year survival rates, respectively, when adequate tumor doses (≥4500 rad) were given.

While there is consensus that ependymomas should be irradiated there is controversy whether craniospinal irradiation is necessary. There is no doubt that ependymomas occasionally seed within the nervous system but the incidence is probably small. Svien et al. [60] stated that none of 162 patients with ependymoma had clinical evidence of spinal metastases. Fokes and Earle [61] reported 14 cases of seeding in 127 patients whose pathologic material was reviewed at autopsy. At the University of California, San Francisco there were two instances of spinal seeding among 42 patients [59]. Thus, the overall incidence of seeding from ependymomas is hardly sufficient to justify the morbidity from routine craniospinal irradiation. The exception to this is undifferentiated (high grade) ependymoma of the posterior fossa where seeding can occur in 20-30% of cases [59, 60, 62].

Table 3. Surgery and irradiation for ependymoma.

Author	5-yr survival rate (%)	10-yr survival rate (%)
Cushing — Surgery alone	20	
Ringertz and Reymond — surgery alone	27	
Bouchard and Peirce — surgery and irradiation*	58	50
Phillips et al. — surgery and irradiation*	87	62

* Tumor dose ≥ 4500 rad

5. MEDULLOBLASTOMA

The cerebellar medulloblastoma accounts for 15-20% of childhood intracranial tumors [63]. Frequently it infiltrates the subarachnoid space and has a pronounced tendency to spread via cerebrospinal fluid (CSF) pathways. Presently, craniospinal irradiation is the standard treatment of choice after as much tumor as possible has been resected. McFarland et al. [64] reported that 33% of 430 patients developed metastases to the central nervous system (CNS) when treated with localized radiation portals.

Although there is agreement that the entire cerebrospinal axis must be irradiated, the optimum dose to provide control in various areas of the CNS is uncertain and the primary site of failure, even after 5500 rad tumor dose, is a local recurrence in the posterior fossa [63, 64]. Older series in the literature with craniospinal irradiation have yielded 5-year and 10-year recurrence-free rates of 35 and 25%, respectively [63–65]. With modern techniques and maximum doses to all areas of the CNS, we have increased the 5-year survival rate to 40–50% [66]. With this increased survival, effects on growth, endocrine function and intellectual development now must be taken into consideration in treating these patients.

In order to determine the effect of adjuvant chemotherapy (CCNU, Vincristine and prednisone) on patients with medulloblastomas, Childrens Cancer Study Group (CCSG) initiated a randomized study in 1975 to compare the addition of chemotherapy to standard craniospinal irradiation. This study was designed to parallel a European study (International Society of Paediatric Oncology, SIOP) so that more patients would be available for analysis. Preliminary results reveal a trend toward improved survival in the chemotherapy group which is not yet significant. Of interest is the fact the group treated with irradiation alone is projected to have a higher disease-free rate than previous historical controls [67].

Future protocols in the planning stages propose to give less irradiation to low risk patients who have had gross surgical removal and negative myelograms, thereby minimizing treatment morbidity. High risk patients (intracranial metastases and/or spinal metastases) will be treated with more aggressive chemotherapy (Table 4). As more effective drugs become available adjuvant chemotherapy will be placed into new protocols, especially with the malignant tumors in which the historical results are poor.

Table 4. Proposed new medulloblastoma protocol (CCG 982).

All patients would have a myelogram before irradiation for staging:	
Low risk (negative myelogram) 50%	High risk (positive myelogram) 50%

Standard irradiation
  5500 rad posterior fossa
  4000 rad whole brain
  3500–4000 rad spine
  versus
  5500 rad posterior fossa
  2500 rad whole brain
  2500 rad spine
Maintenance: best arm current protocol
	* Pre-irradiation chemotherapy
	  Standard irradiation
	  Best arm current protocol
	
	CT scan before and after chemotherapy,
	  week 1 and 4
	
	* Drug priority
	  1) Cytoxan
	  2) BCNU
	  3) Dibromoducital
	  4) Vincristine
	  5) Nitrogen mustard
	  6) Methotrexate

REFERENCES

1. Rubinstein LJ: Tumors of the central nervous system. Atlas of tumor pathology, ser. 2, fasc. 6. Washington, DC: Armed Forces Institute of Pathology, 1972.
2. Caveness WF: Pathology of radiation damage to the normal brain of the monkey. Natl Cancer Inst Monogr 46:57–76, 1977.
3. Jones A: Transient radiation myelopathy (with reference to Lhermitte's sign of electrical paresthesia). Br J Radiol 37:727–744, 1964.
4. Boldrey E, Sheline G: Delayed transitory clinical manifestations after radiation treatment of intracranial tumors. Acta Radiol 5:5–10, 1967.
5. Gangji D, Reaman GH, Cohen SR, Bleyer WA, Ladisch S, Poplack DG: Elevated basic myelin protein in the cerebrospinal fluid of acute lymphoblastic leukemia patients with leukoencephalopathy. Proc Am Assoc Cancer Res Am Assoc Clin Oncol 20:353, 1979.
6. Harrop JS, Davies TJ, Capra LG, Marks V: Hypothalamic–pituitary function following successful treatment of intracranial tumours. Clin Endocrinol 5:313–321, 1976.
7. Richards GE, Wara WM, Grumbach MM, Kaplan SL, Sheline GE, Conte FA: Delayed onset of hypopituitarism: sequelae of therapeutic irradiation of central nervous system, eye, and middle ear tumors. J Pediat 89:553–559, 1976.
8. Samaan, NA, Bakdash MM, Caderao JB, Cangir A, Jesse RH, Ballantyne AJ: Hypopituitarism after external irradiation: evidence for both hypothalamic and pituitary origin. Ann Intern Med 83:771–777, 1975.
9. Shalet SM, Beardwell CG, Morris-Jones PH, Pearson D: Pituitary function after treatment of intracranial tumors in children. The Lancet July 19, 1975, pp 104–107.
10. Shalet SM, Price DA, Beardwell CG, Morris-Jones PH, Pearson D: Normal growth despite abnormalities of growth hormone secretion in children treated for acute leukemia. J Pediat 94:719–722, 1979.
11. Soni SS, Marten GW, Pitner SE, Duenas DA, Powazek M: Effects of central-nervous-system irradiation on neuropsychologic functioning of children with acute lymphocytic leukemia. N Engl J Med 293:113–118, 1975.
12. Bamford FN, Morris-Jones P, Pearson D, Ribeiro GG, Shalet SM, Beardwell CG: Residual disabilities in children treated for intracranial space-occupying lesions. Cancer 37:1149–1151, 1976.
13. Hirsch JF, Pierre-Kahn A, Benveniste L, George B: Les médulloblastomes de l'enfant. Survie et résultats fonctionnels. Neurochirurgie 24:391–397, 1978.
14. Obetz SW, Smithson WA, Groove RV, House OW, Klass DW, Ivnik RJ, Colligan RC, Burgert O, Gilchrist GS: Neuropsychological follow-up study of central nervous system function in children with acute lymphocytic leukemia. Proc Am Assoc Cancer Res Am Soc Clin Oncol 20:342, 1979.
15. Raimondi, AJ, Tomita T: The disadvantages of prophylactic whole CNS postoperative radiation therapy for medulloblastoma. In: Multidisciplinary aspects of brain tumor therapy, Paoletti P, Walker MD, Butti G, Knerich R (eds). New York: Elsevier/North Holland, 1979, pp 209–218.
16. Eisner C: Intellectual abilities among survivors of childhood leukaemia as a function of CNS irradiation. Arch Dis Childh 53:391–395, 1978.
17. Allen JC: The effects of cancer therapy on the nervous system. J Pediat 93:903–909, 1978.
18. Allen JC, Rosen G: Transient cerebral dysfunction following chemotherapy for osteogenic sarcoma. Ann Neurol 3:441–444, 1978.

19. Allen JC, Thaler HT, Deck MDF, Rottenberg DA: Leukoencephalopathy following high-dose intravenous methotrexate chemotherapy: quantitative assessment of white matter attenuation using computed tomography. Neuroradiology 16:44–47, 1978.

20. McIntosh S, Fischer DB, Rothman S, Rosenfield N, Lobel JS, O'Brien RT: Intracranial calcifications in childhood leukemia. J Pediat 91:909–913, 1977.

21. Norrell H, Wilson CB, Slagel DE, Clark DB: Leukoencephalopathy following the administration of methotrexate into the cerebrospinal fluid in the treatment of primary brain tumors. Cancer 33:923–932, 1974.

22. Shapiro WR, Chernik NL, Posner JG: Necrotizing encephalopathy following intraventricular installation of methotrexate. Arch Neurol 28:96–102, 1973.

23. Smith B: Brain damage after intrathecal methotrexate, J Neurol Neurosurg Psychiat 38:810–815, 1975.

24. Fusner J, Poplack DG, Pizzo PA, DeChiro G: Leukoencephalopathy following chemotherapy for rhabdomyosarcoma; reversibility of cerebral changes demonstrated by computed tomography. J Pediat 91:77–79, 1977.

25. Kay HEM, Knapton PJ, O'Sullivan JP, Harris RF, Innes EM, Stuart J, Schwartz FCM, Thompson EN: Encephalopathy in acute leukemia associated with methotrexate therapy. Arch Dis Childh 47:344–353, 1972.

26. Meadows AT, Evans AE: Effects of chemotherapy on the CNS: A study of parenteral MTX in long term survivors of leukemia and lymphoma in childhood. Cancer 37:1079–1085, 1976.

27. Phillips TL, FU KK: Quantitation of combined radiation therapy and chemotherapy effects on critical normal tissues. Cancer 37:1186–1200. 1976.

28. Pratt RA, DeChiro G, Weed JC: Cerebral necrosis following irradiation and chemotherapy for metastatic choriocarcinoma. Surg Neurol 7:117–120, 1977.

29. Burger PC, Mahaley MS, Dudka L, Vogel FS: The morphological effects of radiation administered therapeutically for intracranial gliomas. A postmortem study of 25 cases. Cancer 44:1256–1272, 1979.

30. Bouchard J: Central nervous system. In: Textbook of radiotherapy, 2nd ed, Fletcher J (ed.). Philadelphia: Lea & Febiger, 1973 pp 336–418.

31. Kramer S, Southard M, Mansfield C: Radiation effect and tolerance of the central nervous system. Front Radium Ther Oncol 6:332, 1972.

32. Richmond J: Malignant tumours of the central nervous system. In: Cancer 5, Raven R (ed.). London: Butterworth, 1959, pp 375–389.

33. Sheline G, Boldrey E, Karlsberg P, Phillips T: Therapeutic considerations in tumors affecting the central nervous system: oligodendrogliomas. Radiology 82:84, 1964.

34. Leibel S, Sheline G, Wara W, Boldrey E, Neilsen B: The role of radiation therapy in the treatment of astrocytomas. Cancer 35:1551–1557, 1975.

35. Fazekas JT: Treatment of grades I and II brain astrocytomas. The role of radiation therapy. Int J Radiat Oncol Biol Phys 2:661, 1977.

36. Uihlein A, Colby M, Layton D, et al.: Comparison of surgery and surgery plus irradiation in the treatment of supratentorial gliomas. Acta Radiol 5:67, 1966.

37. Stage W, Stein J: Treatment of malignant astrocytomas. Am J Roentgenol 120:7, 1974.

38. Kramer S: Radiation therapy in the management of malignant gliomas. In: 7th Natl Cancer Conf Proc. Philadelphia: Lippincott, 1973, pp 823–826.

39. Sheline G: Conventional radiation therapy of gliomas. In: Gliomas: current concepts in Biology, diagnosis, and therapy: proceedings. New York: Springer-Verlag, 1975, pp 123–234.

40. Walker MD, Alexander E Jr, Hunt WE, *et al.*: An evaluation of BCNU and/or radiotherapy in the treatment of anaplastic gliomas: a cooperative clinical trial. J Neurosurg 49:333, 1978.

41. Walker MG, Strike TA, Sheline GE (for the Brain Tumor Study Group): A dose–effect relationship of radiotherapy in the treatment of malignant glioma. Int J Radiat Oncol Biol Phys (in press).

42. Bloom HJG, Peckham MJ, Richardson AE, et al: Glioblastoma multiforme: a controlled trial to assess the value of specific active immunotherapy in patients treated by radical surgery and radiotherapy. Br J Cancer 27:253, 1973.

43. Urtasun R, Band P. Chapman D, *et al.*: Radiation and high dose metronidazole (Flagyl) in supratentorial glioblastomas. N Engl J Med 294:1364, 1976.

44. Douglas BJ: Preliminary results using superfractionation in the treatment of glioblastoma multiforme. Personal communication.

45. Childrens Cancer Study Group: Brain tumor survey. Unpublished data.

46. Panitch HS, Berg BO: Brain stem tumors of childhood and adolescence. Am J Dis Child 119:465–472, 1970.

47. Ingraham FD, Matson DD: Neurosurgery of infancy and childhood. Springfield. Ill.: Charles C. Thomas, 1969.

48. Bray PF, Carter S, Taveras JM: Brain stem tumors in children. Neurology 8:1–7, 1958.

49. Lassman LP, Arjona VE: Pontine gliomas of childhood. Lancet 1:913–915, 1967.

50. Hittle RE, Anderson F, Fishman LS: Unpublished data. Children's Hospital of Los Angeles.

51. Marsa GW, Probert JC, Rubenstein LF, Bagshaw MA: Radiation therapy in the treatment of childhood astrocytic gliomas. Cancer 32:646–655, 1973.

52. Bouchard J: Radiation therapy of tumors and diseases of the nervous system. Philadelphia: Lea & Febiger, 1966.

53. Smart CR, *et al.*: Clinical experience with vincristine (NSC067574) in tumors of the central nervous system and other malignant diseases. Cancer Chemother Rep 52:733–737, 1968.

54. Lassman LP, Pearce GW, Gang J: Effects of vincristine sulfate on intracranial gliomas of childhood. Br J Surg 52:774–777, 1966.

55. Fewer D, Wilson CB, Boldrey EB, Enot JK: Phase II Study of CCNU in the treatment of brain tumors. Cancer Chemother Rep 56:421, 1972.

56. Levin VA, Hoffman WF, Pischer TL, Crafts DC, Enot JK, Seager ML, Boldrey EB, Wilson CB: BCNU-5-fluorouracil combination in the treatment of recurrent malignant brain tumors. Cancer Treatment Rep 62:2071–2079, 1979.

57. Levin VA, Wilson CB, Davis R, Wara W, Pischer TA, Irwin L: A phase III comparison study of BCNU, Hydroxyurea and irradiation for the treatment of primary malignant gliomas. J Neurosurg 51:526–532, 1979.

58. Bouchard J, Peirce C: Radiation therapy in the management of neoplasms of the central nervous system with a special note in regard to children: twenty years' experience, 1939–1958. Am J Roentgenol 84:610, 1960.

59. Phillips T, Sheline G, Boldrey E: Therapeutic considerations in tumors affecting the central nervous system: ependymomas. Radiology 83:98, 1964.

60. Svien H, Mabon R, Kernohan J, Craig M: Ependymoma of the brain: pathologic aspects. Neurology 3:1, 1953.

61. Fokes E, Jr, Earle K: Ependymomas: clinical and pathological aspects. J Neurosurg 30:585, 1969.

62. Kim Y, Fayos J: Intracranial ependymomas. Radiology 124:805, 1977.

63. Bloom HJG, Wallace ENK, Henk JM: The treatment and prognosis of medulloblastoma in children—a study of 82 verified cases. Am J Roentgenol 105:43–62, 1969.

64. McFarland DR, Horwitz H, Saenger EL, Bahr GK: Medulloblastoma—a review of prognosis and survival. Br J Radiol 42:198–214, 1969.
65. Kramer S: Radiation therapy in the management of brain tumors in children—part II. Diagnostic and therapeutic aspects of brain tumors. Ann NY Acad Sci 159:571–584, 1969 (2nd article).
66. Cumberlin RL, Luk KH, Wara WM, Sheline GE, Wilson CB: Medulloblastoma: treatment results and effect on normal tissues. Cancer 43:1014–1020, 1979.
67. Evans AE, Anderson J, Chang C, Jenkin RDT, Kramer S, Schoenfeld D, Wilson C: Adjuvant chemotherapy for medulloblastoma and ependymoma. In: Multidisciplinary aspects of brain tumor therapy, Paoletti P, Walker MD, Butti G, Knerich R (eds). Amsterdam: Elsevier/North Holland, 1979.

II. Rare Tumors of the Central Nervous System

8. Primitive Neuroectodermal Tumors of Brain in Childhood: Literature Review and the M. D. Anderson Experience

JOHN KNAPP, DAISY FRANCINI, JAN VAN EYS and AYTEN CANGIR

1. INTRODUCTION

Brain tumors with a prominent component of undifferentiated 'small cells' have appeared in various series as 'cerebral medulloblastoma,' 'central or cerebral neuroblastoma,' or 'undifferentiated glioma'[1–3]. Such neoplasms are rarely encountered but mainly occur in children[1] and occasionally in young adults in the cerebrum and, less frequently, the spinal cord[1, 4]. There is apparent multipotentiality for differentiation into neuronal and glial components focally or diffusely[1, 4]. Both the undifferentiated character and more mature elements imply resemblance to the germinal or matrix cells of primitive neuroectoderm[1]. The cytogenetic considerations of the relationship to embryonal precursors has been reviewed by Rubenstein[5]. He discussed the distinct tumor entities in early life which consist predominantly or exclusively of primitive elements corresponding to cell types at various stages in development. These neoplasms were designated as cerebral neuroblastoma, true polar spongioblastoma, ependymoblastoma, and medulloblastoma. The somewhat controversial medulloepithelioma as a special example of primitive central nervous system tumors was also discussed by Rubenstein[5]. Less predictable in appearance is the 'small cell' group with wide ranges of differentiation and also a mesenchymal component[1]. For this reason such cases are collectively categorized under the designation of primitive neuroectodermal tumors[1–3].

The clinical summaries of three series of PNET[1–3] have been tabulated (Table 1). Two other series together with a composite collection of related entities in the neuroblastoma and neuronal tumor groups are also included. Microscopic criteria restricting the pattern of the PNET to 90–95% of undifferentiated cells[1] has been applied by Kosnik et al.[2] and Parker et al.[3]. Further, the other features common to PNET as noted by Hart et al.[1] were also evident. Namely, these were predominant in early life, malignant biologic

G. B. Humphrey et al. (eds.), Pediatric oncology 1, 215–224. All rights reserved.
Copyright © 1981 Martinus Nijhoff Publishers bv, The Hague/Boston/London.

Table 1. Clinical histories of undifferentiated and neuronal differentiating embryonal tumors in brain, primitive neuroectodermal tumors in brain.

Series	Hart et al. [1]	Kosnik et al. [2]	Parket et al. [3]	Horten et al. [9]	Feigen et al[7] Pearson et al. [8]	Others [6, 10, 11]
No. of patients	23	18	7	31	6	4
Microscopic diagnosis	Undifferentiated small cell	Undifferentiated small cell	Undifferentiated small cell	Neuro-blastoma	Anaplastic neuroma	Primary cerebral neuro-blastoma
Average age (yr)/range (yr)	8.1/0–24	3.1/0.5–10	4.6/0.3–9	4/0.2–11	7.5/4.5–13	9.4/1.5–6
Sex (F/M)	8/15	10/8	5/2	14/17	5/1	2/2
Presenting signs and symptoms						
Headache	9	8		4	4	3
Vomiting and/or nausea	6	9		4	3	2
Seizures	5	5		2	2	1
Eye signs	4			1	3	3
Motor signs	4	8		2	3	1
Papilledema		4		2	4	3
Lethargy		3				
Anorexia		2				
Head enlargement	2				1	
Hydrocephalus				1		
Subdural hematoma						1
Diabetes insipitus						1
Lymphadenopathy						1
Separated skull sutures						1
Comatose						1

Table 1. (continued)

Series	Hart et al. [1]	Kosnik et al. [2]	Parket et al. [3]	Horten et al. [9]	Feigen et al. [7] Pearson et al. [8]	Others [6, 10, 11]
No. of patients	23	18	7	31	6	4
Average time of duration of signs and symptoms prior to diagnosis	4.8 mo.	3 weeks†			2.7 yr	
Survival (%)/No. cases		<10%, 1 yr 14%	14%	37%/20	20%/5	0%/4
Average time of survival following initial treatment (surgery, radiation, chemotherapy) (yr/range)	1.5 (6 cases)		0.5/-1.7	3.8/0.4-13	2/0.5-4.5	1.9/0-6
Average time of recurrence following 1st surgery (yr/range)				2.8/0.5-7		2.2/0.25-6
Location R/L				12/19	5/0	3/0
Frontal	9	3		19	2	
Parietal	4	3	6	14	2	2
Temporal	4	3	2	7	3	1
Occipital	2	2	2	2	2	
Bilateral hemispheres	1					
3rd ventricle		4	1			
Lateral ventricle						1
Cerebellum	1				1	
Foramen of Munro	1					1
Corpus callosum						
Spinal cord		3				
Intraventricular					1	

behavior, location in the cerebrum, discrete gross borders, hemorrhages and cysts, and undifferentiated cells. There were also focal and diffuse areas with early maturation into glial or neuronal cells and a prominent mesenchymal component.

A recent electron microscopic study by Markesbery and Challa [4] of three cases of PNET has revealed evidence of potential differentiation into ependymal, neuronal, and astrocytic elements. The conclusion is that the precursor cell is a primitive multipotential cell and not a neuroblast. It was pointed out by these authors that others who had performed ultrastructural studies of cerebral neuroblastomas found many immature cells in addition to differentiated neurons and glia. The relationship between these two tumors was apparent and similarities in fine structure demonstrated by these studies made the two neoplasms comparable.

The clinical features of 31 cases of cerebral neuroblastoma [9] have been summarized in Table 1. In this study by Horton and Rubinstein [5], the children ranged in age from 3 months to 11 years. They observed microscopically that the tumors were densely cellular and composed of primitive cells. Because of difficulty in the precise characterization of tumor cells by histologic techniques, three microscopic criteria were utilized. These were distinctive Homer-Wright pseudorosettes, maturation to ganglion cells, and neuroblastic forms as demonstrated by silver impregnation. The latter was present in only seven of their 31 cases. Twenty-four cases had Homer-Wright pseudorosettes and 10 tumors showed maturation to ganglion cells. The composite series cited as 'other,' are cases from the literature accepted by Horton and Rubenstein as consistent with their criteria (Table 1). A more recent example contributed by Azzarelli et al. [6] was included. The combined series of Feigen et al. [7] and Pearson et al. [8] represent six pediatric cases included for comparison. The criteria are not equivalent to those of PNET and cerebral neuroblastoma. These latter tumors were composed of neurons and their multipotential precursors. They noted evidence of progressive maturation and anaplasia. Feigen et al. [7] commented that the tumors did not resemble neuroblastomas. However, Horton et al. [9] accepted two cases from the 10 described by Feigen et al. [7] as consistent with their criteria for cerebral neuroblastoma.

2. CASE REPORTS

Two cases of childhood PNET are described from the M.D. Anderson Hospital who were admitted after initial diagnosis and treatment.

2.1. Case 1

The patient was a 2 year old white female admitted to the Pediatric Clinic with a diagnosis of neuroblastoma of the right parietal lobe. She had a 2 week history of headache, projectile vomiting, and unsteady gait. A brain scan revealed a mass in the right parietal region displacing the ventricles to the left. Right craniotomy was performed with excision of a necrotic tumor which was diagnosed as cerebral neuroblastoma. One month following surgery she was seen at M.D. Anderson Hospital on medications including decadron, dilantin, and apresoline. Physical examination revealed no neurologic deficit. Residual tumor was detected on CT scans performed 3 weeks postoperatively. She was begun on radiotherapy with 3500 rads to whole brain, 2800 rads to the spine, and 1600 rads boost to the right temporoparietal area over 7 weeks. Three months after radiotherapy, recurrent disease was diagnosed on CT scan. She returned to M.D. Anderson one month later and received two courses of chemotherapy, vincristine-high dose cytoxan-trifluorodeoxythimidine protocol given one month apart. During her last admission to begin the second course of chemotherapy it was noted that her gait had become broad based and nodules were noted on the scalp in the site of the craniotomy scar. These regressed before discharge. She died one month later in the emergency room of another hospital.

2.1.1. Microscopic Findings.

The tumor was very cellular with a moderately abundant stromal component composed of fibrous septa. Fragmentation precluded a careful evaluation of the relationship of the brain to the surrounding brain. The small cells had little visible cytoplasm and the vesicular nuclei were oval, round or irregular with dispersed chromatin, and prominent single or double nucleoli. Mitoses were present at a range of 3–4/HPF. Solid sheets without a particular arrangement characterized the overall pattern. In some foci, however, groups of cells radiated from large septa and vessels. The cells were somewhat polar with a small amount of cytoplasm in these areas. Pleomorphism and giant cells were not present. Multiple foci of necrosis were scattered throughout the tumor. Vascular and endothelial proliferation were present, but not striking. Areas of differentiation included ependymal-like foci with elongated cells having terminal bars and cilia and forming perivascular rosettes. Neuronal differentiation was suggested by large cells with clear cytoplasm in a circular arrangement around a central fibrillary tangle.

2.2. Case 2

The patient was a 20 month old white male when he presented with a left hemiparesis. Partial resection of a right parietal tumor was performed, and the diagnosis was a primitive neuroectodermal tumor with ependymal and astroglial elements. He received 3000 rads over 6 weeks and an additional 2000 rads. Recurrence of tumor was diagnosed on a CT scan four months after surgical treatment. Two months later he had progressive left hemiparesis and seizure activity. At this time he was started on vincristine and BCNU. There was improvement neurologically, but progression on CT scan was noted. He was referred to M.D. Anderson Hospital for further treatment. On admission his gait was unsteady, favoring the left side. A CT scan showed a mass in the right parietal lobe. He was begun on the vincristine-high dose cytoxan-trifluorodeoxythymidine protocol. Three courses one month apart were given. There was persistence of the left hemiparesis. He could not walk during his visit for the third course of treatment. One month after returning home he was hospitalized with fever which responded to antibiotics. A white blood cell transfusion was given before transfer to M.D. Anderson three days later. On admission he had fever, rash and pancytopenia. The patient died one day later.

2.2.1. Postmortem Examination. Serial horizontal sections of the brain showed a large tumor measuring $6 \times 1.5 \times 6$ cm and occupying the entire right parietal lobe. It was necrotic with areas of cystic degeneration. The basal ganglia were destroyed by the mass which extended over the midline and into the right lateral ventricle, the substantia nigra, and right hippocampus. The left cerebral hemisphere was intact except for dilation of the left lateral ventricle. There was no involvement of the midbrain, brainstem, cerebellum and spinal cord.

2.2.2. Microscopic Findings. The tumor was highly cellular with prominent rosettes and a trabecular pattern in many areas. Cytologically, the cells were very similar to Case 1. Mitoses were numerous. In many foci, perivascular rosettes were striking and the cells had elongated cytoplasm. There was marked vascular proliferation. Large areas of necrosis were scattered through-out the tumor. An infiltrative pattern of invasion of the adjacent brain and dura was present. There was extension through the subarachnoidal space with secondary deposits along the meninges and spinal cord.

3. REVIEW OF CLINICAL AND PATHOLOGICAL FEATURES FROM TABLE 1 AND REVIEW OF LITERATURE

3.1. Age

The average age of the patients with a diagnosis of PNET inclusive of the three series of 48 cases show is 5.3 years. A slightly older age (6.7) was obtained from the series of Horton and Rubinstein[9] and the composite group.

3.2. Sex

The sex ratio for the PNET group is 22 females to 26 males and 16 females to 19 males in patients with neuroblastoma.

3.3 Presenting Signs and Symptoms

All studies show signs of increased intracranial pressure occurring at a higher frequency than localizing signs or seizures. The two cases presenting with anorexia reported by Kosnik et al. [2] had third ventricular lesions. Head enlargement and hydrocephalus were present in three cases including all series. Lymphadenopathy presented as the initial sign of disease in a case of cerebral neuroblastoma with extraneural metastases [10]. Diabetes insipidus was present in a case described by Kernohan et al. [11] which was diagnosed as gangliocytoma in a third ventricular location.

3.4. Survival

Three of the seven cases of PNET reported by Parker et al. [3] survived 2 weeks, 21 months, and 18 months following surgery. One other patient was still alive 3 years later. In the 18 cases of Kosnik et al. [2] less than 40% were alive in 6 months and less than 10% at one year. The average postoperative survival time for the patients of Parker et al. [3] was 7 months. Of the neuroblastoma cases collected by Horton and Rubinstein [9], 57% of 28 patients who had surgery died during or shortly after the procedure. Twelve patients (43%) were alive at the time of the report with survivals from 5 months to 15 years after surgery.

3.5. Recurrence

In the neuroblastoma group [9], 40% of 22 patients surviving surgery had recurrence of disease during the interval from 6 months to 7 years. Only one was alive at the time of the report. Published data are not available for recurrent disease in the PNET group.

3.6. Location

As shown in Table 1, PNET is not limited to the supratentorial location. Spinal cord tumors were reported in the cases of Kosnik et al. [2] and also one case with lung metastases is mentioned by Smith et al. [12] in their series of metastasizing neuroectodermal tumors.

3.7. Metastases

Parker et al. [3] reported meningeal gliomatosis in all four cases of PNET with postmortem examinations. The second case described from M.D. Anderson Hospital had extensive subarachnoid spread and spinal meningeal implants. Horton and Rubinstein [9] noted that metastatic spread as leptomeningeal and ventricular implants occurred in 8% of their fatal cases. One patient developed metastases to the liver. Henriquez et al. [10] reported a case with metastases in cervical lymph nodes, meninges and posterior nerve roots at presentation.

3.8. Treatment

The cases from M.D. Anderson Hospital reported in this review both received radiotherapy following surgery. Radiation to the whole brain and spinal cord was given in the first case (Case 1). Both patients received chemotherapy on the vincristine-high dose cytoxan–F_3TdR protocol after progression of disease was apparent. Parker et al. [3] noted that two of their autopsy cases received irradiation after surgery. Each child except one reported by Kosnik et al. [2] was given radiotherapy in the range of 4000–6000 rads following subtotal resection. They also indicated chemotherapy was used including intrathecal methotrexate in past cases and a combination of vincristine, prednisone, and 1-(2-chlorethyl)-3-cyclohexyl-1-nitrosourea (CCNU). Horton and Rubinstein [9] stated that 12 cases of neuroblastoma in their study received radiation to the whole brain and the entire neuraxis following surgery. The case of Henriquez et al. [10] was given radiotherapy following initial surgery and again after the appearance of spinal disease. Cytoxan was also given at this later time.

3.9. Histologic Findings

Both tumors in the M.D. Anderson experience were highly cellular and infiltrative neoplasms (Cases 1 and 2). When dura and adjacent brain were present for evaluation, invasion was present. The tumor cells were arranged in a solid pattern but in some areas, there was a suggestion of nests and cords, trabeculae and rosettes. Most tumor cells were small with little visible cytoplasm. The nuclei for the most part were oval to round, usually dispersed chromatin and prominent single or double nucleoli. Mitoses were frequent with both normal and abnormal figures.

Differentiation suggesting glial, ependymal and/or neuronal elements in focal areas was seen. Perivascular rosettes with polarity of the cells and terminal bars suggested ependyma. Glial elements were represented by large cells with fibrillary cytoplasm and occasional Rosenthal fibers, better demonstrated by PTAH and Holzer stains. Pseudorosettes, represented by cells arranged in a circle around a central fibrillary tangle, characterized neuronal or neuroblastic differentiation. The stroma was formed by fibrous septa with abundant vascularity. Capillary and endothelial proliferation were prominent.

4. DISCUSSION

Primitive neuroectodermal tumors of childhood are rare mainly supratentorial neoplasms that are probably related cytogenetically to the multipotential cells of the primitive neuroepithelium [1]. The specific types have been classified by Rubenstein [5], but they are a spectrum which merge imperceptibly and are classified according to specific cell type [2]. Markesberg and Challa [4] have indicated the subtle difference between cerebral neuroblastoma and PNET from their electron microscopic studies. This enigma of classification was present in the two cases examined at M.D. Anderson Hospital. They reflected the predominance of the undifferentiated cells, differentiation suggesting glial, ependymal or neuronal cells, and obvious malignant features. The occurrence of such tumors only in early life remains unclear. It is of biologic interest that the tumor cells demonstrate to some extent the characteristics of the progenitor developing tissue, such as divergent differentiation. Interesting also is that tumors of embryonal origin outside the central nervous system exhibit spontaneous regression or maturation in a number of instances [5].

The clinical onset is no different than other space occupying lesions with signs of increased intracranial pressure and, less frequently, seizure activity and/or localizing eye signs and motor defects. The number of sites this tumor can occupy shows that locations are diverse, although mainly supratentorial. As a primary site, the spinal cord was significant at 16% in the cases of Kosnik et al. [2] but was not seen in the other series of PNET. These tumors are highly lethal.

There was a tendency for this tumor to spread through the subarachnoid route. All autopsied cases reported by Parker et al. [3] demonstrated meningeal involvement. Horton and Rubinstein [9] noted leptomeningeal or ventricular sites as selective areas of implantation for neuroblastoma. An example of extraneural metastasis for PNET occurred only in the case of Smith et al. [12] with a lung lesion from a primary neoplasm in the spinal cord. There were two instances of neuroblastoma with metastases to lymph nodes and liver [9, 10].

Postoperative treatment has been attempted with both radiation and chemotherapy. Clinical studies to evaluate the response of both modes of therapy for PNET and neuroblastoma are not available perhaps because of the rarity and the brief period of recognition of the PNET. The patients treated at M.D. Anderson Hospital both showed progressive disease shortly after cessation of their courses of radiotherapy. Subsequent chemotherapy was ineffective in slowing the process. Parker et al. [3] have suggested that radiotherapy should be given to the entire neuraxis because of the evidence of meningeal involvement.

5. SUMMARY AND CONCLUSIONS

Three series reporting cases of primitive neuroectodermal tumors in children and young adults were reviewed for their clinical and pathological findings. Two cases of this entity treated at M.D. Anderson Hospital have been described with respect to the clinical presentation and histopathology. Some generalizations from the survey of the literature and the case studies can be made:

1) PNET is a tumor of young individuals with a mean age at diagnosis of 5.3 years.
2) The differential diagnosis is an enigma on histologic grounds because of the high degree of undifferentiation and neuroglial elements showing divergent lines of differentiation.
3) The tumor occurs largely in the supratentorial region of the brain and metastases occur through the subarachnoid spaces.
4) The tumor produces a high mortality. Following partial surgical excision, therapy with radiation and/or chemotherapy has not been successful to prevent progression.
5) It has been suggested that because of the biologic behavior toward leptomeningeal implantation that radiation be given to the entire neuraxis.

REFERENCES

1. Hart N, Earle KM: Primitive neuroectodermal tumors of brain in children. Cancer 32:890–897, 1973.
2. Kosnik EJ, Boesel MD, Bay J, Sayers MP: Primitive neuroectodermal tumors of the central nervous system in children. J Neurosurg 48:741–746, 1978.
3. Parker JC, Mortara RH, McCloskey JJ: Biologic behavior of the primitive neuroectodermal tumors: significant supratentorial childhood gliomas. Surg Neurol 4:383–388, 1975.
4. Markesbery WR, Challa VR: Electron microscrope findings in primitive neuroectodermal tumors of the cerebrum. Cancer 44:141–147, 1979.
5. Rubenstein LJ: Cytogenesis and differentiation of primitive central neuroepithelial tumors. J Neuropath Exp Neurol 31:7–26, 1972.
6. Azzarelli B, Richards DE, Anton AH, Roessman U: Central neuroblastoma. J Neuropath Exp Neurol 36:384–397, 1977.
7. Feigen I, Budzilovich GN: Tumors of neurons and their precursors. J Neuropath exp Neurol 33:483–506, 1974.
8. Pearson J, Milstoc M, Harris J, Budzilovich G, Feigen I: Anaplastic neuronal tumors of the brain. Cancer 38:1424–1437, 1976.
9. Horten BC, Rubenstein LJ: Primary cerebral neuroblastoma. A clinicopathological study of 35 cases. Brain 99:735–756.
10. Henriquez AS, Robertson DM, Marshall WJS: Primary neuroblastoma of the central nervous system with spontaneous extracranial metastases. Case report. J Neurosurg 38:226–231, 1973.
11. Kernohan JW, Learmonth JR, Doyle JB: Neuroblastomas and gangliocytomas of the central nervous system. Brain 55:287–314, 1932.
12. Smith DR, Hardman JM, Earle KM: Metastasizing neuroectodermal Tumors of the central nervous system. J Neurosurg 31:50–58, 1968.

9. Primary Cerebral Neuroblastomas

WILLIAM M. WARA, MICHAEL S. EDWARDS, NERGESH R. SURTI,
GLENN E. SHELINE, VICTOR A. LEVIN and CHARLES B. WILSON

1. INTRODUCTION

The entity of primary cerebral neuroblastoma has only recently been described [1]. These tumors arise mainly in children and young adults as opposed to the more common peripheral neuroblastoma which usually occurs in a younger pediatric age group. They have the same clinical presentation as other brain tumors of childhood but are quite different histologically [2].

Horten and Rubinstein published the largest clinicopathologic study of this

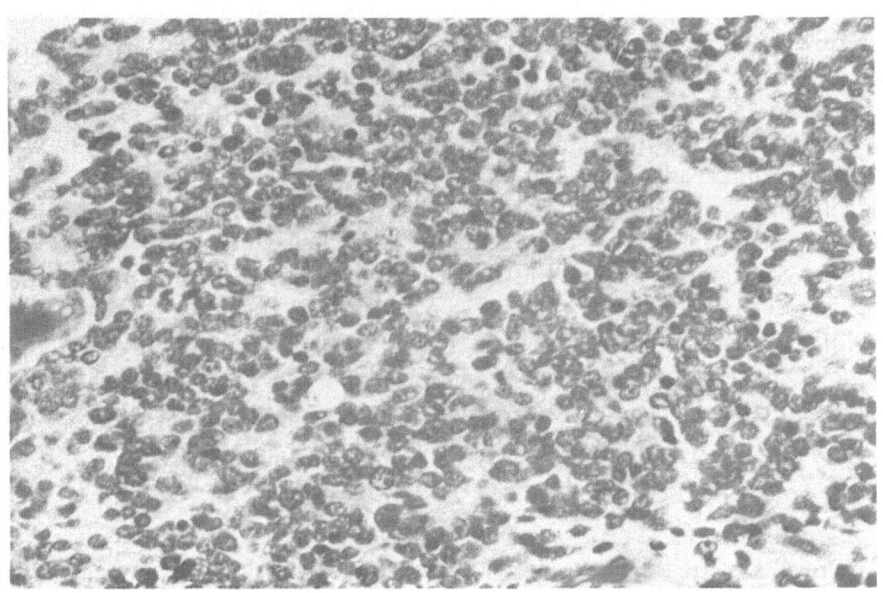

Figure 1. Photomicrograph of biopsy specimen from primary cerebral neuroblastoma, demonstrating Homer-Wright rosettes, cellularity, and neuronal maturation characteristic of tumor.

G. B. Humphrey et al. (eds.), Pediatric oncology 1, 225–228. All rights reserved.
Copyright © 1981 Martinus Nijhoff Publishers bv, The Hague/Boston/London.

tumor (35 cases), most of which were seen for diagnostic consultation or autopsy review[1]. They described histopathologically dense cellular tumors, composed of primitive cells arranged in variable patterns, with intense mitotic activity, formation of Homer-Wright rosettes, and areas of advanced neural maturation. While the pathology is similar to other peripheral neuroblastomas, they do not behave clinically like other neuroblastomas, nor do they secrete increased amounts of catecholamines. Searches for a primary extracerebral site for these tumors has been unsuccessful, hence they are described as primary cerebral neuroblastomas.

Since previous reports suggested a poor prognosis for these patients, with frequent spinal metastases, necessitating craniospinal axis irradiation, we elected to review our experience at the University of California, San Francisco (UCSF), in order to determine a rational treatment regimen[3–5].

2. MATERIALS AND METHODS

Ten patients have been diagnosed as having primary cerebral neuroblastoma at UCSF in the last ten years. All patients had pathologic confirmation of the diagnosis by the same neuropathologist and some have been previously reported by Horten and Rubinstein. As detailed in the table, our experience consists of five males and five females, aged 2–26 years, the last being an achondroplegic dwarf. Five of the ten cases were over 10 years of age at presentation and only two patients were less than 7 years of age. Lesions were distributed randomly throughout the cerebral cortex (four parietal, three occipital, two frontal, and one basal ganglion).

Treatment consisted of surgical biopsy or conservative subtotal removal followed by postoperative irradiation given with megavoltage equipment, either a ^{60}Co apparatus or a 4 MeV linear accelerator. Primary tumor doses ranged from 4500 rad/25 fractions to 6000 rad/30 fractions with a median dose of 5040 rad/28 fractions given to the tumor volume with a generous margin. Only two patients received craniospinal axis irradiation with spinal doses of 4000 rad and 3000 rad (patients # 1 and # 2).

3. RESULTS

The results of treatment along with the patient characteristics are shown in the table. One patient died of local recurrence, 2 years and $8\frac{1}{2}$ months after diagnosis. He was treated postoperatively with irradiation and chemotherapy. Eight of nine live patients have been followed from 2 to 8 years after diagnosis. All patients have been treated with irradiation alone or in combi-

Table 1. Primary cerebral neuroblastoma — patient characteristics and treatment.

Case	Sex	Age	Anatomic lesion	Surgery	Irradiation (rad)	Chemotherapy	Outcome
1	M	8	R. parietal	Subtotal	5940 (brain) 4000 (spine)	Procarbazine, CCNU, Vincristine	Expired 2 yr, 8½ months
2	F	2	R. frontal	Subtotal	4500 (brain) 3000 (spine)	Cytoxan DTIC	Expired 2 yr
3	M	14	R. frontal	Subtotal	5040 (brain)	—	NED 2 yr
4	F	9	R. occipital	Subtotal	5040 (brain)	—	NED 2 yr
5	F	11	L. occipital	Subtotal	5040 (brain)	—	NED 5 yr
6	M	26	R. occipital	Subtotal	5400 (brain)	—	Recurrence 1 yr with complete excision; NED 2 yr
7	F	7	L. basal ganglion	Biopsy	5040 (brain)	Hydroxyurea	NED 2 yr
8	M	12	R. parietal	Biopsy	5100 (brain — 1975)	—	Recurrence 1978
9	M	14	L. parietal	Subtotal	3000 (brain — 1978) 6000 (brain)	Procarbazine, CCNU, Vincristine	NED 2 yr
10	F	2	R. parietal	Biopsy	5040 (brain)	Procarbazine, CCNU, Vincristine —	NED 3 yr NED 8 yr

nation with chemotherapy. One other patient expired due to disseminated CNS disease.

Of the remainder, six patients are free of disease and two have recurrences with surgical and irradiation salvage. Four of the six patients received local field irradiation alone and all are disease free at present. Two of the patients received adjunctive chemotherapy (patients # 7 and # 9) and are free of disease at 2 and 3 years, respectively. One recurrent patient (# 6) was reoperated with complete excision and is disease free for 2 years; one (# 8) was reirradiated with chemotherapy and is disease free at 2 years.

4. DISCUSSION

Our 10 patients' pathologic specimens reveal a combination of Homer-Wright rosettes, intense cellular mitotic activity and areas of neuronal maturation which clearly establishes the diagnosis of cerebral neuroblastoma. All of our patients had extensive roentgenographic and biochemical examinations to exclude a peripheral tumor. All patients had solitary cerebral lesions and only recurrent patients demonstrated spinal metastases.

Our experience suggests that the spectrum of these patients is extremely variable but that local treatment with surgery and irradiation is adequate as initial treatment. We now recommend spinal fluid examination at diagnosis and complete myelogram to determine whether spinal metastases are present. If these studies are negative and brain scans (computerized tomographic and nuclide) show a solitary lesion we recommend local irradiation to the tumor volume with a generous margin to a dose of 5000 rad/6 weeks. While several recurrent patients have had limited responses to chemotherapy, until a more adequate regimen is discovered, routine adjuvant chemotherapy is not recommended.

REFERENCES

1. Horten BC, Rubinstein LJ: Primary cerebral neuroblastoma: A clinicopathological study of 35 cases. Brain 99:735–756, 1976.
2. Yagishita S, Itoh Y, Chiba Y, Yuda K: Cerebral neuroblastoma. Virchows Arch A Path Anat Histol 381:1–11, 1978.
3. Kosnik EJ, Boesel CP, Bay J, Sayers MP: Primitive neuroectodermal tumors of the central nervous system in children. J Neurosurg 48:741–746, 1978.
4. Henriquez AS, Robertson DM, Marshall WJS: Primary neuroblastoma of the central nervous system with spontaneous extracranial metastases. J Neurosurg 38:226–231, 1973.
5. Parker JC, Mortara RH, McCloskey JJ: Biological behavior of the primitive neuroectodermal tumors: Significant supratentorial childhood gliomas. Surg Neurol 4:383–388, 1975.

10. Cerebral Primitive Neuroectodermal Tumor (Primary Cerebral Neuroblastoma): CHLA Experience

BARTON WALD, STUART E. SIEGEL, HART ISAACS, JR. and PHILIP STANLEY

1. INTRODUCTION

Primitive neuroectodermal tumors (PNET) of the central nervous system are very rare tumors of childhood. They were defined by Hart and Earle as tumors of undifferentiated cells resembling germinal or matrix cells of the embryonal neural tube [1]. Histologically these tumors are similar to medulloblastomas; however, PNETs that occur above the tentorium, usually in the cerebral cortex, are considered a separate group, often called cerebral neuroblastomas. This paper reviews the experience of the Children's Hospital of Los Angeles with these cerebral PNETs over the past 25 years.

2. MATERIALS AND METHODS

The diagnosis of cerebral PNET or neuroblastoma was established in these patients by a retrospective review of pathology specimens from all unusual cerebral neoplasms at the Children's Hospital of Los Angeles between the periods 1953 through 1979. All histological specimens were reviewed by one of the authors (H.I.), a total of nine patients were identified by this review and are listed in Table 1. The initial diagnoses in patients 1 through 7 were of other brain tumors, including astrocytoma, cerebral medulloblastoma, ependymoma and gangliogioma. In all cases the diagnosis of cerebral PNET or neuroblastoma was based on the criteria of Horton and Rubinstein [2].

3. RESULTS

Of the nine patients with PNET, there were three males and six females. All of our patients were under 10 years of age at diagnosis. Presenting

G. B. Humphrey et al. (eds.), Pediatric oncology 1, 229–234. All rights reserved.
Copyright © 1981 Martinus Nijhoff Publishers bv, The Hague/Boston/London.

Table 1. Primary PNET-intracerebral neuroblastomas. Patient characteristics, treatment and outcome.

Patient No.	Year diagnosed	Age	Sex	Presenting symptoms	Site	Surgery	Radiotherapy	Chemotherapy	CNS metastases	Metastases outside CNS	Outcome
1	1953	4 yr	F	4 months headache, vomiting, lethargy	Right parietal	Biopsy and subtotal excision	None	None	No	No	Died at surgery
2	1957	8 yr	F	2 months headache, vomiting	Right parietal	Biopsy and subtotal excision	5000 R whole brain 3600 R— spinal	None	No	No	Alive and well, 8 yr post-op. Lost to follow-up subsequently
3	1960	3 yr	M	1 month headache, vomiting, ptosis, incontinence	Left frontal	Biopsy and subtotal excision	None	None	Yes, gross spinal cord	Yes, solitary pulmonary	Died 3 weeks post-op
4	1961	7 yr	F	1 month headache, personality change	Left parietal	Biopsy and subtotal excision	None	None	Unknown	No	Died at surgery
5	1965	1 yr	F	2 weeks vomiting, lethargy, seizures coma	Right parietal	Biopsy only	4000 R whole brain	None	Unknown	No	Died 3 months post-op
6	1966	4 yr	F	1 month left arm weakness	Right parietal	Biopsy only	5000 R to tumor	None	Unknown	No	Died 3 yr post-op

Table 1. (continued)

Patient No.	Year diagnosed	Age	Sex	Presenting symptoms	Site	Surgery	Radiotherapy	Chemotherapy	CNS metastases	Metastases outside CNS	Outcome
7	1967	6 yr	F	1 year headache, vomiting, 1 week	Right temporal	Biopsy and subtotal excision	5200 R to tumor	None	Yes+LP	No	Recurrence 18 months post-op; died 19 months post-op
8	1977	8 yr	M	3 weeks lethargy, ataxia	Brain stem and left frontal	Biopsy only	5000 R to tumor	Vincristine, CCNU, Procarbazine, Cyclophosphamide, Prednisone	Yes+LP, cerebral mass	No	Recurrence left frontal area, 22 months post-op; died 24 months post-op
9	1979	4 yr	M	3 weeks ptosis, mydriasis	Right temporal	Biopsy and subtotal excision	4000 R whole brain; 1000 R boost to tumor	Vincristine cyclophosphamide DTIC	No	No	Alive, NED 9 months post-op

symptoms included headache (six patients), vomiting (six patients), specific neurological deficits (four patients), seizures (one patient), and nuchal rigidity (one patient). The site of the tumor was the parietal lobe in five patients, the temporal lobe in two patients, the frontal lobe in one patient and the brain stem in one patient. The latter patient subsequently noted a second lesion in the frontal lobe.

Initial therapy included biopsy in all nine patients, with subtotal excision of the primary mass in six of the patients. Three patients, all seen prior to 1965, died either at surgery or within one month of the surgical procedure and received no therapy. Six patients received radiotherapy to the primary tumor and two patients received additional radiotherapy to the spinal axis. The radiotherapy dose was 4000–5200 R to the primary tumor and, in the case of the patients receiving spinal axis radiation, 3600–4000 R to the whole axis. Four of these six patients received radiation only. Four of the six radiated children died of progressive disease 3 months to 3 years after initial diagnosis. One of the four patients noted initial evidence of recurrence in the spinal fluid. The two surviving patients both received radiation to the spinal axis as well as the whole brain.

Two of the six patients receiving radiation therapy also received combination chemotherapy. Patient # 8 received vincristine, prednisone and CCNU. Appearance of second tumor mass in the cerebrum distinct from the primary brain stem lesion was noted 22 months after initial diagnosis and the patient was treated with vincristine, cyclophosphamide, procarbazine and prednisone. Despite the therapy, the patient expired 24 months after initial diagnosis with progressive disease. Patient # 9 received vincristine, cyclophosphamide and DTIC following radiation therapy and currently is alive and well, without any evidence of active disease 9 months following initial diagnosis.

Three patients had evidence of metastatic spread in the central nervous system during the course of their disease. Patients # 7 and # 8 had tumor cells present on cytological examination of spinal fluid obtained at lumbar puncture, and patient # 3 had gross tumor involvement of the spinal cord noted at autopsy. Only one patient in our series was found to have metastatic disease outside of the central nervous system. Patient # 3 was found to have a small pulmonary metastasis at autopsy.

4. DISCUSSION

The diagnosis of cerebral neuroblastoma or PNET has been a controversial one due to its similarity to other tumors which may occur in the central nervous system. Horton and Rubinstein in their review of 35 cases, list six features which are useful in separating cerebral neuroblastomas from other central neuroepithelial tumors of childhood. They include: (a) circumscribed tumor growth, (b) intense stromal response, (c) presence of distinctive Homer-Wright rosettes, (d) maturation of ganglion cells, (e) demonstration of neuroblastic cell forms with silver impregnation techniques, and (f) conspicuous hypertrophic astrocytic glial reaction along the margins of the desmoblastic variant [2]. The histologic patterns of the tumors in our patients was consistent with these criteria and other published reports [1-3].

The clinical picture of the tumor emerging from our patients is similar to that described in the literature [1-3]. The tumor was encountered in younger children, all in the first decade of life and showed no sex predilection. Symptoms were those of an intracranial mass and were frequently short in duration, indicating a rapidly growing tumor. Symptoms occurred for less than 2 months prior to diagnosis in all of our patients with the exception of patients # 1 and # 7. Finally, the primary tumor arose from a wide variety of sites throughout the cerebral cortex.

Historically, treatment has consisted of surgical resection, if possible, followed by radiation to the tumor or whole brain. In our group of seven patients diagnosed prior to 1967, there were four early deaths occurring either intraoperatively or within the first month following surgery, usually related to hemorrhage and/or tumor progression. With the appreciation that this tumor has the capability of seeding throughout the central nervous system, spinal irradiation has been added to the therapeutic program. Two patients in our series received craniospinal radiation and both were alive, without disease 9 months and 8 years respectively, following diagnosis. Spread outside the central nervous system has occasionally been demonstrated [2, 4] and, in our study, was noted at autopsy in one patient.

The use of combination chemotherapy in addition to radiation therapy has been a recent development. In general, the agents employed have been similar to those utilized for other central nervous system tumors such as medulloblastoma or astrocytoma or those employed in neuroblastoma. In our series, patient # 8 was treated with drugs now being utilized for other central nervous system tumors and noted a recurrence within 2 years of initial diagnosis. Patient # 9 is being treated with agents utilized primarily for neuroblastoma outside the central nervous system, but the effectiveness of these agents cannot be adequately evaluated at this early date in his course.

We currently recommend that, at the time of diagnosis of cerebral neuroblastoma or PNET, the diagnostic and metastatic work-up should include a lumbar puncture with spinal fluid cytology, computerized tomography and radio-nucleide brain scans, skeletal survey and a chest X-ray. If no evidence of seeding is found within the central nervous system or distant metastases, treatment should include, at a minimum, radiation to the entire tumor volume to a dose of 5000 R given over a 5-6 week period. The role of chemotherapy in this disease is not yet determined and should be subject to an appropriately designed clinical trial which would permit an evaluation of the relative contribution of radiation versus chemotherapy to ultimate outcome.

REFERENCES

1. Hart M, Earle K: Primitive neuroectodermal tumors of the brain in children. Cancer 32:890–897, 1976.
2. Horton B, Rubinstein L: Primary cerebral neuroblastoma. Brain 99:735–756, 1976.
3. Kosnick E, Boesel C, Bay J, Sayers M: Primitive neuroectodermal of the central nervous system in children. J Neurosurg 48:741–746, 1978.
4. Henriquez A, Robertson O, Marshall J: Primary neuroblastoma of the central nervous system with spontaneous extracranial metastases. J Neurosurg 38:226–231,1973.

11. Supratentorial Primitive Neuroectodermal Tumor: Clinical Response of a Single Case to Vincristine, Cyclophosphamide, and BCNU

CHARLES L. SEXAUER, HENRY F. KROUS, RALPH J. KAPLAN, PATRICK D. BARNES and G. BENNETT HUMPHREY

1. INTRODUCTION

In the treatment of primitive neuroectodermal tumors of the brain, chemotherapy has thus far shown little effect [1, 2]. Since the cure rate from surgery and radiation therapy remains low, continued experimentation with chemical agents holds the greatest hope for improved survival. To stimulate such clinical investigation, we report the clinical response of a patient with this uncommon neoplasm.

2. CASE REPORT

A 15 year old white male had undergone a craniotomy with partial resection of a right frontal brain tumor in October 1972, $2\frac{1}{2}$ years prior to being seen at OCMH. Initial therapy included central nervous system radiation of 2000 rads (Table 1). In May 1973, he received an additional 1600 rads because of a recurrence. In December 1974, 2 months prior to the patients arrival in the State of Oklahoma, he had received cytoxan therapy for tumor recurrence. Details of the earlier clinical response could not be obtained due to an unfortunate family situation. On admission, the patient had multiple neurological problems (inappropriate affect, urine and fecal incontinence, slurred speech, left homonymous hemianopsia, and left hemiparesis).

In March 1975, he was started on monthly courses of: vincristine (VCR) 1.5 mg/m^2 IV on day 1, cyclophosphamide (CP) 450 mg/m^2 IV on days 2 and 3, and BCNU 50 mg/m^2 on days 2 and 3. After four courses of therapy, the patient described himself as 'asymptomatic'. However, detailed examination revealed persistent left side weakness and no change in the homonymous hemianopsia. These two neurological signs remained unchanged for the next 2 years. No radiologic studies were implemented during

G. B. Humphrey et al. (eds.), Pediatric oncology 1, 235–237. All rights reserved.

Table 1. Clinical characteristics, treatment, and response.

Date	Clinical status	Therapy	Response	Duration
Oct. 1972	L. hemiparesis	Surgery 2000 R CNS	'Asymptomatic'	6 months
May 1973	L. hemiparesis	1600 R CNS	Lost to followup	—
Dec. 1974	L. hemiparesis	VCR, CP	No progression	—
March 1975	Multiple problems	VCR, CP, BCNU	Progressive improvement with four courses	—
July 1975	Asymptomatic	VCR, CP, BCNU	'Asymptomatic'	24 months
Feb. 1976	Severe hemorrhagic cystitis	Discontinue Rx	'Asymptomatic'	—
Aug. 1977	Disoriented	Ventriculoperitoneal shunt	Improved	4 months
Jan. 1978	L. hemiparesis, multiple problems	Surgery CNS (biopsy)	No response	—
Feb. 1978	L. hemiparesis	CCNU	No response	—
June 1978	L. hemiparesis, disoriented	VCR, PRED, PROC	No response	—
Sept. 1978	Expired	—	—	—

this period to document tumor residual or regression. In February 1976, therapy was discontinued due to cyclophosphamide induced cystitis. His clinical status remained unchanged (Table 1) until August 1977, when he became disoriented secondary to increased intracranial pressure. Radiologic studies (cranial CT and isotope cisternography) demonstrated right cerebral porencephaly and hydrocephalus but no definite evidence of tumor residual or recurrence. The placement of ventriculoperitoneal shunt resulted in clinical improvement. In late December 1977, a definite tumor mass was identified by cranial CT and biopsy reconfirmed the diagnosis of primitive neuroectodermal tumor. The patient failed to respond to additional trials of chemotherapy (Table 1) and expired. Permission was not given for necropsy examination.

The histologic and ultrastructural features of the initial biopsy taken in 1972 were very similar to those of the recurrent tumor evaluated in 1978. The circumscribed tumor was composed of medium sized cells which had little cytoplasm. Rosettes and neurofibrillary stromia were not found. No neurosecretory granules, cytoplasmic processes, or microtubules were identified by ultrastructural examination. A diagnosis of primitive neuroectodermal tumor was made on both original and recurrent tumor.

3. DISCUSSION

Our patient experienced a dramatic and prolonged clinical response following the treatment of his recurrent brain tumor with VCR, CP, and BCNU. These drugs were chosen on the basis of their efficacy as demonstrated in an animal model [3, 4]. The results of the animal experiments prompted in 1974 a pilot study by our group for the Pediatric Division of the Southwest Oncology Group wherein the effect of VCR, CP, and BCNU was evaluated in children with Stage IV neuroblastoma. Since primitive neuroectodermal tumors of the central nervous system have certain histogenetic and morphologic features of neuroblastoma, it was our opinion that antitumor activity might occur.

It is impossible to judge the relative efficacy of these three drugs in our patient. It is possible that any one agent used alone may have been just as effective. It is also possible the drugs had no direct effect on tumor size since computerized axial tomography was not available at our institution in 1974 and reduction in tumor mass could not be documented. The latter possibility seems unlikely since clinical remission was achieved for 24 months.

We are aware that little success has thus far been achieved with drug therapy of this uncommon tumor, but this anecdotal experience clearly implies that continued experimentation is indicated.

REFERENCES

1. Kosnik EJ, Boesel CP, Bay J, Sayers MP: Primitive neuroectodermal tumors of the central nervous system in children. J Neurosurg 48:741–746, 1978.
2. Parker JC, Mortara RIT, McCloskey JJ: Biologic behavior of the primitive neuroectodermal tumors: significant supratentorial childhood gliomas. Surg Neurol 4:383–387, 1975.
3. Valeriote FA, Bruce WR, Meeker BE: Synergistic action of cyclophosphamide and 1,3-bis (2-chloroethyl)-1-nitrosourea on a transplant murine lymphoma. J Natl Cancer Inst 935–944, 1968.
4. Razek A, Vietti T, Valeriote F: Optimum Time Sequence for administration of vincristine and cyclophosphamide *in vivo*. Cancer Res 34:1857–1861, 1974.

12. Review of Experience with Primitive Neuroectodermal Tumors of Childhood

EDWARD S. BAUM, ELAINE R. MORGAN, MAURO C. DAL CANTO and
PATRICE M. WEST

Neuroectodermal tumors of the central nervous system (CNS) are rare
tumors in children. Review of the pathology of CNS tumors biopsied or
removed at Children's Memorial Hospital in the last 10 years has revealed
seven cases which were confirmed to be of primitive neuroectodermal origin.

1. PATHOLOGY

1.1. Gross Appearance

Biopsy specimens from these tumors generally appeared as fragments of
gray soft tissue. In the larger tumors yellowish areas of necrosis were also
present.

1.2. Histologic Appearance

The most common feature of these tumors was their extreme cellularity.
Cells were generally arranged in sheets without any particular architecture on
a scanty stroma made up of fine vessels which were surrounded by moderate
amounts of reticulum fibers. The neoplastic cells had the appearance of undifferentiated elements, i.e. round to oval nuclei with abundant finely distributed chromatin and occasional nucleoli surrounded by scanty cytoplasm with
no or very few short processes. Occasionally, cells with very large lobulated
nuclei were observed. Mitoses varied in number from scanty to very numerous. The overall appearance of these tumors was similar, if not identical to
that of cerebellar medulloblastoma. Special stains for neural fibers and glial
fibers gave generally poor results. Most portions of all tumors were negative
for these stains whereas in isolated areas, and especially at the periphery of
the tumors, a few wisps of both type of fibers could be seen. It was always
difficult to decide whether such fibers were really produced by tumor cells or

G. B. Humphrey et al. (eds.), Pediatric oncology 1, 239–242. All rights reserved.
Copyright © 1981 Martinus Nijhoff Publishers bv, The Hague/Boston/London.

Table 1. Clinical characteristics, treatment, and response.

Pt.	Date Dx.	Age sex/race	Site	Presentation	Initial Rx	Duration of response	Subsequent Rx	Present status
EC	8/72	8 yr/ F/W	Frontal lobes, corpus callosum	Increased intracranial pressure, hydrocephalus	V-P shunt	6 months	Partial resection, C-S XRT	Expired 4/74
EV	11/74	3½ yr/ F/SA	Rt. frontal (mediocentral)	Increased intracranial pressure, seizures, coma	Rt. frontal lobectomy, total excision, C-S XRT	3 yr	High dose MTX, 100% resection	NED 6 months, P̄ resection, lt. frontal lobe sarcoma (2nd malignancy)
JM	11/77	2 yr/ M/W	Lt. cerebral hemisphere; extends to 4th ventricle	Ataxia, increased intracranial pressure, hydrocephalus	V-P shunt, 50% excision C-S XRT	7 months	Vincristine, CCNU, Procarbazine	Expired 8/78
AM	5/78	10 months/ M/W	Rt. temporo-parietal; ext. to thalamus	Dilated rt. pupil; Lt. hemiparesis	V-P shunt, 95–98% excision C-S XRT	6 months		Expired 1/79
DC	5/78	16 days/ M/B	Epidural L_1–L_5	Lumbosacral mass, paraparesis	Laminectomy, 90–95% excision XT (lumbosac spine)	12+ months		NED 5/79
EVa	5/79	8 months/ M/W	Post. fossa (4th ventricle)	Kidney tumor (sarcoma), increased intracranial pressure	V-P shunt, 90% excision C-S XRT	0		Expired 8/79
AW	11/79	5 yr/ M/W	Lt. frontal	Strabismus, papilledema, optic atrophy, visual loss	Subtotal surgical excision	Too early		Too early

were rather derived from pre-existing structures invaded by tumor. In no case did we see only one type of fiber represented.

1.3. Ultrastructural Appearance

This was only studied in two cases. Cells showed rather pleomorphic dense nuclei with one or more small nucleoli and small amounts of cytoplasm with primitive appearance. They showed, in fact, a very scanty endoplasmic reticulum, few diffusely distributed ribosomes and a moderate number of mitochondria. Very few tubules and filaments could be observed. Except for sporadic puncta adhaerentia, no cellular specializations indicating a particular cellular lineage were observed. In one of the two tumors, abundant glycogen was observed inside most of the tumor cells.

2. CLINICAL

The clinical presentations, treatment and course of these seven patients is indicated in the table.

Overall, the survival of our patients has been poor and is similar to that of patients previously reported[1]. Four of the seven patients (EC, EVa, JM, AM) died from progressive tumor from 3 to 20 months after diagnosis. Three patients (AW, DC, EV) are currently alive 1 week, 18 months and 5 years post diagnosis. One of these (AW) has just been diagnosed; (DC) had an epidural lesion; and (EV) had a recurrence first treated with high dose Methotrexate without a response and subsequently resected. One and a half years following excision of her recurrent tumor this last patient (EV) developed a sarcomatous lesion in the right frontal lobe which is histologically different than the original tumor and recurrence.

In general, it has not been feasible to achieve total tumor resection in these children. Interestingly, the single long term survivor in this group of patients is the only patient in whom total tumor resections were apparently accomplished in each of three procedures. All of these patients received cranial spinal (C-S) radiation (XRT) (or spinal XRT in one patient). The administered dose to the primary tumor area was approximately 5000 rads. Despite this, early tumor recurrence or absence of initial response was noted in five of six evaluable patients. Chemotherapy administered preterminally in one patient (JM) did not arrest a rapid downhill course.

On the basis of this limited experience and a limited review of the literature, it appears that the prognosis for patients with primitive neuroectodermal tumors of the CNS is extremely poor. In the majority of patients, complete excision appears to be unachievable and C-S XRT administered postoperatively does not salvage these patients. It appears that presently the treatment of these tumors is surgical. The poor prognosis when complete surgical excision is not possible would seem to warrant a more aggressive approach employing chemotherapy and/or radiosensitizers combined with XRT. Future clinical trials could perhaps yield some information as to the usefulness of such a combined modality approach as well as to the most effective drugs and route of administration of chemotherapy.

REFERENCES

1. Kosnik EJ, Boesel CP, Bay J, Sayers MP: Primitive neuroectodermal tumors of the central nervous system in children. J Neurosurg 48:741–746, 1978.

13. Primitive Neuroectodermal Tumour

DEREK JENKIN

1. INTRODUCTION

Primitive neuroectodermal tumour (PNT) at some site in the brain was diagnosed in only five children referred for radiation treatment to the Ontario Cancer Institute 1958–78. The years of registration of these patients were limited to 1973–78 since this tumour classification was not utilized in earlier years.

The principal features of these patients are given in Table 1.

2. SITE

The involved sites are in the cerebral hemispheres in all five patients. This distribution was influenced by a reluctance to classify midline posterior fossa tumours or posterior third ventricle tumours as PNT rather than a variant of medulloblastoma or pineoblastoma.

3. SURGERY

All five patients underwent a gross resection of the tumour which was considered to be at least 90% complete. One patient underwent ventriculoperitoneal shunting prior to resection and one patient required a lumboperitoneal shunt post-operatively to control the complications of excessive CSF production.

G. B. Humphrey et al. (eds.), Pediatric oncology 1, 243–246. All rights reserved.
Copyright © 1981 Martinus Nijhoff Publishers bv, The Hague/Boston/London.

Table 1. Clinical characteristics, treatment and response.

Pt #	Year Dx	Age/ sex	Site	Resection	Shunt	Radiation			Time (months) to		Status	Site first relapse	CNS seeding	Adjuvant chemo
						Field (cm)	Dose (rad)	# Fraction	Relapse	Last follow up				
1	73	10 F	L. frontal	Sub-total	L-P	15×15	5250	28	7	13	Dead	Local	No	No
2	74	11 F	R. temporal	Sub-total	—	10×10	5100	26	38	62	Alive with disease	Local	Yes	No
3	74	3 M	R. parieto-occipital	Sub-total	V-P	15×12	5000	28	46	60	Dead	Local	No	No
4	77	5 M	R. parietal	Complete	—	10×10	5250	28	—	17	Alive	—	No	No
5	78	12 M	L. temporal	Sub-total	—	8×8	5250	28	10	14	Dead	Local	Yes	CCNU VCR

4. RADIATION

All patients underwent local irradiation to a generous volume to 5000–5250 rads at approximately 1000 rad/week using parallel opposed radiation fields.

5. INITIAL TUMOUR CONTROL

Following resection and irradiation, all patients had initial disease control. The time from diagnosis to first relapse was 7, 10, 38 and 46 months. One patient remains in a first remission at 17 months from diagnosis. The mode of first relapse was primary tumour recurrence in all four patients. The time from first relapse to death was respectively 6, 4, 24 and 14 months.

6. CNS SEEDING

Two patients developed CNS seeding: Patient 2 was found to have positive CSF cytology 14 months after primary tumour recurrence and developed gross symptoms of cord compression one month later. Symptomatic improvement occurred following spinal irradiation, but progressive disease in the spine occurred 5 months later. Patient 5 developed spinal seeding 3 months following primary tumour recurrence. There was no response to spinal irradiation.

7. CHEMOTHERAPY

Patient 1 received two cycles of vincristine, procarbazine and CCNU as treatment for first relapse without evidence of response. Patient 2 received 3000 rads in 15 fractions to the locally recurrent primary tumour and this was combined with vincristine and two cycles of CCNU. Disease control was obtained for 14 months. Patient 3 underwent partial excision of the recurrent primary tumour followed by CCNU. The primary tumour relapse was 3 months later. Patient 5 received adjuvant treatment with vincristine and CCNU cyclically for 10 months prior to recurrence of the primary tumour. The recurrent primary tumour was treated with 3000 rads in 10 fractions and misonidazole. CNS seeding occurred 3 months later. At autopsy while there was gross spinal cord disease there was only microscopic disease in the cerebral hemispheres.

Overall this data is not evaluable. There was no evidence that these agents had a strong influence on this tumour.

There was some evidence that re-irradiation was of palliative value.

8. DISCUSSION

In the cerebral hemispheres it is clearly possible to delineate a primitive neuroectodermal tumour, but it is not clear in what fashion the tumour is related to the commoner childhood brain tumours. In two of our five patients while PNT was dominant there was evidence histologically of mixed ancestry.

Empirically it would appear that the surgical and radiation treatment of this tumour should follow the pattern for the common tumours: excision if possible followed by radiation treatment of the primary site to not less than 5000 rad. Four of our patients developed locally recurrent tumour following such treatment, but the duration of initial control suggested a positive effect. Should craniospinal axis irradiation be undertaken? Two of our four patients relapsed in the CNS following first relapse. On balance, the author now favours such treatment given as for a medulloblastoma. Our fragmentary data on chemotherapy is not helpful. Certainly we had no evidence that vincristine or CCNU exerted a strong effect on this tumour.

14. Primitive Neuroectodermal Tumors (Embryonal Gliomas) of Childhood. A Clinicopathologic Study of 12 Cases

JOHN PRIEST, LOUIS P. DEHNER, JOO-HO SUNG and MARK E. NESBIT

One of the more characteristic morphologic findings in some of the common solid malignancies of childhood is a recapitulation of the embryologic stages but in a disorganized neoplastic fashion. Most of these tumors such as the retinoblastoma, neuroblastoma and nephroblastoma occur in characteristic sites and have sufficiently differentiated histologic features and in the case of the classic or peripheral neuroblastoma produce biogenic amines that an unequivocal pathologic diagnosis is possible. Light and even electron microscopy in some of these and other malignant tumors of childhood may reveal highly primitive, undifferentiated cells. The medulloblastoma, one of the commonest tumors of the central nervous system in the pediatric age group, is a poorly differentiated embryonic neoplasm arising in the region of the cerebellar vermis whose cytogenesis still remains a subject of controversy [1]. Exclusive of the tumors which most pathologists would accept as medulloblastoma because of the typical location and consistent histopathologic findings, there is a less well defined group of tumors usually but not exclusively occurring above the tentorium cerebilli with the collective rubric of 'primitive neuroectodermal tumors of the central nervous system' [2]. These neoplasms in part or *en toto* resemble the cells of the neural tube or germinal layer. With these various considerations in mind, we undertook a review of primitive neuroectodermal tumors (or as we would prefer to designate them 'embryonal gliomas') seen at the University of Minnesota Hospitals.

1. MATERIALS AND METHODS

A systematic search of the files and records of children admitted to the University Hospitals, University of Minnesota, Minneapolis from 1969 to 1979 with the diagnosis of a central nervous system tumor was conducted. Additional case material was identified in the Department of Therapeutic

G. B. Humphrey et al. (eds.), Pediatric oncology 1, 247–264. All rights reserved.
Copyright © 1981 Martinus Nijhoff Publishers bv, The Hague/Boston/London.

Radiology (1969–1979) and the Divisions of Neuropathology and Surgical Pathology, Department of Laboratory Medicine and Pathology (1962–1979). Some of the cases from the latter sources were in fact referral material from other hospitals which had been reviewed in consultation. The basic qualifications for inclusion in this study were the following: a patient 15 years of age or less at diagnosis; a primary tumor of the central nervous system; adequate histologic material for examination; complete clinical follow-up and finally a tumor with histologic features which were agreeable to two of us (JHS and LPD).

After the exclusion of cerebellar medulloblastomas, astrocytomas and some metastatic lesions such as retinoblastoma, melanotic neuroectodermal tumor of infancy, neuroblastoma and embryonal rhabdomyosarcoma, we were left with a final study group of 12 cases. It became apparent after the scrupulous screening process that some morphologic heterogeneity still existed and even some controversy between the two of us (JHS and LPD) about the acceptability of a particular case. The one essential histologic feature in each neoplasm was the presence of a pattern consisting of sheets or nests of small dark primitive cells resembling neuroblasts, medulloepithelium or ependymoblasts with or without astroglial, ependymal or oligodendroglial differentiation. Difficulty was encountered in those cases where differentiation was found in the primary tumor or in a recurrence. Five tumors fulfilled the criteria for either a medulloepithelioma (one case) or ependymoblastoma (four cases).

2. RESULTS

2.1. Clinical Features

The 12 patients ranged in age from 5 months to 13 years (mean age, 5 years) at the time of presentation and diagnosis. There were nine females and three males and all patients were caucasian. Hemiparesis, headache, vomiting, cranial nerve dysfunction and papilledema were the initial clinical features and findings in these children (Table 1). The duration of symptoms ranged from two days to 10 months (median, one month). One patient (Case 5, Table 1) had been treated for myoclonic seizures for 10 months before the diagnosis of a deep left cerebral hemisphere mass.

A resumé of the clinical course and management of the 12 children is compiled in Table 1. After a variety of diagnostic roentgenographic techniques, all patients eventually came to some form of surgical intervention which in two cases represented only biopsies (Cases 11 and 12, Table 1). The initial resections were judged as complete in four patients (Cases 2, 3, 9, 10, Table 1) and subtotal in the remaining six children (Cases 1, 4–8, Table 1). There was one post-operative death (Case 5, Table 1). Radiation therapy was

Table 1. Clinicopathologic summary of embryonal gliomas.

Pt.	Age (yr)	Sex	Presenting signs or symptoms*	Tumor location	Surgery	Radiation therapy† Dose	Fractionation	Course and subsequent therapy §
1	3	F	HP,I,P	L frontoparietal lobe	Subtotal	WB 4000 T 5075	(23/30) (29/38)	Alive with tumor at 22 months; VCR and CCNU for first 12 months; then massive recurrence with no response to HDMTX and DAHG.
2	9	F	HP,HA,V	L frontoparietal lobe	Gross total	WB 5000	(25/48)	Doing well at 9 years; seizures
3	11	F	HA,V,P	R frontal lobe	Gross total	WB 3500 T 5000	(20/36) (31/43)	Doing well at 63 months
4	5	F	HP,HA	R parietal lobe	Subtotal	WB 4425	(unknown)	Died of tumor at 11 months; recurrence at 10 months removed surgically.
5	3	F	HP,CN,S	L frontotemporal lobe	Subtotal	none		Died from postoperative bleeding at 1 day
6	1	M	HP,V,CN	R frontoparietal lobe	Subtotal	WB 4800	(30/45)	Died postoperatively at 13 months following hemispherectomy for massive recurrence
7	2	M	S,P	L cerebral hemisphere	Subtotal	WB 3000	(15/19)	Died of tumor at 4 years; extensive local recurrence at 3.5 years removed surgically

* HP = hemiparesis, HA = headache, V = vomiting, I = incontinence, P = papilledema, CN = cranial nerve palsies, S = seizures.
† In all cases, given post-operatively as primary therapy; WB = whole brain, T = tumor dose, CS = craniospinal axis; doses in rads; numbers in parenthesis indicate (number of fractions/total time of radiation in days).
§ All times are following the first surgery: VCR = vincristine, CCNU = lomustine, HDMTX = high dose methotrexate, DAHG = dianhydrogalactitol, CPM = cyclophosphamide.

Table 1. (continued).

Pt.	Age (yr)	Sex	Presenting signs or symptoms *	Tumor location	Surgery	Radiation therapy † Dose	Fractionation	Course and subsequent therapy §
8	13	F	HP,HA,V,P	L parietal lobe	Subtotal	WB 3850	(22/29)	Died of tumor at 14 months; surgical decompression for massive recurrence at 11 months
9	6	F	HP,HA,V,CN,P	L frontoparietal lobe	Gross total	WB 5300	(29/38)	Doing well at 12 years; slight hemiparesis
10	4	F	HA,V,CN,P	L parietal lobe	Gross total	WB 3050 T 3500	(22/35) (25/38)	Died of tumor at 25 months; local recurrence at 10 months removed surgically and treated with additional 3000 rads (20/30)
11	7	F	V,P, scalp masses	Pineal-quadrigeminal plate	Biopsy	WB 3900	(26/40)	Died of tumor at 29 months; see text for further details
12	5	M	I, flaccid legs	Spinal cord	Biopsy	CS 2100 T 2550	(14/22) (17/27)	Died of spinal and intracranial tumor at 3 months; no response to VCR and CPM

* HP = hemiparesis, HA = headache, V = vomiting, I = incontinence, P = papilledema, CN = cranial nerve palsies, S = seizures.

† In all cases, given post-operatively as primary therapy; WB = whole brain, T = tumor dose, CS = craniospinal axis; doses in rads; numbers in parenthesis indicate (number of fractions/total time of radiation in days).

§ All times are following the first surgery; VCR = vincristine, CCNU = lomustine, HDMTX = high dose methotrexate, DAHG = dianhydrogalactitol, CPM = cyclophosphamide.

administered following surgery to 11 patients; the doses and fractionations are summarized in Table 1. Chemotherapy was given to those individuals who developed recurrent disease not considered amenable to re-excision.

There were three long-term survivors beyond 63 months (Cases 2, 3, 9, Table 1). These children had in common the fact that the surgical extirpation of the tumor was judged as complete in each case. With exception of one case, all patients who died had tumor confined to the central nervous system as determined by clinical evaluation or verified at autopsy. That exception is sufficiently unique and instructive in regard to the potential behavior of this group of neoplasms that the clinical features have been described in some detail.

Case 11 (Table 1). The patient presented at seven years of age with the complaints of vomiting and scalp masses. She had been well previously except for mild psychomotor retardation. Physical examination revealed a $5 \times 5 \times 1$ cm painless, immobile firm scalp mass on the upper occiput and a similar but smaller mass ($2 \times 2 \times 1$ cm) on the low occiput. There was no evidence of lymphadenopathy nor abdominal masses. The hemogram and urinanalysis showed no abnormalities. Bilateral bone marrow trephine biopsies and aspirations were unremarkable. Laboratory determinations of 24-hr urinary catecholamines yielded the following results: vanylmandelic acid (VMA), 15 μg VMA/mg creatinine (repeat determination 8.3 μg/mg) (normal for age: 0.5–5.5 μg VMA/mg creatinine); normetanephrine (NMN), 0.6 μg/mg (normal for age: 0.4–2.7 μg creatinine); homovanillic acid (HVA), 21 μg HVA/mg creatinine (normal for age: 0–9.0 μg HVA/mg creatinine) and catecholamines (epinephrine and norepinephrine) 59 μg/24 hr (normal for age: 0–135 μg/24 hr). Roentgenographic studies showed on intravenous pyelography slight lateral deviation of the proximal left ureter and normal computerized tomography (CT), echography and lymphangiography of the abdominal and retroperitoneal contents. Radionuclide scan of the liver–spleen was likewise unremarkable. A bone scan revealed the cranial lesions. Skull radiographs, CT scan of the head and four-vessel cartoid and vertebral angiography demonstrated osteolytic lesions of the skull underlying the scalp masses, mild ventricular enlargement and a diffusely infiltrating, hypervascular mass in the region of the quadrigeminal plate, superior vermis space and posterior thalami. A biopsy of the scalp mass was performed and it revealed a 'small cell tumor' consistent with a primitive neuroepithelial neoplasm. It was a primary tumor of the central nervous system. She was given radiation to the whole brain (3900 rads; 26 treatments in 40 days).

Following the radiation therapy and two months after the diagnosis, marked shrinkage of tumor was confirmed with the CT scan. A neuroblastoma chemotherapy protocol was initiated consisting of vincristine, cyclophosphamide and dacarbazine at intervals of 3 weeks.

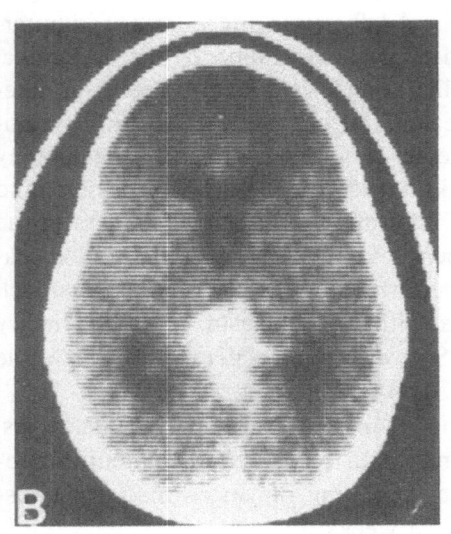

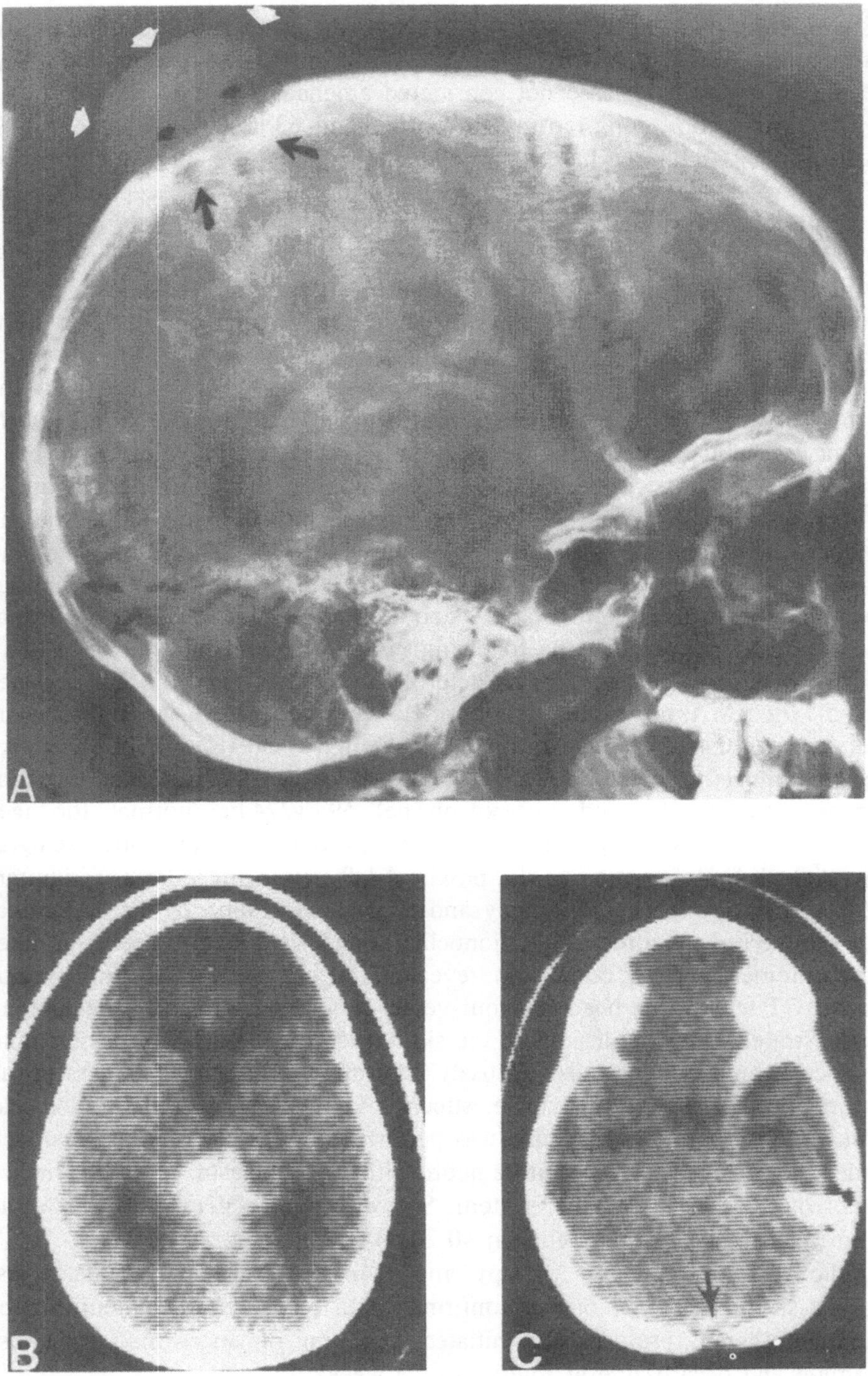

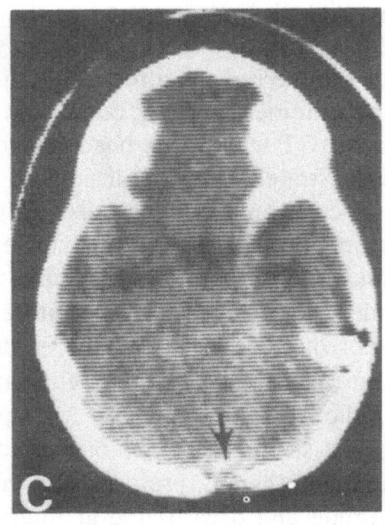

Four months after diagnosis, an osteolytic lesion of the left pedicle of vertebra L_5 was identified. Chemotherapy was continued for the next seven months with no improvement in the vertebral lesion. Abdominal echograms, bone and CT scans were normal but the persistent questionable left ureteral deviation was pursued by an exploratory laparotomy. The operative findings were entirely negative.

Approximately 15 months into her clinical course, a lytic defect of the right tibia was recognized and 1800 rads were administered to the area. Spinal cord compression at the level of T_{9-10} produced paraplegia. There was temporary response to VM-26 and cisplatinum but the patient died from progressive disease 29 months after diagnosis. The findings at autopsy are discussed in the next section.

3. MORPHOLOGIC FEATURES AND CLINICOPATHOLOGIC CORRELATION

With the cerebellar medulloblastoma excluded from the study, there was a predominance of supratentorial neoplasms except for the one apparent primary spinal cord tumor (Case 12, Table 1). The frontoparietal lobes were involved in four cases; the parietal lobe alone in three and the frontal or frontotemporal lobes in one case each. A holohemispheric neoplasm was documented in one child (Case 7, Table 1). The patient whose tumor metastasized outside of the central nervous system had a mass in the pineal-quadrigeminal plate region (Case 11, Table 1). There was a predilection to the left side of the brain (seven cases).

A description of the macroscopic qualities of the tumor was most readily available from the operative report since usually only small irregular fragments of tissue were submitted for pathologic examination. Discrete demarcation and circumscription from the surrounding brain (pseudocapsule) were noted in six cases (Cases 2–4, 6, 7, 9, Table 2). Partial cystification was a frequent feature and invariably associated with evidence of hemorrhage and necrosis. One tumor was commented upon as having evidence of some attachment to the dura (Case 10, Table 2) but microscopically, it was not a meningioma or at least a conventional one. Although a specific dimension

←

Figure 1. A: Primitive neuroectodermal tumor (Case 11, Table 1) at the time of diagnosis showing multiple lytic lesions involving vertex and occipital regions (dark arrows) and soft tissue mass at vertex (white arrows). There is thinning of the floor of the sella turcica and slight spreading of the sutures. B: Computerized tomographic scan showing enhanced lesion in the region of the quadrigeminal plate and slight ventricular dilatation. C: Inferior cut of tomographic scan showing lytic occipital lesion.

Table 2. Major pathologic findings of primitive neuroectodermal tumors (embryonal gliomas).

Case	Gross features	Microscopic features					Interpretation and comment
		Primitive small cells	Astroglia	Oligodendroglia	Medullary and/or ependymal canals	Stroma	
1	Partially cystic and solid mass with focal papillary appearance	2+	–	–	4+	–	Medulloepithelioma
2	Sharply demarcated, partially cystic and necrotic mass	2+	–	–	4+	–	Ependymoblastoma
3	Circumscribed, partially cystic mass, 3×3×2 cm	2+	–	–	4+	–	Ependymoblastoma
4	Circumscribed cystic mass, 6 cm (recurrence)	1+	–	–	4+	–	Ependymoblastoma
5	Large firm grayish-white to soft purplish mass	2+	–	–	4+	–	Ependymoblastoma
6	Circumscribed multicystic mass, grayish-brown color, 12 cm	2+	2+	–	2+	3+	Mixed neoplastic pattern with massive connective tissue
7	Left cerebral hemispheric mass, circumscribed, solid and cystic	2+	2+	–	2+	3+	Mixed neoplastic pattern with differentiation noted in recurrence three years later
8	Grayish-white, soft mass with necrotic cavity, 4 cm	3+	2+	–	–	–	Primitive neuroepithelial pattern with glioblastomatous appearance in recurrence one year later
9	Circumscribed, yellowish multicystic mass	3+	–	1+	–	–	Primitive neuroepithelial pattern with differentiation
10	Soft gelatinous tumor with dural attachment	4+	–	2+	1+	–	Primitive neuroepithelial pattern with differentiation
11	Quadrigeminal-pineal mass (Acta scan), skull, soft tissue masses	4+	–	–	–	–	Primitive neuroepithelial pattern with spinal and tibial metastases
12	Biopsy of spinal mass	4+	–	–	–	–	Primitive neuroepithelial pattern

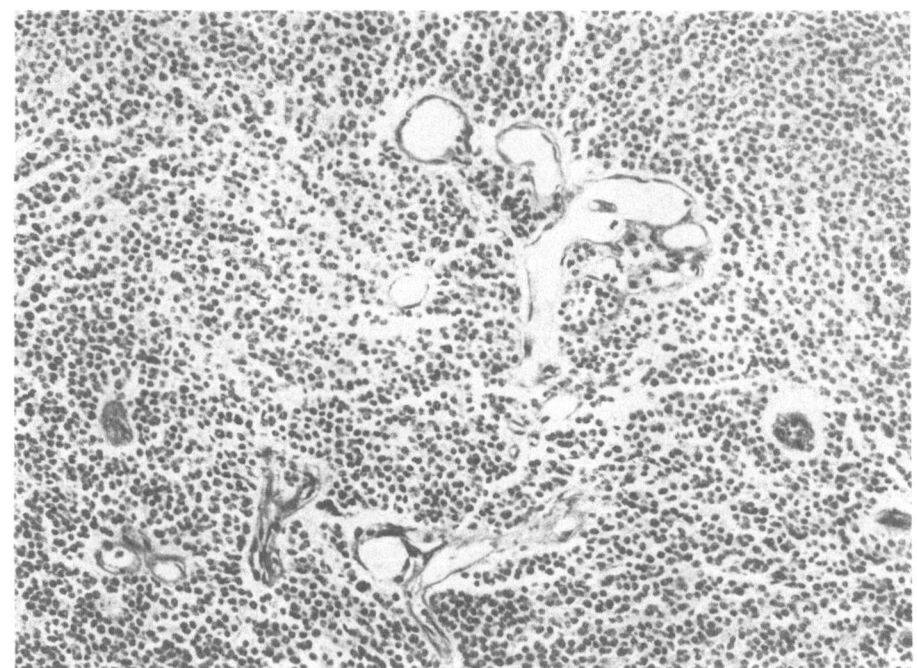

Figure 2. The typical appearance of the primitive neuroectodermal tumor (embryonal glioma) consisting of small uniform cells with or without a fibrillary eosinophilic background.

was not given for the hemispheric tumor, it was undoubtedly the largest one in the series but estimates for some of the neoplasms ranged from 3 to 12 cm in greatest dimension.

As previously noted in Material and Methods, each tumor in the study group had a primitive, small cell component as part of the histologic pattern. It was not a requirement for the primitive cells to be the exclusive component. These small dark cells were present as diffusely infiltrating sheets, forming cords, tubules or canals or interspersed as aggregates among differentiated glial elements and stroma. Various cytologic analogies or even homologies could be drawn between the primitive cells and their similarity to the subependymal germinal plate, medulloblasts and neuroblasts.

Four tumors were interpreted as ependymoblastomas. They were composed of anastomosing columns and cords of small, hyperchromatic cells forming perivascular festoons (Cases 2–5, Table 2). Luminal formation was quite prominent in one of these tumors (Case 4, Table 2). Occasional blepharoplasts were identified. Mitotic activity was relatively abundant in these neoplasms and focal necrosis was also noted. A fifth, somewhat similar appearing tumor from the standpoint of a tubular and papillary pattern, was a neoplasm from the frontoparietal lobe (Case 1, Table 2). The cells resting on the limiting

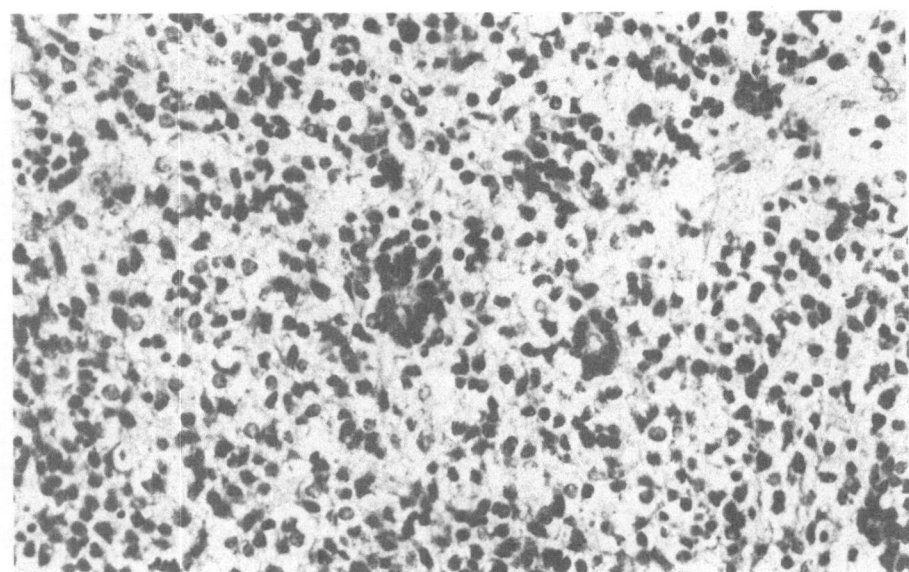

Figure 3. Ependymoblastoma composed of columns and cords of cells which individually are indistinguishable from the PNET.

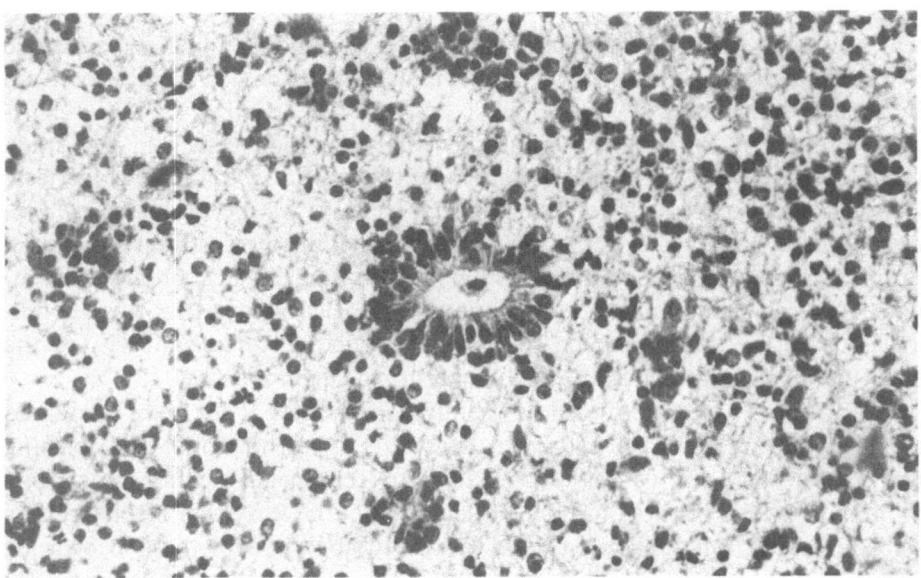

Figure 4. Ependymoblastoma with luminal formation, a feature in common with the better differentiated ependymal neoplasms.

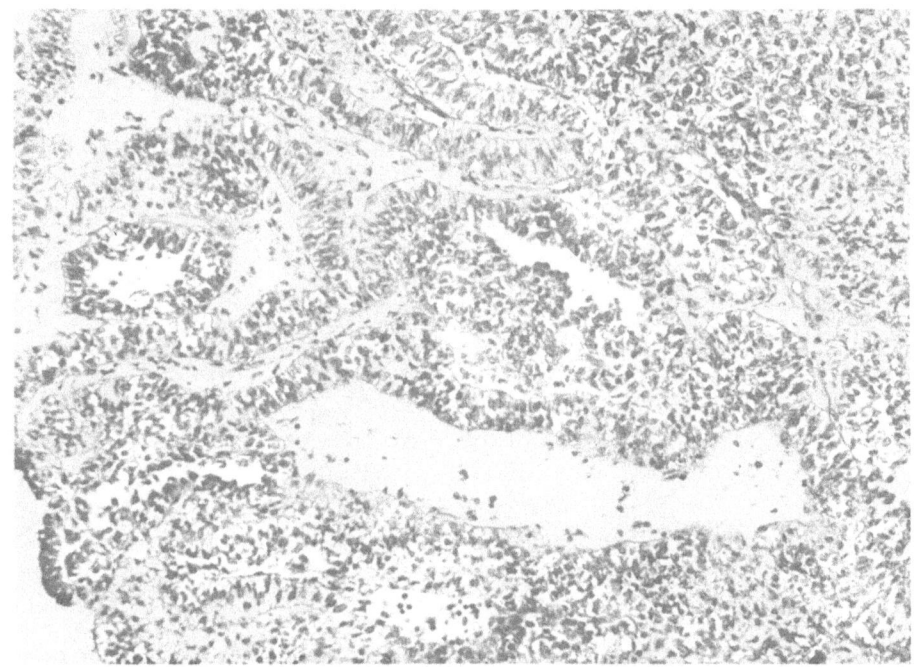

Figure 5. Medulloepithelioma characterized by elongated neural canals lined by columnar to cuboidal cells. In other foci, the tumor had a papillary appearance and small dark cells.

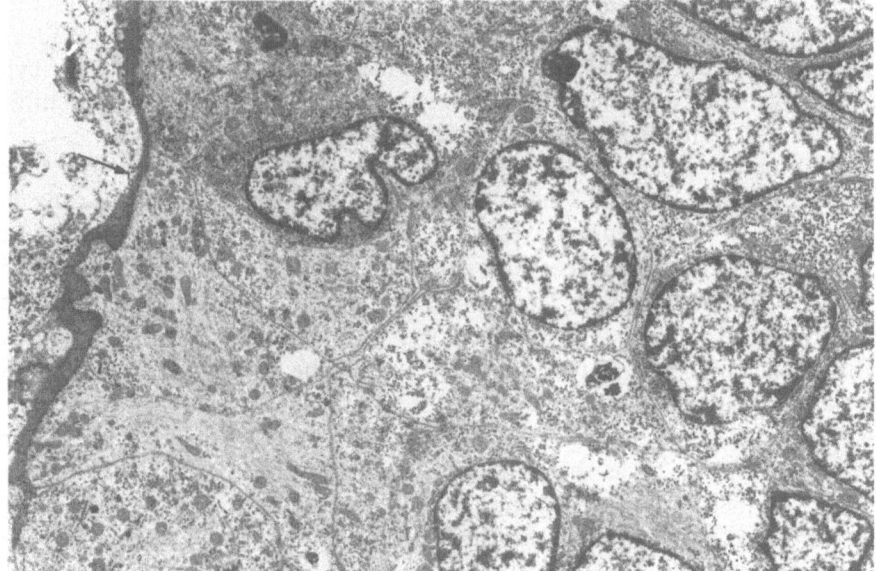

Figure 6. Tumor cells of the medulloepithelioma resting on a basal lamina or basement membrane (arrow). Delicate fibrils are present in the cytoplasm of some cells ($\times 3300$).

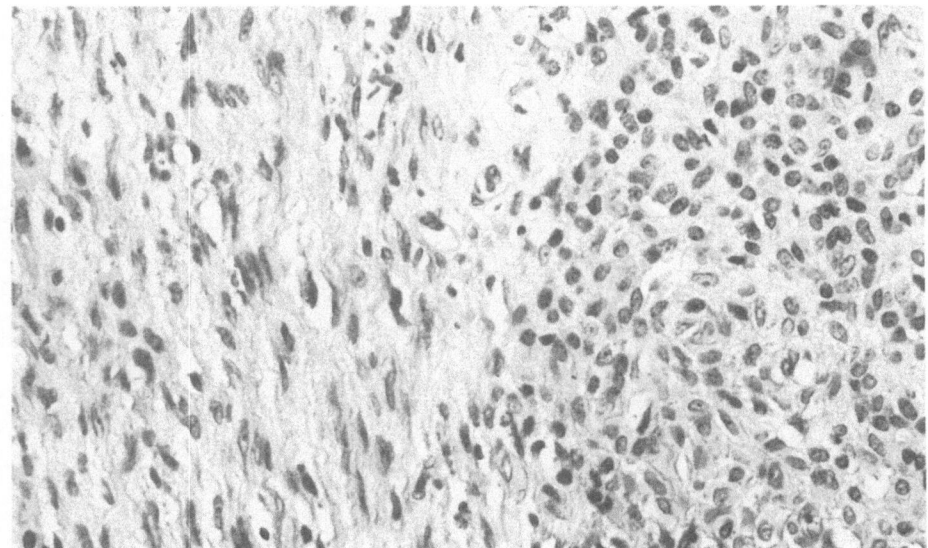

Figure 7. Desmoplastic stroma of a PNET may be a prominent feature.

membrane were for the most part tall columnar in type. There were definite attempts at the formation of canal-like structures resembling the primitive medullary canal of the embryo. Mitotic activity was not as abundant nor the cells as densely hyperchromatic as the cases of ependymoblastoma. Small dark cells were present in those solid foci devoid of medullary canal formation. Ultrastructurally, the epithelial cells had zonula adherens, scanty cytoplasmic organelles and microfilaments. A definite basal lamina was identified on which the tumor cells rested (Figure 6, arrow).

The connective tissue or stroma was quite remarkable in two tumors which demonstrated not only the nests and clusters of small primitive cells but evidence of differentiation (Cases 6, 7, Table 2). Astroglial and ependymal differentiation was seen three years after the first operation in Case 7 (Table 2) but the connective tissue stroma was there originally and unaltered later. The stroma had a fibrous, hyalin and focal vascular appearance. Isolated nests of the epithelial component were present within the stroma. The cellularity of the stroma was not reminiscent of a fibrosarcoma.

A similarity between the preceding two cases (Cases 6, 7, Table 2) and Cases 8–10 (Table 2) was the primitive nature of the tumor cells. The fibrous stroma was inapparent and the margin of the tumor was ill-defined in the latter tumors. One case (Case 8, Table 2) initially showed a highly undifferentiated appearance but had glioblastomatous features in the recurrence. Ependymal and oligodendrogliomatous foci were present in the primitive background in Cases 9 and 10 (Table 2).

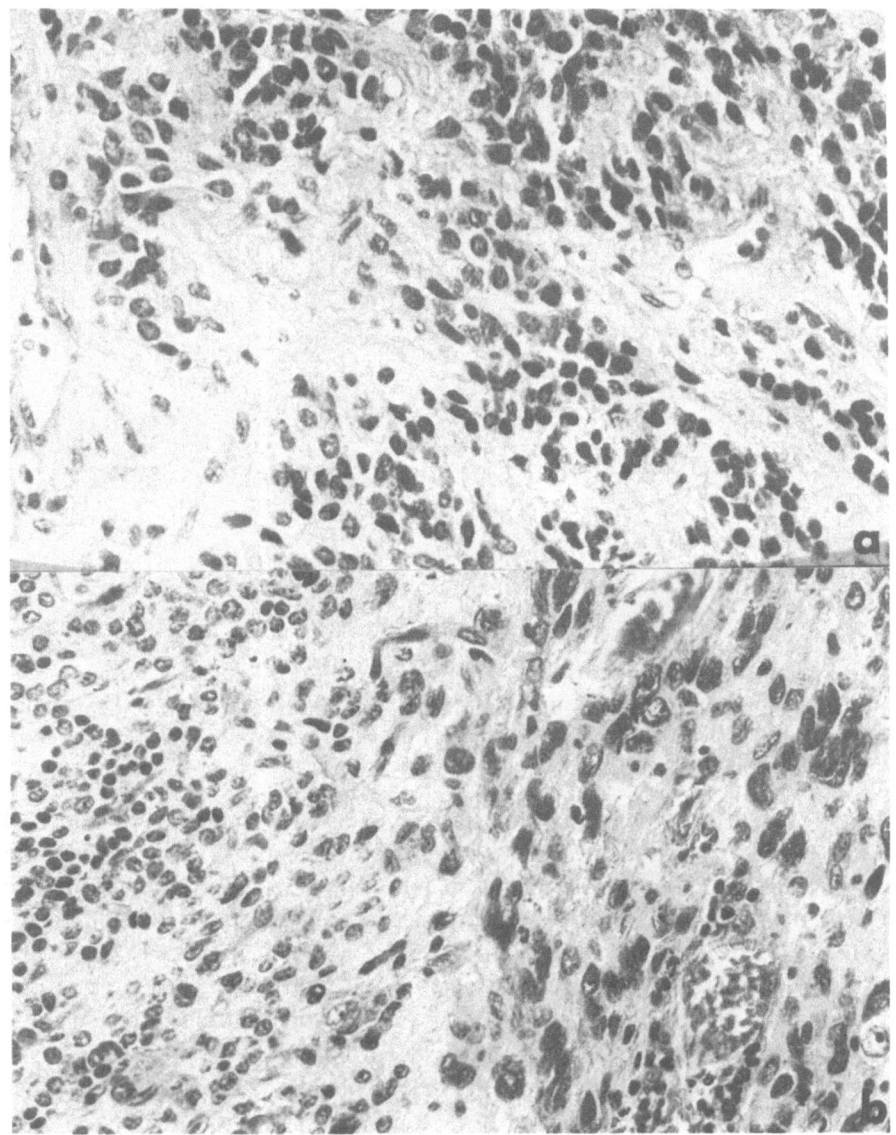

Figure 8. A: Small dark cell pattern of PNET. B: The recurrence revealed palisading of cells, endothelial hyperplasia and necrosis typical of a glioblastoma multiforme.

A monotypic histologic appearance characterized the final two cases (Cases 11, 12, Table 2). These neoplasms consisted of small dark cells which were quite suggestive of neuroblasts yet neither patient had evidence of abnormal catecholamine synthesis. The associated histologic features of neuroblastoma

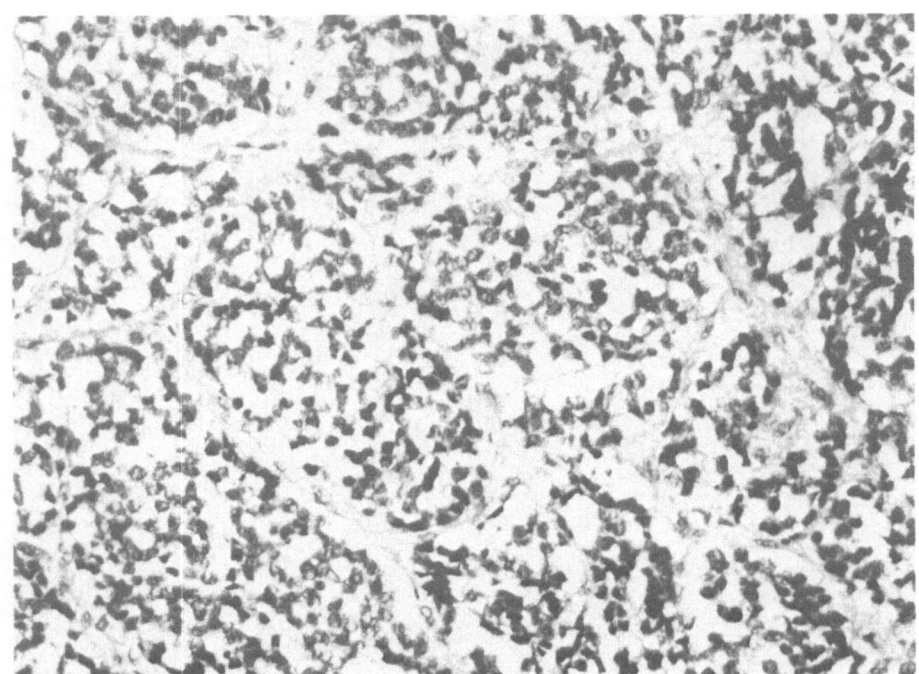

Figure 9. Nests and sheets of small dark cells in this field separated by delicate fibrovascular septa. Embryonal or alveolar rhabdomyosarcoma and Ewing's sarcoma were considerations in the differential diagnosis. Glycogen was not demonstrated in the cytoplasm.

were not evident in either case. At autopsy in Case 11, there was evidence of residual tumor in the central nervous system including the cervical and lumbar spinal cord. There was also metastatic tumor in lumbosacral vertebrae and proximal tibia but no involvement of the adrenal glands, lymph nodes and liver. By electron microscopy the small dark cells in Case 11 revealed occasional junction-like structures indicative of its epithelial differentiation. Some dendritic processes, microtubules and dense core granules attested to its neuroectodermal and more specifically its neuroblastic differentiation.

In such a small series, conclusive clinicopathologic correlations were very difficult to establish but two of the three long-term survivors had ependymoblastomas (Case 2, 3, Table 1). Neither of these neoplasms recurred after apparent complete excision and radiation therapy. The other survivor had a primitive neuroepithelial tumor with evidence of glial differentiation (Case 9, Table 1). Local recurrence within 12–14 months was the behavior of most of the other tumors. There was one delayed recurrence of 3.5 years after treatment (Case 7, Table 1). The most notable neoplasm was the primitive small cell tumor of the pineal-quadrigeminal region which presented with osteolytic lesions in the skull and soft tissue masses of the scalp (Case 11, Table 1).

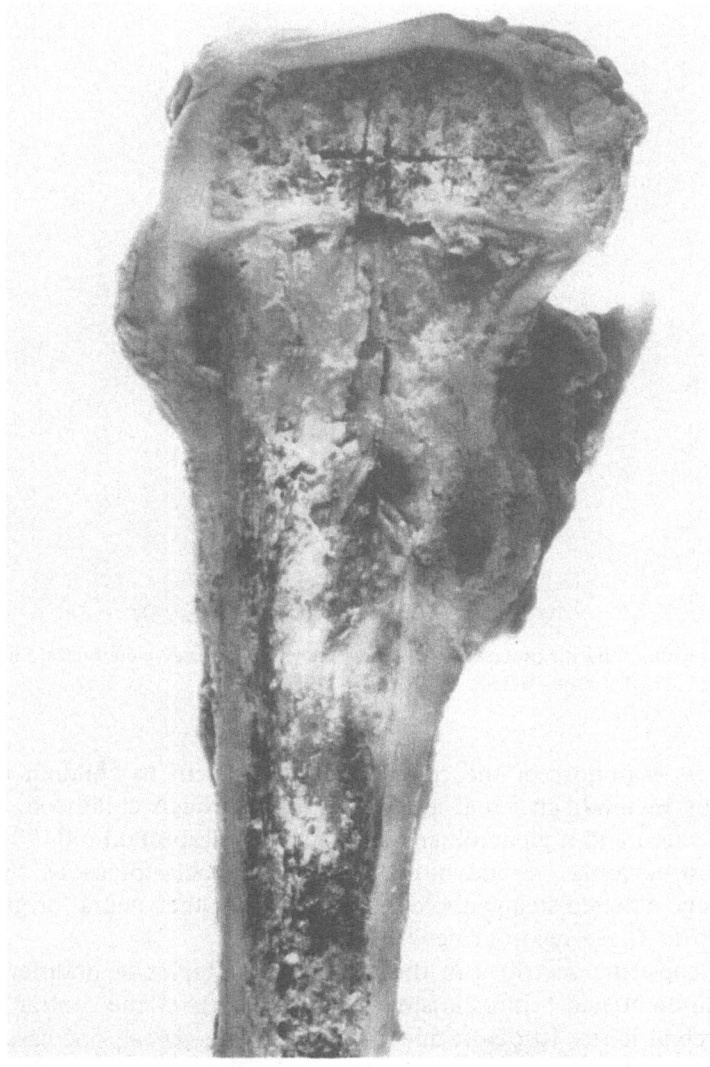

Figure 10. Tibia at autopsy showing a destructive lesion in the medullary region of the metaphysis.

4. DISCUSSION

Tumors of the brain and less commonly the spinal cord constitute an extremely important aspect of pediatric oncology. Most epidemiologic surveys show that neoplasms of the central nervous system are second in frequency to the hematopoietic malignancies in childhood. A more or less common

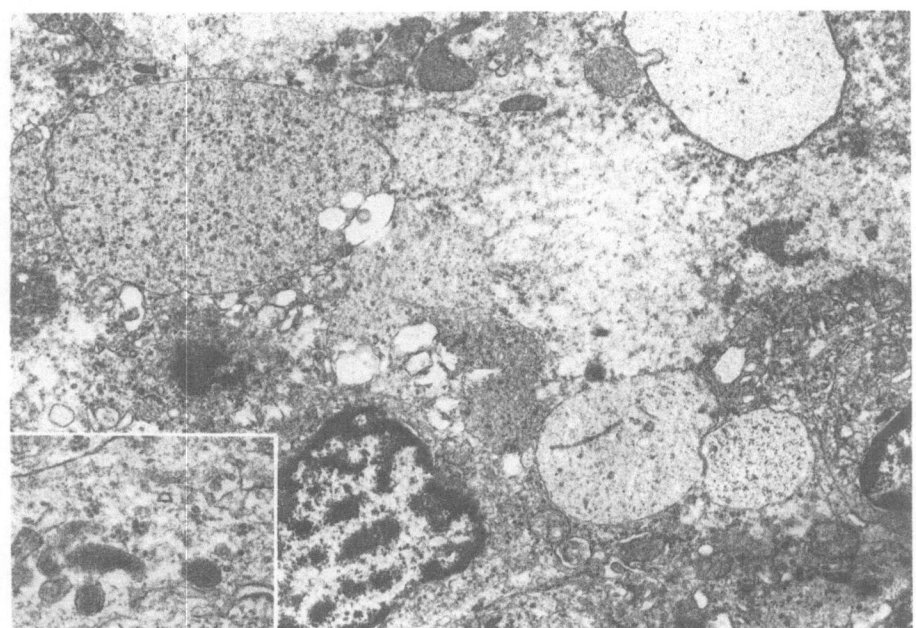

Figure 11. Numerous dendritic processes and dense core granules (inset) were typical findings of a neuroblastoma (×7850; inset, 37,350).

experience with tumors of the central nervous system in children emerges from various reviews: an equal age distribution through childhood, a slight male predilection and a predominant infratentorial localization (60–70%) with cerebellar astrocytomas, ependymomas and medulloblastomas as the most frequently encountered histopathologic types [4–7]. Other neural or glial neoplasms such as those reported here are rare.

The 12 neoplasms described in this study are examples of undifferentiated or poorly differentiated tumors arising in various parts of the central nervous system (cerebral lobes, 10 cases; quadrigemenal plate–pineal, one case; spinal cord, one case). At least two generic designations have been applied to this type of neoplasm: 'primitive central neuroepithelial tumors'; [8] and 'primitive neuroectodermal tumors of the brain' [2]. These descriptions convey the impression that the progenitor cell(s) remains arrested at the stage of replication itself with little tendency to differentiate into a cell identifiable as a neuron, astrocyte, ependymal cell or oligodendroglia. Although there were two such cases essentially composed of small dark cells resembling germinal (progenitor) cells in our study the other ten tumors displayed some tendency toward one or more lines of differentiation at some stage in the evolution of the disease. It does not seem inappropriate to consider these tumors as 'embryonal gliomas' with predominant ependymal differentiation (ependymo-blastoma), neural plate or tube formation (medulloepithelioma), neuroblastic or ganglioneuroblastic features (neuroblastoma) or as in five cases in our study, some form of glial differentiation in the primary tumor or recurrence with or without radiation therapy. This conceptual relationship is depicted by Kosnik et al. [9] in their diagram of the 'primitive neuroectodermal tumor' and the other immature neoplasms of the central nervous system.

The cases of embryonal gliomas reviewed here conform closely to the descriptions of primitive neuroectodermal tumor of children by Hart and Earle [2] and of primitive central neuroepithelial tumors by Rubenstein [8]. The important features are that they are 1) found in children, 2) located usually deep in cerebral hemispheres, 3) clinically aggressive, 4) often well demarcated from surrounding brain, 5) often cystic and hemorrhagic, 6) histologically comprised of primitive cells with areas of either neuronal or glial differentiation or both, and 7) characterized by prominent stromal compo-nent.

Our experience was similar to some of the previous published reports in that these tumors are quite uncommon, representing less than 5% of any one institution's experience with central nervous system tumors in children. There is one notable exception from the University of Kentucky Medical Center in which 35% of the supratentorial gliomas in children were diagnosed as 'poorly differentiated primitive neuroectodermal tumors' [10].

Hemiparesis, headache and vomiting were the most frequent initial clinical features in these children with an average age at diagnosis of 5 years. An interesting and as yet inexplicable finding was the marked female predilection (75%) which was also noted but less overwhelmingly in two other ser-ies [9, 10]. There was a male preponderance in Hart and Earle's study from the Armed Forces Institute of Pathology [2]. A slight male predilection or an equal sex ratio is encountered in larger epidemiologic surveys of childhood brain tumors of all histologic types [5–7]. Surgical excision was attempted in ten of the 12 cases. There were three long-term survivors, two of whom had ependymoblastomas. In each the potential to differentiate along various lines was present, which is not surprising considering the primordial nature of the cell. One major problem in the approach to this group remains the rarity and thus confusion and perplexity in the nosology, classification and manage-ment.

ACKNOWLEDGEMENTS

The authors express their appreciation to the following for their help in collecting information on these cases: Robert Kruger, M.D. and David Gnarra, M.D. of Childrens Memorial Hospital of Omaha, Nebraska; Douglas Perkins, M.D., Alexandria, Minnesota; John Cich, M.D., Minneapolis, Minnesota; and Thomas K. Jones, M.D. and Tae H. Kim, M.D. of the Department of Therapeutic Radiology, University of Minnesota Hospitals.

REFERENCES

1. Rubinstein LJ, Northfield DWC: The medulloblastoma and the so-called 'arachnoidal cerebellar sarcoma.' Brain 87:379–412, 1964.
2. Hart MN, Earle KM: Primitive neuroectodermal tumors of the brain in children. Cancer 32:890–897, 1973.
3. Young JL Jr, Miller RW: Incidence of malignant tumors in U.S. children. J Pediatr 86:254–258, 1975.
4. Dastur DK, Lalitha VS: Pathological analysis of intracranial space-occupying lesions in 1000 cases including children. Part 2. Incidence, types and unusual cases of glioma, J Neurol Sci 8:143–170, 1968.
5. Heiskanen O: Intracranial tumors of children. Child's Brain 3:69–78, 1977.
6. Yates AJ, Becker LE, Sachs LA: Brain tumors in childhood. Child's Brain 5:31–39, 1979.
7. Schoenberg BS, Schoenberg DG, Christine BW, Gomez MR: The epidemiology primary intracranial neoplasms of childhood. A population study. Mayo Clin Proc 51:51–56, 1976.
8. Rubinstein LJ: Cytogenesis and differentiation of primitive central neuroepithelial tumors. J Neuropathol Exp Neurol 31:7–26, 1972.
9. Kosnik EJ, Boesel CP, Bay J, Sayers MP: Primitive neuroectodermal tumors of the central nervous system in children. J Neurosurg 48:741–746, 1978.
10. Parker JC Jr. Mortara RH, McCloskey JJ: Biological behavior of the primitive neuroectodermal tumors: significant supratentorial childhood gliomas. Surg Neurol 4:383–388, 1975.
11. Hendriquez AS, Robertson DM, Marshall WJS: Primary neuroblastoma of the central nervous system with spontaneous extracranial metastases. Case report. J Neurosurg 38:226–231, 1973.
12. Horton B, Rubinstein L: Primary cerebral neuroblastoma. Brain 99:735–756, 1976.
13. Ahdevaara P, Kalimo H, Torma T, Haltia M: Differentiating intracerebral neuroblastoma. Report of a case and review of the literature. Cancer 40:784–788, 1977.

15. Primitive Neuroectodermal Tumors of Infancy and Childhood

LEONARD A. BRUNO, LUCY B. RORKE and DONALD G. NORRIS

We have reviewed the Children's Hospital of Philadelphia's experience with poorly undifferentiated small cell tumors of the central nervous system that are *not* medulloblastoma from 1968 through 1978. Using purely histologic criteria for diagnosis (i.e., small cell tumors with fields of deeply basophilic cells showing scant cytoplasm, some nuclear atypia, occasionally prominent nucleoli, endothelial hyperplasia, no secondary structures and in general reminiscent of germinal matrix tissue of the developing brain) we have been able to recognize 19 primitive neuroectodermal tumors (PNET) in children from 237 histologically verified brain tumors. This total excludes all unbiopsied tumors (e.g., thalamic tumors, brain stem tumors and some dominant parietal lobe lesions) which would increase the number of tumor patients seen by about 30%. Of these 19 PNETs, 11 were posterior fossa tumors and although they showed evidence of divergent differentiation were diagnosed in most instances as medulloblastoma. The remaining eight tumors included two pineal area lesions, which would qualify as pineoblastoma. Six met criteria to be diagnosed as PNETs as described by Hart and Earle[1] and recently again reviewed by Kosnik et al. [2]. Our incidence of PNET in 10 years is, therefore, 2.5% (6 of 237) but would be less (approximately 1.9%) if unbiopsied patients were included. A summary of the patient data is included below.

As the patient data catalogued indicate, the Children's Hospital of Philadelphia experience has not been good. Although our patient group is small, three interesting points appear to emerge from this group.

First, most PNET patients present with a precipitous downhill neurologic course often whith no preceding sentinel neurologic complaints. Our two patients who remain alive with no evidence of tumor 1 year and $3\frac{1}{2}$ years since diagnosis both had long histories of headache and lethargy.

Second, both long-term survivors had truly intraventricular tumors at surgery. It is certainly possible that poorly differentiated small cell tumors arising within the cerebral ventricles are biologically more analogous to medulloblas-

Table 1. PNET patient data.

Name	Age	Sex	Race	Diagnosis	Date of Dx	Presentation	Initial therapy of response	Duration	Second therapy survival
K.R.	14 yr	F	B	Spinal PNET	5/74	Pain and weakness in lower extremities, incontinence	Laminectomy 5/74, RT-6000 rads to low spine	month	Chemo.RX 11/74 — Died 12/75 19 months
A.M.	9 yr	M	B	Central neuro-blastoma	1/76	Aqueductal stenosis '74, r. ventricular tumor	Biopsy 1/76, RT-4000 rads head+spine, RT-1200 rads tumor 3/76	3½ yr	VCN, CCNU, Prednisone ×2 yr — Alive 45 months CAT* 5/79 No tumor
S.R.	10 yr	F	B	R.temporal PNET	5/77	2 days prior to admission, headache, vomiting, walking problems	Craniotomy 5/77, steroids, mannitol	1 day	None — Died 5/77
E.T.	2 yr	M	W	R.fronto-temp. PNET	3/78	5 days prior to admission fell fown-stairs, then increasing lethargy	Resuscitation, craniotomy 3/78 following arrest, steroids, mannitol	3 days	None — Died 3/78
R.J.	8 yr	M	B	L.atrium of vent. PNET	8/78	3 months headache, vomited on day of admission and lapsed into coma	Craniotomy 8/78, RT-3780 rads to brain; 1800 rads l.atrium; 2400 rads spine 9–11/78	1 yr	None — Alive EMI 9/79 No tumor
D.D.	6 days	F	W	L.cerebral hemis. PNET	9/78	Coma at 2 days of age, R/O meningitis vs SAH	Resuscitation	4 days	None — Died 9/78

toma of the IV ventricle than they are to hemispheric PNET. If this is so, clinical response of cerebral intraventricular PNET may also be quite analogous to that of IV ventricular medulloblastoma.

Finally, from our patient group there does not appear to be any age, sex or racial predominance which correlates with development of PNET. Our youngest patient was 2 days old at diagnosis, whereas our oldest patient was 14 years.

It is possible that patients with cerebral intraventricular PNET was present with a subacute clinical course may have a relatively good overall prognosis with respect to all other PNET patients. These patients appear to respond to radiation therapy and possible to adjunctive chemotherapy as well.

Earlier diagnosis of patients with cerebral intrahemispheric PNET may improve their prognosis, presuming a satisfactory course of radiation therapy can be delivered before irreversible neurologic compromise and fatal intracranial hypertension develop.

REFERENCES

1. Hart MN and Earle KM: Primitive neuroectodermal tumors of the brain in children. Cancer 32:890–897, 1973.
2. Kosnik EJ, Goegel CP, Bay J and Sayer MP: Primitive neuroectodermal tumors of the central nervous system in children. J Neurosurg 48:741, 1978.

16. Poorly Differentiated Small Cell Tumours of the Central Nervous System that Are Not Medulloblastomas

K.D. WATERS, C.W. CHOW and P.E. CAMPBELL

From July 1969 to June 1979, 25 cases of non-medulloblastomatous poorly differentiated small cell tumours of the central nervous system were seen at the Royal Children's Hospital. During the same period of time there were 84 astrocytomas and 35 medulloblastomas.

1. CRITERIA OF DIAGNOSIS

The selection of types of tumours for the category 'poorly differentiated small cell tumours' was rather arbitrary. Thus highly cellular malignant ependymomas were included, but the less cellular subependymomas were excluded, although there were cases showing a mixture of patterns. The ones showing a predominantly highly cellular pattern were included. Also germinomas were strictly speaking not small cell tumours although there may be a predominance of lymphocytes and granulomatous tissue. It was felt, however, this group of tumours was pertinent to the present topic.

Of the 25 cases, there were 14 malignant ependymomas, six germinomas, two malignant lymphomas, two pinealoblastomas and one choroid plexus carcinoma. The diagnoses in all cases were mainly based on histological features. In some of the later cases in the series, ultrastructural studies were performed. The anatomical distribution of the lesion was of particular importance in some tumours.

The malignant ependymomas were highly cellular tumours with numerous mitoses. Pseudorosettes around small vessels were prominent and these were often obvious in squash preparations. Also frequently present were genuine rosettes with lumens. Moderate amounts of glycogen were present in the cytoplasm. Ultrastructurally there were small lumens bound by cells joined together by zonula adherens type cell junctions. Numerous microvilli were seen.

G.B. Humphrey et al. (eds.), Pediatric oncology 1, 269–276. All rights reserved.
Copyright © 1981 Martinus Nijhoff Publishers bv, The Hague/Boston/London.

The germinomas were composed of nests of cells with vesicular nuclei, prominent nucleoli and clear to pale eosinophilic cytoplasm which was heavily loaded with glycogen. Sometimes tumour cells were scanty and the bulk of the lesion was composed of stromal elements with varying numbers of lymphocytes and histiocytes. A very prominent filamentous portion of te nucleoli was seen in ultrastructure.

Of the malignant lymphomas, the diagnosis in one case was based entirely on cytological examination of the cerebral spinal fluid on two occasions. Both specimens showed a uniform population of lymphoblasts. There was no evidence of a malignant lymphoma outside the CNS. In the other case the diagnosis was based on a cerebellar biopsy. This showed large masses of a polymorphous mixture of round cells. The predominant cells had oval nuclei with a fine chromatin pattern and prominent nucleoli. Cytoplasm varied from eosinophilic to foamy. These were mixed with moderate numbers of lymphocytes and a few plasma cells. There was diffuse infiltration into the adjacent brain. Also the perivascular spaces were markedly distended with similar cells with abundant reticulin fibres.

The pinealoblastomas were cellular small cell lesions with occasional rosettes containing fibrillary material. Occasional larger cells resembling immature neurons were seen. The anatomical location was of particular significance in the diagnosis of these tumours which on histological grounds were difficult to differentiate from medulloblastomas.

The single case of choroid plexus carcinomas was a highly cellular tumour with numerous mitoses composed in most areas of papillary structures with a vascular core surrounded by columnar epithelium. Ultrastructurally numerous microvilli and occasional cilia were seen on the surface of the tumour cells. An occasional tight junction was seen between adjacent tumour cells. The basal lamina of the tumour cells and that of the capillary were separated by a space containing a few collagen fibres. Most of the vessels were fenestrated.

2. CLINICAL FEATURES, TREATMENT AND RESULTS

A summary of the clinical features, diagnosis, treatment and survival is presented in Table 1. The patients within each group are listed according to the age at diagnosis rather than the chronological order of presentation.

Of the 14 patients with *malignant ependymomas,* one was lost to follow-up after completion of post-operative irradiation therapy and is excluded from further discussion. Twelve of the other 13 patients had subtotal surgical removal of the tumour. In one, the tumour was biopsied only. Four patients, aged less than one year at diagnosis, received no further treatment. All four

Table 1. Clinical characteristics, treatment and response.

Patient	Sex	Age	Presenting symptoms	Surgery	Irradiation therapy	Chemotherapy	Survival
				Malignant ependymoma			
A.A.	M	1 month	Hydrocephalus	Subtotal removal	Nil	Nil	2 months
T.C.	F	1 month	Hydrocephalus	Subtotal removal	Nil	Nil	8 months
B.C.	M	8 months	Vomiting Ataxia	Subtotal removal	Nil	Nil	6 months
A.S.	M	9 months	Hydrocephalus	Subtotal removal	Nil	Nil	5 months
M.H.	M	1 year	Vomiting Lethargy	Subtotal removal	Cranial irradiation 3000 rad	A	7 month →
P.L.	M	2 years	Vomiting Drowsy Ataxia	Subtotal removal	Cranial irradiation 4000 rad	Nil	7 years →
G.P.	M	2 years	Ataxia Vomiting Head tilt	Subtotal removal	Cranio-spinal 3000 rad	Nil	9 months
K.W.	F	2 years	Vomiting	Biopsy	Cranio-spinal 3000 rad	B	8 month

Abbreviations—Chemotherapy A : vincristine, prednisolone, procarbezine, chlorambucil
Chemotherapy B : vincristine, chloro-ethyl-cyclohexyl-nitrosurea (CCNU)
I.T.MTX   : intrathecal methotrexate
CPA   : cyclophosphamide
6MP   : 6mercaptopurine
MTX   : methotrexate
L.T.F.U.   : lost to follow-up

Table 1. (continued).

Patient	Sex	Age	Presenting symptoms	Surgery	Irradiation therapy	Chemo-therapy	Survival
C.L.	M	2 years	Vomiting Drowsy	Subtotal removal	Cranio-spinal 3000 rad	Nil	8 months
D.R.	M	4 years	Headache Vomiting	Subtotal removal	Cranio-spinal irradiation 4500 rad	B	2 years →
S.F.	F	5 years	Ataxia Vomiting Headache	Subtotal removal	Cranio-spinal 3500 rad	Nil	5 years →
P.J.	F	9 years	Headache Vomiting	Subtotal removal	Cranio-spinal 4750 rad	B	4 years →
B.G.	M	11 years	Diplopia Headache	Subtotal removal	Cranial 5000 rad Spinal 3500 rad	A	1 year →
W.M.	M	4 years	Headache Vomiting	Subtotal removal	Cranio-spinal 4500 rad	Nil	L.T.F.U.
Germinoma							
C.S.	M	10 years	Growth failure Polyuria	Biopsy	Cranial 4600 rad	Nil	6 months →
T.R.	F	11 years	Anorexia Ptosis	Biopsy	Cranial 4500 rad	Nil	1 year *

* Local recurrence at 12 months, retreated with irradiation therapy.

Table 1. (continued).

Patient	Sex	Age	Presenting symptoms	Surgery	Irradiation therapy	Chemotherapy	Survival
S.J.	M	12 years	Headache Vomiting Diplopia	Biopsy	Cranial 4750 rad	Nil	1 year †
P.K.	M	12 years	Diabetes insipidus Headache Vomiting	Subtotal removal	Cranial 4500 rad	Nil	5 years ‡
G.B.	M	13 years	Diabetes insipidus	Partial removal	Cranial 4000 rad	Nil	3 years §
G.B.	M	14 years	Diabetes insipidus Growth failure Visual failure	Biopsy	Cranial 4200 rad	B	8 months →
Malignant lymphoma							
J.H.	F	1 year	Ataxia Vomiting	Biopsy	Nil	I.T.MTX	Died **
P.M.	F	9 years	Blurred vision Intermittent vomiting	Nil	Cranio-spinal 350 rad	I.T.MTX CPA, MTX, 6MP	1 year →

† Spinal recurrence at 5 months, treated with irradiation therapy.
‡ No evidence of tumour at post-mortem.
§ Spinal recurrence at 12 months, treated with irradiation therapy.
** Died suddenly following intrathecal methotrexate, post-mortem refused.

Table 1. (continued).

Patient	Sex	Age	Presenting symptoms	Surgery	Irradiation therapy	Chemo-therapy	Survival
				Pinealoblastoma			
C.R.	M	8 months	Hydrocephalus	Subtotal removal	Nil	Nil	Died ††
M.J.	M	7 years	Headache Vomiting	Partial removal	Cranio-spinal 5000 rad	B	1 year →
				Choroid plexus carcinoma			
J.O.	M	5 months	Hydrocephalus Irritability	Biopsy	Nil	A	3 months

†† Died suddenly 24 hours following surgery, post-mortem refused.

died of recurrent tumour, between 2 and 8 months from diagnosis. The other nine patients all received irradiation therapy. In two of these, aged 13 and 24 months, cranial irradiation alone was given. In the remaining seven, all aged over 24 months, cranio-spinal irradiation was given. Five of the nine patients treated with irradiation were also treated with chemotherapy. The chemotherapy consisted of weekly vincristine during irradiation therapy, followed 4 weeks later by intermittent courses of either vincristine and C.C.N.U., or vincristine, prednisolone, procarbazine and chlorambucil for 12 months. Of these nine patients, six survive tumour free. Of these six, four received chemotherapy in addition to irradiation therapy. The median follow-up is 27 months, with a range from 7 to 93 months.

Of the six *germinomas,* two were from the pineal region, and the other four were from the pituitary suprasellar area. Two were partially removed, the remaining four were biopsied only. All six patients were treated with cranial but not spinal irradiation. One patient was also treated with vincristine and C.C.N.U. Two patients, including the one who received chemotherapy, survive tumour-free, 6 and 8 months from diagnosis respectively. Three died from tumour recurrence and in two of these the first recurrence was in the spinal cord. The last patient died out of hospital following intractable fitting 5 years after diagnosis. Autopsy performed outside hospital showed no residual tumour and the cause of death was not established.

One patient with *primary CNS lymphoma* had a cerebellar lesion and did not have free tumour cells in the CSF. She died suddenly two hours after intrathecal methotrexate. The other had free tumour cells circulating in the CSF but no mass lesion could be demonstrated. She was treated with intrathecal methotrexate to clear the CSF followed by cranio-spinal irradiation and systemic chemotherapy. She remains well and tumour free 14 months from the time of diagnosis.

One patient with *pinealoblastoma* died 24 hours post-operatively. The other had partial surgical removal followed by cranial irradiation and vincristine and C.C.N.U. for 12 months. He remains tumour free 20 months from diagnosis.

The only patient with *choroid plexus carcinoma* had a large tumour which involved the right parietal and occipital lobes. This was biopsied only. There was no clinical response to a single course of vincristine, prednisolone, procarbazine and chlorambucil. She died of progressive tumour 3 months from diagnosis.

3. MANAGEMENT IN FUTURE

The future management of patients with these tumours will continue to involve the combined approach of surgery, radiotherapy and chemotherapy.

It has been the surgical policy here to remove as much tumour as possible, the extent of surgery being limited by accessibility and risk of damaging vital structures. This policy will probably continue due to previous experience that the survival following total or subtotal surgery was better than that following biopsy alone.

Cranio-spinal irradiation continues to be an essential part of management of these patients. However, due to severe long-term side-effects, particularly on the growth of the spine, this will be reserved for patients aged 2 years or more. Radiotherapy will be avoided in patients who are aged less than 1 year at the time of diagnosis. For those between 1 and 2 years, cranial irradiation will be given. The high incidence of recurrence in the spinal cord among patients with germinoma certainly strongly suggests that these cases should be given cranio-spinal irradiation as for the other malignant tumours.

The experience with chemotherapy is the management of central nervous system tumours at this hospital is limited to just over 4 years. At the moment, patients with malignant central nervous system tumours are randomized into two chemotherapy programmes. However, due to the small number of cases and the short periods of follow-up, no statement can be made on the exact role and usefulness. It is hoped that this will be of particular value in the management of patients less than 1 year of age, for whom radiotherapy is not considered.

17. Primitive Neuroectodermal Tumors of the Central Nervous System in Childhood. Retrospective and Overview

LOUIS P. DEHNER

The pediatric pathologist and oncologist have long since become accustomed to the histologic common denominator which characterizes so many of the solid malignant tumors in childhood. Since the individual cytologic features regardless of the specific developing organ in early embryonic development seem to be dominated by a small dark cell, it is not surprising that the embryonic tumors of childhood (medulloblastoma, retinoblastoma, neuroblastoma, etc.) have an exclusive or predominant pattern of undifferentiated or poorly differentiated hyperchromatic diminutive cells by light microscopy. Most of these tumors, however, have foci of morphologic differentiation or produce a biochemical product that permits a specific pathologic diagnosis beyond the point of 'small blue cell tumor' in a child. Within the spectrum of some of the solid childhood tumors, there are identifiable grades of histopathologic differentiation, i.e., neuroblastoma, differentiating neuroblastoma and ganglioneuroblstoma. Retinoblastoma, neophroblastoma and hepatoblastoma likewise demonstrate phases of differentiation with some prognostic significance when integrated with the clinical stage of the tumor.

This preamble thus leads into a consideration of the primitive neuroectodermal tumors (PNET) of the central nervous system which have remained an enigma for neuropathologist because of the uncertainty about the nature of the progenitor cell. The controversy initially centered upon the prototypic example of a primitive neuroectodermal tumor, the medulloblastoma. During the 55 years that have lapsed since this tumor was initially described by Bailey and Cushing[1], the medulloblast remains the elusive embryonic cell. Ultrastructural and *in vitro* studies of the medulloblastoma indicate that the neoplastic cell has the potential for neuronal (neuroblastic) and astroglial differentiation[2]. The versatility of this cell is even broader when one considers the rare examples of medulloblastoma with myoid cells or melanocytes[3–5]. It may be overly generous to consider the cell of the medulloblastoma as totipotential but it is certainly multipotential. An interesting experi-

G. B. Humphrey et al. (eds.), Pediatric oncology 1, 277–288. All rights reserved.

ment of nature was reported by Kadin *et al.* [6] of a neonatal medulloblastoma which originated from the external granular layer of Obersteiner of the cerebellar cortex. These cells are progenitors for neuronal and glial elements.

If uncertainty still shrouds the cytogenesis of the medulloblastoma after a half century, is it reasonable to expect less, the same or greater understanding of the supratentorial and spinal primitive neuroectodermal tumors? Rubinstein [7], in an address to the American Association of Neuropthologists which was published in 1972, reviewed the topic of primitive central neuroepithelial tumors with the designations into subtypes of medulloepithelioma, cerebral neuroblastoma, polar spongioblastoma, ependymoblastoma, pineoblastoma and cerebellar medulloblastoma. The implication was that each of these neoplasms had some morphological feature(s) which permitted the pathologist to make a catergorical diagnosis. Hart and Earle [8] indicated that the waters were less clear and that there existed in their experience certain tumors predominantly of the cerebral hemispheres in individuals between stillbirth and 24 years with essentially undifferentiated features. These tumors were soft, oftentimes cystic and well demarcated from the adjacent brain. Microscopically, an undifferentiated pattern of small dark cells was the dominant finding. Approximately 90–95% of any one tumor had to have this appearance in order to qualify as a PNET. Mesenchymal stroma, mainly collagenous bands, was present in nine of the 23 cases. Some differentiation was noted in their cases including focal glial formation only (three cases), focal neuronal differentiation only (six cases) and both in six cases. They also alluded to rosette formation. There have appeared two subsequent studies, one from the University of Kentucky Medical Center [9] and the other from the Children's Hospital, Columbus, Ohio [10] with a total of 25 cases. From a variety of institutions, an additional 27 cases and individual case studies have been compiled in this section [11–16]. Only the series have been summarized and tabulated (Table 1). Waters *et al.* [17] have not been included because most of their 25 cases do not qualify as primitive neuroectodermal tumors but attention is drawn to the very important differential diagnostic problem for the pathologist. With the possible exception of the choroid plexus carcinoma, the other tumors reported by Waters *et al.* [17] consist for the most part of small dark cells which could be readily interpreted as PNET or cerebral neuroblastoma.

Areas of conformity and discordance become all too apparent when 85 cases are collated from eight different institutions and the neoplasm(s) in question is as controversial and incompletely defined as the PNET. Some relatively noncontroversial points which emerged from the various institutional experiences are that the tumors occur almost exclusively in childhood with mean age ranges of 3–10 years. The youngest case was diagnosed at autopsy in a stillborn infant and the oldest in a 26 year old male [8, 14]. Although

Table 1. Summary of 85 cases of primitive neuroectodermal tumors of central nervous system.

Authors	No. of cases	Age range	Sex	Site	Follow-up
Hart and Earle [8]	23	Still-birth–24 (8 yr)	15 M 8 F	Frontal—9 Temporal—4 Parietal—4 Occipital—2 Bihemisphere—1 Corpus callosum—2 Foramen of Munro—1	Average survival 18 months (six cases)
Parker et al. [9]	7	4 months-4 yr (4.6 yr)	2 M 5 F	Parieto-occipital—2 Temporo-parietal—2 Parietal—2 3rd vent.—1	Operative deaths (four) Dead of tumor (two, 18 months, 21 months) Alive (one, 3 yr)
Kosnik et al. [10]	18	6 months–10 yr (3.1 yr)	8 M 10 F	Frontal—3 Temporal—3 Parietal—3 Occipital—2 3rd vent.—4 Spinal cord—3	Dead of tumor—12 cases in 2 yr
Bruno et al. [11]	6	2 days–14 yr (7 yr)	3 M 3 F	Ventricle—2 Cerebral hemisphere—1 Temporal—1 Fronto-temporal—1 Spinal cord—1	Dead of tumor—four Alive (one, 3½ yr)
Jenkin [12]	5	3–12 yr (8 yr)	3 M 2 F	Temporal—2 Frontal—1 Parietal—1 Parieto-occipital—1	Dead of tumor—three (1–5 yr) Alive with tumor—one Alive—one (17 months
Wald et al. [13]	9 *	1–8 yr (5 yr)	3 M 6 F	Parietal—5 Temporal—2 Frontal—2 (incl. brain stem-1)	Dead of tumor—four (3 months–3 yr) Operative deaths—three Alive—two (9 months, 8 yr)
Wara et al. [14]	10 *	2–26 yr (10½ yr)	5 M 5 F	Parietal—4 Occipital—3 Frontal—2 Basal ganglion—1	Dead of tumor—two Alive—eight (two recurrences) (2–8 yr)
Priest et al. [15]	7 **	5 months–13 yr (4.8 yr)	3 M 4 F	Parietal—2 Fronto-parietal—2 Hemisphere—1 Quadrigeminal plate-pineal—1 Spinal cord—1	Dead of tumor—six (3–48 months) Alive—one (12 yr)

* Series diagnosed as cerebral neuroblastoma.

** Five cases excluded from this summary because of the diagnoses of medulloepithelioma (one case) and ependymoblastoma (four cases).

some series reflected a female predilecion, it appeared that none existed overall. Symptoms of an enlarging intracranial mass brought most of these children to clinical attention within a few days to weeks after the onset. Bruno et al. [11], suggested that a prolonged history and an intraventricular localization were favorable prognostic features. The experience with one case from the University of Minnesota [15] was unique in that the child presented with not only intracranial signs but metastatic lesions in the skull and soft tissue masses on the scalp. Only one other patient developed a metastasis outside of the cranio-spinal axis among the 85 cases but later in the course of the disease [13]. The diagnostic techniques in the pre-operative evaluation and post-operative follow-up interval should obviously take into consideration the potential for such behavior. If there is no immediate risk to the patient, a cerebrospinal fluid cytology is warranted since seeding is a definite mode of spread which, for instance, Wald et al. [13] note in one-third of their cases.

By definition, convention and the admitted difficulties in the differentiation of the cerebellar medulloblastoma from PNET, if there is any real difference in the first place, the PNET is predominantly a supratentorial neoplasm. The parietal and/or temporal lobes were the most frequent sites although holo-hemispheric and even bihemispheric involvement was reported in a total of three cases (Table 1). There were eight instances (10%) of tumors which were located in a ventricle or the foramen of Munro. The spinal cord was the presumed primary site in five cases (6%) including one case from the University of Minnesota [15].

Macroscopic descriptions were inconsistently documented in the various reports but the impression existed that many of these neoplasms were well circumscribed and even encapsulated in some instances. This feature would presumably facilitate total excision but the size and multilobe involvement often precluded such extirpations. Cystic formation secondary to necrosis was another common feature but was notably absent in those tumors with a marked desmoplastic reaction.

A perusal of the current studies and those previously published indicate some level of perplexity in the morphologic criteria for the acceptibility of a neoplasm as a PNET. Hart and Earle [8] stated the problem and followed with their basic criterion, 'At what point a tumor should cease to be considered a "primitive neuroectodermal tumor" and named according to its avenue of predominant differentiation is arbitrary; for our purposes, we have restricted the present series to those tumors appearing at least 90–95% undifferentiated.' An immediate enigma is the cerebral neuroblastoma. There is probably little disagreement that it is closely related to the PNET and used synonymously in the series from the University of California, San Francisco [14] and the Children's Hospital of Los Angeles [13]. The study of 12 cases from the University of Minnesota [15] drifted even further with the inclusion

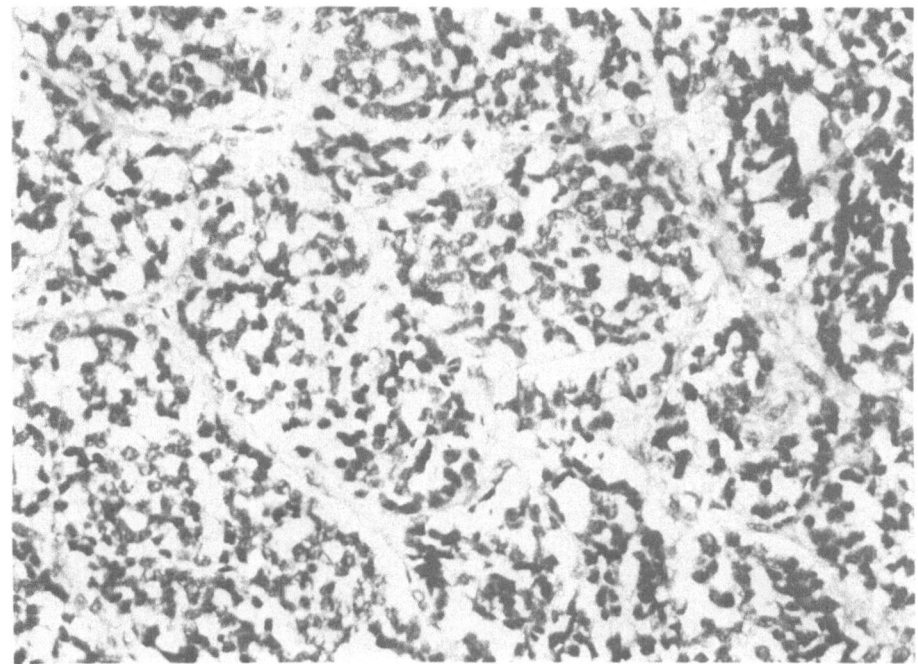

Figure 1. Small dark tumor cells arranged into nests by thin fibrovascular septa.

of one medulloepithelioma[18] and four ependymoblastomas[19] Obviously, Hart and Earle[8] would have deleted these latter five tumors as examples of PNET.

A sense of arbitrariness then emerges when the sampling problem alone is contemplated. The pathologist oftentimes receives but small portion of a large neoplasm. Given these and other overlooked qualifications, the basic microscopic appearance is initially dominated by small dark tumor cells arranged in dense cohesive nests and sheets. The cells are uniform in size and shape. There is mitotic activity, but cellular anaplasia is uncommon. Neuronal differentiation is recognizable as enlargement of individual cells and amphophilic cytoplasm. A delicate fibrillary background is indicative of neurite or glial differentiation. Desmoplasia was quite prominent in two cases from the University of Minnesota[15]. Hart and Earle[8] noted a mesenchymal stroma in 13 of their 23 cases. There is more than a passing resemblance to the desmoplasia that also occurs in the medulloblastoma. The 'transitional' subgroup of cerebral neuroblastomas as described by Horton and Rubinstein[20] were likewise characterized by a fibrous desmoplastic reaction. In addition to the focal glial differentiation which other authors have commented upon, the experience at the University of Minnesota also disclosed some ependymal and

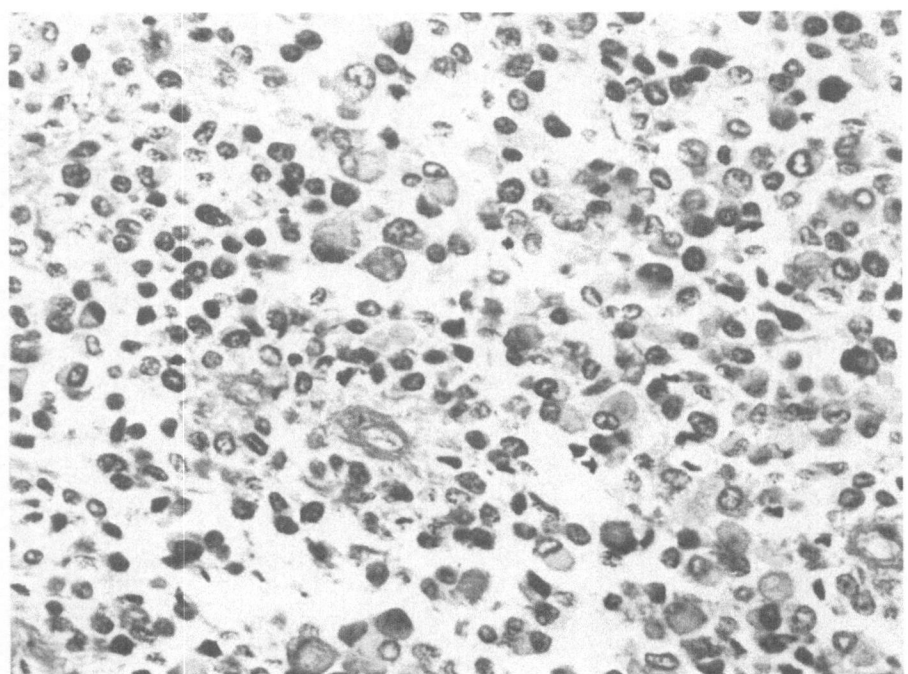

Figure 2. Larger cells with essentrically placed nuclei with prominent nucleoli and amphophilic cytoplasm among smaller tumor cells. The larger cells resemble ganglion cells.

oligodendroglial area [15]. There was a definite impression of a maturational continuum which existed from the small dark cell through various lines of differentiation. Thus, it was felt artificial to eliminate those tumors in the University of Minnesota series with primitive ependymal features (ependymoblastoma) or embryonic medullary canals (medulloepithelioma). Patterns associated with both of these latter neoplasms were identified in some of the other PNETs. The practical consideration is the appropriate diagnostic locution. This exercise is more often based on capriciousness than any basic biologic understanding of the tumor. Kosnik *et al.* [10] have made a cogent statement when referring specifically to the ependymoblastoma: 'Regardless of their predominant histologic features and clinical behavior they are similar to their PNETs.' A cerebral medulloepithelioma in a 12 year old female showing glial and neuronal differentiation also supports the theme of multipotentiality which exists in these tumors [21].

One investigative approach to a more enlightened understanding of these tumors is ultrastructural characterization. Boesel *et al.* [22] have examined six PNETs by electron microscopy and concluded that the cells were poorly differentiated neuroepithelium without neuroblastoic features. In this regard

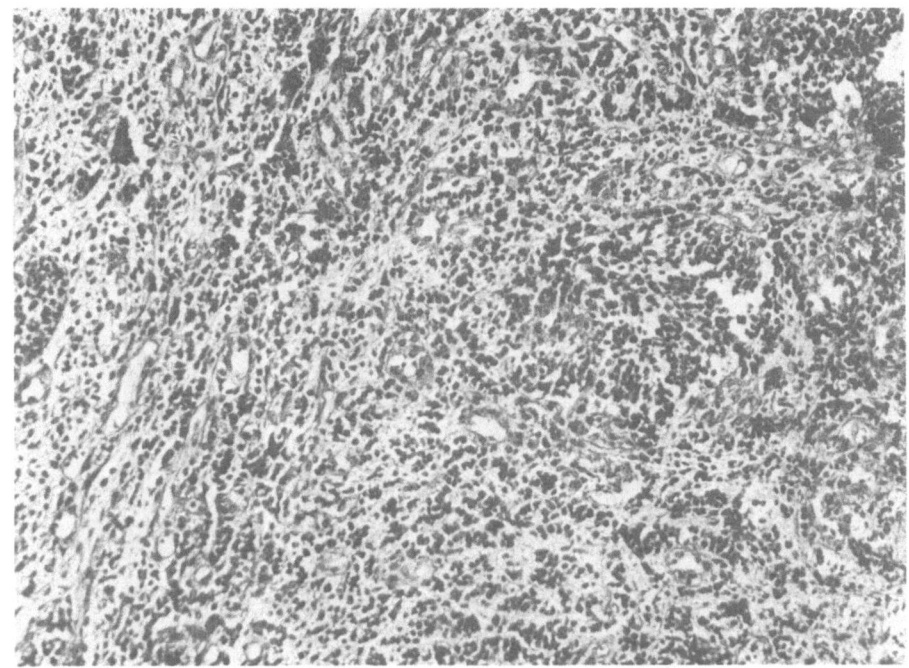

Figure 3. Other lines of differentiation including astroglial and oligodendroglial cells among the small dark cells or as discrete foci within the tumor.

to the absence of ultrastructurally specificity, the PNET is similar to the medulloblastoma [23]. When glial filaments were found, it was unclear whether they were present in tumor cells. Divergent lines of differentiation were detected in a cerebral neuroblastoma studied ultrastructurally by Azzarelli *et al.* [24]. Dense core granules and empty vesicles were present in the cytoplasmic processes of some cells in their case. The one case of a monotonous small cell tumor examined by electron microscopy at the University of Minnesota revealed neurite formation, microtubules and membrane bound electron-dense granules in peripheral processes [15]. Catecholamine production was never documented in this case and at autopsy, there was no evidence of a peripheral neuroblastoma. The only other case in the University of Minnesota series with ultrastructure was a medulloepithelioma. There were similarities to previous examples in the literature [25].

Whatever knowledge may be lacking about the histogenesis of the PNETs, the clinical course is better defined but in unfavorable terms. One impressive feature which emerged from some of the studies was the frequency of intra- and post-operative deaths (Table 1). The size of these tumors and the attempt to completely resect the mass were at least two factors in the surgically

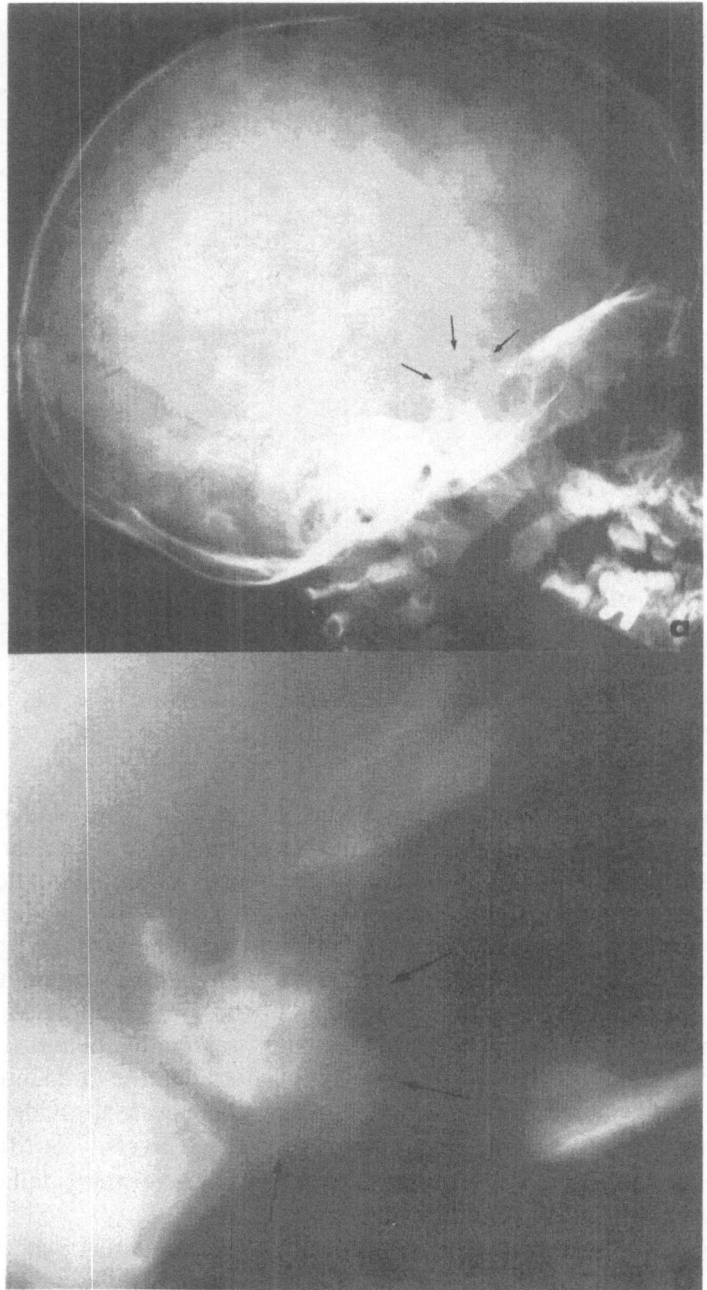

Figure 4. (a) Destructive mass at the base of the brain (arrows) in a child presenting with blindness and intracranial signs. (b) Tomogram revealed the bone destructive properties of the tumor and a mass (arrows).

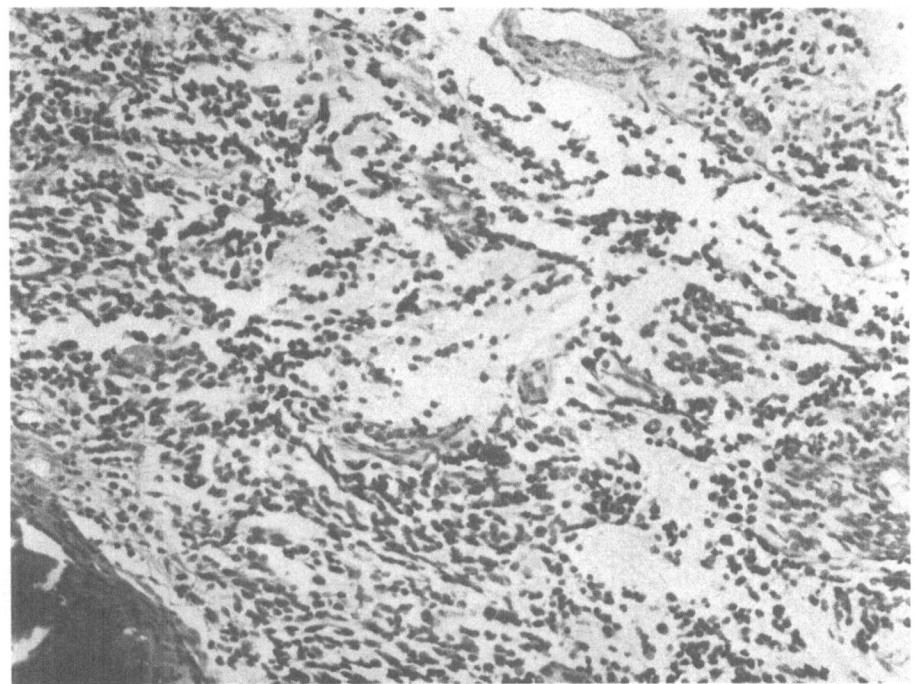

Figure 5. A biopsy of the tumor showed small dark cells loosely arranged in fibrillary background.

related mortality. One or more local recurrences within 12–18 months of the original treatment were the subsequent events in greater than 80% of the patients. As noted previously, the PNET has the potential to spread through the subarachnoid space and infiltrate the spinal cord. The hematogenous route is yet another but less common mode of dissemination.

Finally for the pathologist, the PNET as a 'small cell tumor of childhood' must be included in the differential diagnosis of other neoplasms, i.e. embryonal rhabdomyosarcoma, neuroblastoma, retinoblastoma, Ewing's sarcoma and malignant lymphoma [26]. The clinical context of most cases will provide considerable direction to the pathologist in his interpretation. It is a fact, however, that the various 'embryonic tumors' in children when they metastasize will often lack some or all of the differentiating light microscopic findings. The childhood tumor that most frequently baits the trap is the peripheral or classic neuroblastoma. An example of this problem is illustrated by the case of a 2 year old child who presented with blindness and a destructive and expansile retrochiasmal and suprasellar mass. Following a biopsy showing a primitive neuroectodermal tumor, a roentgenogram of the abdomen demonstrated a left suprarenal mass with punctate calcification. The

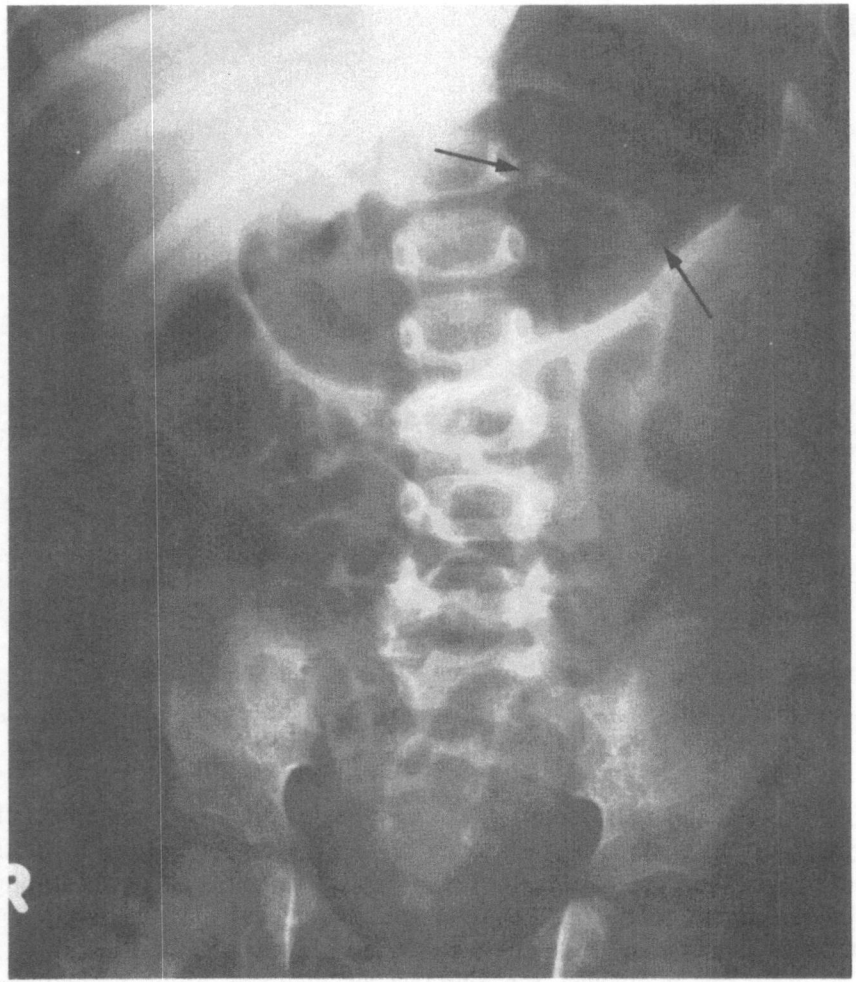

Figure 6. Speckled foci of calcification (arrows) are noted in the left suprarenal area consistent with an adrenal neuroblastoma.

rhabdomyosarcomas of the head and neck region with a parameningeal location can directly seed the subarachnoid space with small dark tumor cells [27]. Water *et al.* [17] have included the malignant ependymoma, malignant lymphoma, pinealoblastoma and choroid plexus carcinoma as neoplasms of the central nervous system which can simulate the medulloblastoma or PNET.

The primitive neuroectodermal tumor of the central nervous system in childhood is a cumbersome and equivocal designation for a poorly differentiated 'small blue cell' neoplasm usually occurring in a supratentorial location. It is a highly malignant process with a fatal outcome in more than 80%

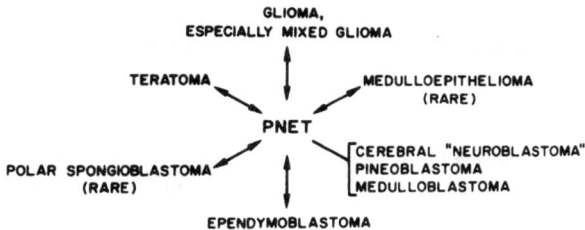

Figure 7. Proposed histogenetic relationship between the PNET and other less primitive tumors of the central nervous system. (From Kosnik *et al.* [10].)

of the patients within one to two years of diagnosis. Unlike a similar appearing and possibly related neoplasm, the peripheral neuroblastoma, there has been no evidence of catecholamine production. There is a suggestion that the cell(s) of PNET is more primitive than the neuroblastoma, i.e. less committed to a particular line of differentiation as the neuroblast. The observation exists that neuronal, astroglial, ependymal and oligodendroglial differentiation occurs in the PNET. In some respects, the PNET shares a biologic affinity to the cerebellar medulloblastoma. The PNET may exist at the histogenetic hub as suggested in the diagrammatic depiction of Kosnik *et al.* [10] (Figure 7). A tumor such as the ganglioglioma [28] may conceivably represent the differentiated end point of the PNET as the ganglioneuroma is the final stage in the maturation of the neuroblastoma.

REFERENCES

1. Bailey P, Cushing H: Medulloblastoma cerebelli—a common type of midcerebellar glioma of childhood. Arch Neurol 14:192–224, 1925.
2. Rubinstein LJ, Herman MM, Hanbery JW: The relationship between differentiating medulloblastoma and dedifferentiating diffuse cerebellar astrocytoma. Light, electron microscopic, tissue and organ culture observations. Cancer 33:675–690, 1974.
3. Stahlberger R, Friede RL: Fine structure of myomedulloblastoma. Acta Neuropathol (Berl) 37:43–48, 1977.
4. Best PV: A medulloblastoma-like tumour with melanin formation. J Pathol 110:109–111, 1973.
5. Hahn JF, Sperber EE, Netsky MG: Melanotic neuroectodermal tumors of the brain and skull. J Neuropathol Exp Neurol 35:508–519, 1976.
6. Kadin ME, Rubinstein LJ, Nelson JS: Neonatal cerebellar medulloblastoma originating from the fetal external granular layer. J Neuropathol Exp Neurol 29:583–600, 1970.
7. Rubinstein LJ: Cytogenesis and differentiation of primitive neuroepithelial tumors. J Neuropathol Exp Neurol 31:7–26, 1972.
8. Hart MN, Earle KM: Primitive neuroectodermal tumors of the brain in children. Cancer 32:890–897, 1973.
9. Parker JC Jr, Mortara RH, McCloskey JJ: Biological behavior of the primitive neuroectodermal tumors: significant supratentorial childhood gliomas. Surg Neurol 4:383–388, 1975.

10. Kosnik EJ, Boesel CP, Bay J, Sayers MP: Primitive neuroectodermal tumors of the central nervous system in children. J Neurosurg 48:741–746, 1978.
11. Bruno LA, Rorke LB, Norris DG: Primitive neuroectodermal tumors of infancy and childhood. In: This volume, chapter 15, pp 265–267.
12. Jenkin D: Primitive neuroectodermal tumour. In: This volume, chapter 13, pp 243–246.
13. Wald B, Siegel SE, Isaacs H Jr, Stanley P: Cerebral primitive neuroectodermal tumor (primary cerebral neuroblastoma): CHLA experience. In: This volume, chapter 10, pp 229–234.
14. Wara WM, Edwards MS, Surti NR, Sheline GE, Levin VA, Wilson CB: Primary cerebral neuroblastomas. In: This volume, chapter 9, pp 225–228.
15. Priest J, Dehner LP, Sung J-H, Nesbit ME: Primitive neuroectodermal tumors (embryonal gliomas) of childhood. A clinicopathologic study of 12 cases. In: This volume, chapter 14, pp 247–264.
16. Sexauer CL, Krous HF, Kaplan RJ, Barnes PD, Humphrey GB: Supratentorial primitive neuroectodermal tumor: clinical response of a single case to vincristine, cyclophosphamide, and BCNU. In: This volume, chapter 11, pp 235–237.
17. Waters KD, Chow CW, Campbell PE: Poorly differentiated small cell tumours of the central nervous system that are not medulloblastomas. In: This volume, chapter 16, pp 269–276.
18. Jellinger K: Cerebral medulloepithelioma. Acta Neuropathol (Berl) 22:95–101, 1972.
19. Rubinstein LJ: The definition of ependymoblastoma. Arch Pathol 90:35–45, 1970.
20. Horten BC, Rubinstein LJ: Primary cerebral neuroblastoma. A clinicopathological study of 35 cases. Brain 99:735–756, 1976.
21. Scheithauer BW, Rubinstein LJ: Cerebral medulloepithelioma. Report of a case with multiple divergent neuroepithelial differentiation. Child's Brain 5:62–71, 1979.
22. Boesel CP, Suhan JP, Bradel EJ: Ultrastructure of primitive neuroectodermal neoplasms of the central nervous system. Cancer 42:194–201, 1978.
23. Matakas F, Cervos-Navarro J: The ultrastructure of medulloblastoma. Acta Neuropathol (Berl) 16:271–284, 1970.
24. Azzarelli B, Richards DE, Anton AH, Roessmann U: Central neuroblastoma. Electron microscopic observations and catecholamine determinations. J Neuropathol Exp Neurol 36:384–397, 1977.
25. Pollak A, Friede RL: Fine structure of medulloepithelioma. J Neuropathol Exp Neurol 36:712–725, 1977.
26. Dehner LP: Soft tissue sarcomas of childhood. The differential diagnostic dilemma of the small blue cell. Cancer Inst Monogr 57:1980 (in press).
27. Tefft M, Fernandez C, Donaldson M, Newton W, Moon TE: Incidence of meningeal involvement by rhabdomyosarcoma of the head and neck in children. A report of the Intergroup Rhabdomyosarcoma Study (IRS). Cancer 42:253–258, 1978.
28. Garrido E, Becker LF, Hoffman JH, Hendrick EB, Humphreys R: Gangliogliomas in children. A clinicopathological study. Child's Brain 4:339–346, 1978.

18. Overview on the Management of Primitive Neuroectodermal Tumors

G. BENNETT HUMPHREY, LOUIS P. DEHNER, RALPH J. KAPLAN, KEITH D. WATERS, R.D.T. JENKIN and WILLIAM M. WARA

1. INTRODUCTION

In this volume of *Pediatric Oncology,* we have collected and reviewed a group of rare CNS tumors of childhood. This management overview will be limited to those tumors grouped under the diagnoses of primitive neuroectodermal tumors (PNET and primary cerebral neuroblastoma. The authors of this overview have reviewed the case material and two of the editors have synthesized this overview from correspondence received from the above authors.

Most of the authors of this overview expressed concern over the possible histologic heterogeneity of the material reviewed. If these tumors are an enigma to the neuropathologists, then we are probably dealing with more than one malignancy or more likely a very primitive neoplasm capable of various lines of morphologic differentiation. Therefore comparisons between series are difficult and any summary of management recommendations must be made with some caution. The suggestions for management in this overview are therefore general guidelines and are in no way definitive recommendations.

2. CLINICAL PRESENTATION

The PNETs and related neoplasms as a whole are characterized by aggressive behavior. A brief clinical course, usually less than a month, is a reflection of the rapid growth and the frequent occurrence of necrosis and cyst formation. The presumed rapid rate of growth produces signs and symptoms of markedly increased intracranial pressures as well as localized neurological signs. In the infant and young child, the yielding skull and compliant brain may allow the tumor to reach massive size prior to diagnosis. Exceptions to

G.B. Humphrey et al. (eds.), Pediatric oncology 1, 289–294. All rights reserved.
Copyright © 1981 Martinus Nijhoff Publishers bv, The Hague/Boston/London.

this characteristic agressive behavior may exist as suggested by Bruno *et al.* [1] and by the single case reported by Sexauer *et al.* [2].

3. PATHOLOGY

In section II of this volume the existing literature has been reviewed as well as the pathologic features of the reported cases [3, 4]. Readers are therefore referred to this section for a detailed discussion of pathology which is not included in this management overview. An interesting point has been raised with regard to whether these tumors should be thought of as one group or whether as subgroups with designation other than PNET. In this context a case can be made that the true primitive neuroectodermal tumor is a highly malignant neoplasm that can seed throughout the entire central nervous system. Whereas, the cerebral neuroblastoma reoccurs locally and is less likely to seed the CNS. This perspective obviously has therapeutic implications which will be discussed later.

A review of all cases reported in this volume emphasizes the need for an accurate deliniation and pathological diagnosis before management decisions are made. The need for outside consultation is obvious for those centers where the experience is quite limited due to the rarity of these tumors.

4. DIAGNOSTIC EVALUATION

The presentation of PNET may be suggested from the history and neurological examination of an obviously aggressive supratentorial hemispheric tumor in an infant or a young child. However, in older children the presumptive diagnosis is usually that of a more indolent CNS tumor. Skull X-rays may reveal evidence of increased intracranial pressure as manifested by split cranial sutures, prominent digital markings or evidence of demineralization of the sella. Computerized axial tomography (C.A.T.), before and after contrast enhancement, will demonstrate the location and size of the tumor as well as the presence of associated cerebral edema and cyst formation. The C.A.T. scan will also reveal the occurrence of hydrocephalus when present in association with intraventricular or paraventricular tumors. If a C.A.T. scan is not available, a nuclear brain scan will usually show the tumor but not its precise location or the associated distortions of the adjacent brain. The necessity for cerebral angiography is determined by the location of the tumor. Lesions in the frontal, temporal, or occipital pole may be surgically managed on the basis of the C.A.T. scan alone. If the tumor is at the base of the brain or in close relationship to the brain stem, or intraventricular in location, angiography must be done to demonstrate the relationship of the mass to the major vessels in the circle of Willis as well as its blood supply. The need for ventriculography or pneumoencephalography has generaly been supplanted by the C.A.T. scan, however, on occasions the intrathecal or intraventricular injection of metrizamide followed by C.A.T. scanning may be required to define the anatomy of intraventricular tumors. Spinal cord tumors are best demonstrated by plain X-rays of the spine followed by myelography. The role of metrizamide and myelography performed in conjunction with C.A.T. scanning of the spine has shown promise in the diagnosis of intraspinal lesions [5].

There was a minor difference among the authors with regard to the role of CSF evaluation in patients with these tumors. On one hand, lumbar puncture to obtain CSF for cytological studies was usually contraindicated in all but the smallest tumors because of the risk of tonsillar or uncal herniation. On the other hand, some authors indicated that a thorough diagnostic evaluation of the central nervous system including lumbar puncture for chemistry, cytology and appropriate biological markers should serve as the basis for proper management of these patients. There was no disagreement as to the value of a complete myelogram to try to determine which patients might benefit from spinal radiation.

5. NEUROSURGICAL APPROACH

The pre-operative management of the patient is directed toward the control of intracranial hypertension. Steroids (Decadron) are used to control cerebral edema. If the patient's level of consciousness is impaired, the intracranial pressure should be reduced by the rapid intravenous infusion of mannitol. If there is evidence of impending cerebral herniation and the C.A.T. scan demonstrates a cyst or hydrocephalus, external drainage may be life-saving.

The goal of the neurosurgical treatment of PNET is the complete excision of the tumor when possible. It is apparent that the size and location of these tumors will modify the surgical approach to them and will influence the potential for surgical excision. The rare long term survivals following treatment have been in those lesions totally excised, especially those which were intraventricular in location. More often a subtotal excision is the best that can be accomplished without increasing the neurological deficit needlessly. This will serve to debulk the tumor and reduce the pressure on the adjacent brain and open CSF pathways if they were blocked by the tumor. In deeply situated tumors of the basal ganglia or thalamus, a needle biopsy is recommended or radiation treatment may be started without pathological confirmation. In tumors of the anterior third ventricle and tuberal region, a biopsy may be obtained by craniotomy or the diagnosis may be made on the basis of CSF cytology in conjunction with C.A.T. scan findings. Treatment with radiation is then started. The response to therapy is monitored by periodic C.A.T. scans and CSF cytology [6]. The same therapeutic approach may be used in tumors of the pineal region although here total tumor excision may be accomplished through the occipital–trans-tentorial route [7].

Long-term survival is seemingly correlated with the extent of resection. While there are only a few cases, most survivors are among those patients with complete resection; fewer are found among patients with only partial resection or biopsy only. The case material presented here does not indicate any differences in survival rate between subtotal resection and biopsy.

6. RADIATION THERAPY

There is a uniform consensus that radiation therapy for all patients with PNET should be the full dose according to the age of the patient. There is less agreement regarding the disposition of the therapeutic fields. Cranial/spinal radiotherapy is recommended by some, radiotherapy to the tumor only by others, and some centers have used both treatment approaches.

Based upon the experience of two institutions, a dose of 5000 rads given in six weeks is appropriate and produces minimal reaction to normal tissues [8]. While no detailed analysis can be performed it is of some interest that none of the patients receiving a radiation dose of <4500 rads survived compared to those patients given doses >4500 rads.

From the therapeutic outcome it is obvious from this review that the definition of the tumor(s) remains uncertain. This is the only reasonable way to explain the excellent survival results in one institution with eight of 10 patients surviving [8]. This institution used essentially identical therapeutic modalities notably unsuccessful in other centers.

7. ADJUVANT CHEMOTHERAPY

Many of the cases reported in this volume show that chemotherapeutic agents may have a role in adjuvant therapy. As the reports are limited to those patients with recurrences, no guidelines for adjuvant therapy can be developed at this time.

One group is currently evaluating adjuvant therapy for PNET following surgery and radiation therapy. Chemotherapy consists of a four drug combination of Vincristine, Prednisone, Procarbazine and Dibromodulcitol. At present, it is too early to evaluate this trial of adjuvant therapy. There is a consensus that patients who relapse after a period of clinical remission should receive a trial of chemotherapy. However, the role of re-excision of recurrent tumor should not be dismissed since in some cases it produced very acceptable palliation.

There is no consensus regarding which chemotherapeutic agent or drug combination should be used in recurrent PNETs. While many centers elected to evaluate drug combinations that included a nitrosourea, other therapeutic approaches not including nitrosourea have also been reported. At present, no guidelines can be made for chemotherapeutic approach to these tumors. A recommendation has been made that patients initially treated with radiation only and who relapsed should receive further courses of radiation therapy but not be given intrathecal or intraventricular Methotrexate in view of the significant risk of leukoencephalopathy. At one center, systemic chemotherapy is currently under evaluation with a four-drug combination that includes Vincristine, Prednisolone, Procarbazine and Chlorambucil. This four-drug combination is different from that under evaluation as adjuvant therapy in that Chlorambucil is substituted for Dibromodulcitol.

Cis-diamino-dichloro platinum may prove to be an effective agent in treatment of PNET. Six of eight children with a variety of CNS malignancies responded favorably to a dose schedule of 50 mg/m^2 given on two consecutive days at monthly intervals [9]. This small series included one child with PNET in whom there was a dramatic clinical response with complete resolution of a frontal lesion demonstrated by C.A.T. scan. Therapy was discontinued after two courses due to kidney toxicity and the patient died due to regrowth of tumor [10].

8. PROGNOSIS

The prognosis for these tumors is very poor. The disease free survival of greater than five years is estimated to be only 20%. The case material emphasized the need for a guarded prognosis for those patients who respond to primary therapy during the first five years after initial therapy. This is based on the number of late re-occurrences observed during the third and fourth year.

9. SPECIAL PROBLEMS: THE CHILD UNDER ONE YEAR OF AGE

In children with PNET who are less than one year of age, the Australian investigators have advocated total surgical resection when possible, obviously considering accessibility and possible damage to vital structure. They would recommend the radiation not be given since curative doses of cranial/spinal radiation would lead to significant growth retardation should the patient become a long-term survivor. Chemotherapy would be given in these cases with intrathecal Methotrexate and systemic Vincristine, Prednisone, Procarbazine and Chlorambucil. If no re-occurrence occurred, then consideration would be given to delayed cranial/spinal radiation once the child reached two years of age.

REFERENCES

1. Bruno LA, Rorke LB, Norris DG: Primitive neuroectodermal tumors of infancy and childhood. In: This volume, chapter 15, pp 265–267.
2. Sexauer CL, Krous HF, Kaplan RJ, Barnes PD, Humphrey GB: Supratentorial primitive neuroectodermal tumor: clinical response of a single case to Vincristine, Cyclophosphamide, and BCNU. In: This volume, chapter 11, pp 235–237.
3. Knapp J, van Eys J, Cangir A: Primitive neuroectodermal tumors of brain in childhood: literature review and the M.D. Anderson experience. In: This volume, chapter 8, pp 215–224.
4. Dehner LP: Primitive neuroectodermal tumors of the central nervous system in childhood. Retrospective and overview. In: This volume, chapter 17, pp 277–288.
5. DiChiro G, Schellinger D: Computed tomography of spinal cord after lumbar intrathecal introduction of metrizamide (computer-assisted myelography). Radiology 120:101–104, 1976.
6. Spiegal AM, DiChiro G, Gorden P, Ommya AK, Kolins J, Pomeroy TC: Diagnosis of radiosensitive hypothalamic tumors without craniotomy. Ann Intern Med 85:290–293, 1976.
7. Jamieson KG: Excision of pineal tumors. J Neurosurg 35:550–553, 1971.
8. Wara WM, Edwards MS, Surti NR, Sheline GE, Levin VA, Wilson CB: Primary cerebral neuroblastomas. In: This volume, chapter 9, pp 225–228.
9. Khan A, McCullough D, Borts F, Sinks LF: Update on use of cis-platinum in CNS malignancies. Proc ASCO, 21(C-283):390, 1980.
10. Sinks LF: Personal communication.

Index